Contemporary Approaches in Stuttering Therapy

Contemporary Approaches in Stuttering Therapy

Edited by

Maryann Peins, Ph.D.

Professor and Chairperson, Department of Speech, Language, and Hearing Sciences, School of Applied Health Sciences, Rutgers, The State University of New Jersey, New Brunswick; Adjunct Professor of Psychiatry, University of Medicine and Dentistry of New Jersey, Rutgers Medical School, Piscataway

Little, Brown and Company
Boston/Toronto

Contents

Contributing Authors

Eugene B. Cooper, Ed.D.
Professor and Chairman, Department of Communicative Disorders, University of Alabama, University

Delva M. Culp, M.A.
Coordinator, Preschool Fluency Development Program, The University of Texas at Dallas, Callier Center, Dallas

Bernard S. Lee, B.S.
Research Associate, Department of Psychiatry, University of Medicine and Dentistry of New Jersey, Rutgers Medical School, Piscataway

W. Edward McGough, M.D.
Professor of Psychiatry, University of Medicine and Dentistry of New Jersey, Rutgers Medical School, Piscataway; Chief, Psychiatric Services, Middlesex General–University Hospital, New Brunswick

Maryann Peins, Ph.D.
Professor and Chairperson, Department of Speech, Language, and Hearing Sciences, School of Applied Health Sciences, Rutgers, The State University of New Jersey, New Brunswick; Adjunct Professor of Psychiatry, University of Medicine and Dentistry of New Jersey, Rutgers Medical School, Piscataway

Glyndon D. Riley, Ph.D.
Professor of Communicative Disorders, California State University, Fullerton; Consultant, Rileys Speech and Language Institute, Santa Ana

Jeanna Riley, Ph.D.
Director, Rileys Speech and Language Institute, Santa Ana, California

Richard E. Shine, Ed.D.
Professor of Speech Pathology, School of Allied Health and Social Professions, East Carolina University, Greenville, North Carolina

Adeline E. Weiner, M.S.
Assistant Professor of Speech, Temple University, Philadelphia, Pennsylvania

Marcel E. Wingate, Ph.D.
Professor of Speech, Washington State University, Pullman

Preface

Stuttering continues to confound and challenge speech-language pathologists, clinicians, researchers, and students. Certainly the problem of stuttering and the treatment of this disorder can pose a lifelong challenge to the stutterer.* The amount of therapy may be quite extensive before the stutterer attains and maintains significant speech improvement.

In spite of the vast amount of research on stuttering, there are still no definitive answers as to the cause or causes of stuttering or to the most effective therapy for stutterers. However, we have come closer to a better understanding of the disorder.

In the past dozen years, many speech-language pathologists have reported success with different methods for the treatment of stuttering, ranging from variations of stuttering modification to fluency-shaping therapies (Guitar and Peters, 1980). Speech clinicians now confront a wide array of therapies as they decide which method will enable stutterers to achieve and maintain an effective speech pattern in the shortest period of time. These and other considerations cause a clinician to deliberate carefully about the choice of an appropriate therapy.

Speech clinicians may feel justifiably wary of therapies that demand a great deal of time and energy for lesson plan preparation. Some therapies require considerable skill on the part of the clinician to plan sessions that maintain client motivation, engender insight and stimulate the client to complete therapy assignments, and transfer speech improvement from the therapy session to the environment outside the clinical setting. Some therapies require the purchase of expensive equipment that can be used only in clinical, research, or university facilities and not in typical school settings; others require intensive training in the administration of the therapy, extensive course work, and knowledge of learning theory as well as the principles of conditioning.

Although Wingate's assertion that most speech therapists are more afraid of stuttering than their clients was true in 1971, the picture has changed. Therapists have overcome many of their hesitations and allayed their fears about treating stutterers, but they now face a complex task when seeking to understand and evaluate the many therapies available to them today.

To facilitate this process, we present in-depth discussions of several distinctive therapies for children and adults who stutter.

*Because of the higher incidence of stuttering in males, masculine pronouns will be used in reference to a single stutterer of either gender throughout the book. Since the majority of speech-language clinicians are female, feminine pronouns will be used to refer to them. To alternate masculine and feminine pronouns, would cause unnecessary confusion.

The contents of this book will broaden the therapy horizons of our readers, particularly speech pathology students who are or will be working with stutterers.

In the initial planning stages of this book, I placed myself in the roles of both the questioning student and experienced clinician and asked, "What kind of book about stuttering therapy would benefit me?" The answer proved to be a book containing a cross section of contemporary stuttering therapies. The next question was, "In what format can I present this information so that students and clinicians will find it practical and useful?" The answer was to design a comprehensive chapter outline for the presentation of each therapy. In following a standardized chapter format, we would (1) provide consistent coverage of topics in every presentation, (2) foster the understanding of each therapy, (3) allow comparison of each therapy, and (4) facilitate future reference to specific aspects of each therapy.

The chapter outline listed below has specific comments or questions under each topic heading to help the speech-language pathology student and the clinician evaluate and compare the treatment approaches.

Overview
    An abstract of the essential features of the therapy.
History of the Therapy
    What is the origin of the therapy?
    Who developed the therapy and when?
    Why was the therapy developed?
Assessment Procedures
    What are the assessment procedures?
    When and how does the speech clinician assess speech progress?
Description of the Therapy
    What are the therapy goals?
    What are the essential features of the therapy?
    Is attention given to the associated physical behaviors of stutterers?
    Is attitudinal work part of the therapy?
    Are transfer and maintenance therapy included?
    Are there follow-up procedures of clients after completion of the therapy?
    Does the clinician need equipment or special materials to administer the therapy?
    Are special skills or training required of speech clinicians?
    What are the client's eligibility requirements?

Evaluation of the Therapy
  Did the author(s) evaluate the therapy?
  How did the author(s) evaluate the therapy?
  What were the results of the research studies?
  Does the research data indicate that the therapy is effective
  with mild, moderate, and severe stutterers?
  How long must a stutterer receive therapy before speech im-
  provement occurs?
  Do follow-up investigations indicate long-term speech im-
  provement?
Reasons for Therapeutic Effectiveness
  Why is the therapy effective?
Advantages of the Therapy
  What are the advantages of the therapy for the clinician and
  the client?
Appendix
  Materials or equipment cited in the text
References
  Sources cited in the text

Who are the authors who contributed chapters to this book?
They are decision-makers who had the creativity to develop new
therapies and the tenacity to persist in their investigation of
them, often in spite of skepticism and, sometimes, adverse criticism from their professional peers. They draw upon a wide variety of training and extensive clinical and research experience
with stutterers. These authors agreed to contribute to this text
because they recognize the need to provide clinicians and students with an organized presentation of several contemporary
stuttering therapies. The authors discuss the specifics of their
therapy approaches and, when possible, document the effectiveness of each therapy with their research data. I neither interpret
nor evaluate the treatment strategies; the authors speak for
themselves and their therapies.

I now turn the challenge to you, the reader. Read, consider,
evaluate, and compare as you make your way to an informed
clinical decision.

                                                          M.P.

References

Guitar, B., and Peters, T. J. *Stuttering: An Integration of
  Contemporary Therapies.* Memphis, Tenn.: Speech Foundation of
  America, 1980.
Wingate, M. E. The fear of stuttering. *ASHA* 13: 3–5, 1971.

Acknowledgments

Many persons deserve thanks and recognition for their contributions to the realization of this book. I wish to acknowledge Barbara O. Ward, Allied Health Editor, Little, Brown and Company, who provided the initial impetus for the book and offered continuous counsel and encouragement, and Carol Snarey, also of Little, Brown, who supervised the copyediting and final production in an efficient and gracious manner. Dr. June Birnbaum receives my deep gratitude for helping me to develop my creative capacities and for providing editorial assistance. Her insightful criticisms and sage counsel, graciously given, greatly influenced my writing. Roseanne Hiatt Harris also deserves special thanks and recognition both for her critical evaluation of the entire manuscript and her adept editing of the text. I wish to express my appreciation to Robert B. Truscott for encouraging the writer in me; to Barbara Knolmeyer Glazewski for her professional partnership and feedback; and to Susan Waters for providing the necessary perspective of the student. I am grateful as well to Helen Goleskie and Betsy Hanlon whose typing assistance greatly facilitated my work.

I happily express my gratitude to many individuals who by their presence and example influenced my personal and professional growth, especially my parents, Marie Hanko Peins and the late Rudolph Manning Peins, and my brother Rudy; my mentors, particularly Dr. James V. Frick, for guiding me into the study of stuttering; Dr. W. Edward McGough and Bernard S. Lee, who gave me the opportunity to collaborate with them in research, writing, and the development of a stuttering therapy; the Sisters of the Cenacle, Lantana Community, who created the quietude and allowed me the space and solitude necessary for creative writing; and those friends, near and far, who freely offered encouragement and support.

Finally, to the chapter authors, I extend special thanks for their talent and time devoted to the book. I know that all of us who worked together on this project shared an invaluable and enriching experience.

*Contemporary
Approaches in
Stuttering Therapy*

1. Personalized Fluency Control Therapy: A Status Report

Eugene B. Cooper

Overview

Personalized Fluency Control Therapy (PFCT), an integrated cognitive and behavior therapy process for stutterers, was developed over a period of more than 20 years. PFCT has four stages: identification and structuring, examination and confrontation, cognition and behavior orientation, and fluency control. Although the specific therapeutic activities employed during any one stage of PFCT vary according to the client's age, abilities, environment, and stuttering problem, the underlying therapeutic process and end goal of therapy (the feeling of fluency control) remain the same.

History of the Therapy

At the beginning of the 1960s, when I was a doctoral student at Pennsylvania State University, most of the authorities then writing on stuttering therapy agreed that a meaningful interpersonal relationship between client and clinician contributed significantly to therapeutic success (Bloodstein, 1958; Sheehan, 1958; Murphy and FitzSimons, 1960; and Van Riper, 1963). They observed that the clinical relationship is critical to the development and maintenance of fluency-enhancing attitudes and feelings in the client. At the same time these clinicians and others (Martin, 1963; and Matthews, 1964) also noted a lack of research into the nature of this relationship and its impact on the therapeutic process. Throughout the 1960s, then, I pursued several studies aimed specifically at investigating the significance of the client-clinician relationship and at describing and defining the therapeutic process (Cooper, 1965a, 1965b; Cooper, 1966; Cooper, 1968a; Cooper and Cooper, 1969; and Manning and Cooper, 1969). At that time I described a therapy procedure labeled "Inter-Personal Communications (IPC) Therapy" (Cooper, 1965b, 1968a), and began a series of "process" studies (Cooper, 1965a, Cooper and Cooper, 1969; and Manning and Cooper, 1969).

During this time I, like almost everyone concerned with changing human behavior, initially embraced the developments in behavior modification with optimism (Daly and Cooper, 1967; Cooper, Cady, and Robbins, 1970). My own research and clinical practice, however, quickly convinced me that behavior modification techniques, while unquestionably efficient and effective in altering behavior, were not, in and of themselves, the answer to the problem of stuttering. By the late 1960s I perceived a need for a treatment program that included psychodynamically oriented procedures attending to the stutterer's feelings and attitudes, as well as to behavior modification, and began describing how behavior therapy and

1

attitude therapy might be integrated in a stuttering therapy process (Cooper, 1968a; Cooper, 1969a, 1969b, 1969c; Cooper, 1971a, 1971b; and Cooper, 1973a).

The name for the therapy procedure, "Inter-Personal Communications Therapy," apparently suggested an exclusive emphasis on the psychodynamic aspects of therapy, since clinicians erroneously interpreted it as suggesting that all stutterers have problems with interpersonal relationships. To avoid that misperception, I changed the name to "Personalized Fluency Control Therapy" and, with my wife, published the program as a kit with assessment and therapy materials (Cooper and Cooper, 1976) and a clinician's manual (Cooper, 1976). Subsequently, we developed *PFCT: Individualized Education Program (IEP)* forms, which include parent and teacher guides (Cooper and Cooper, 1980), and currently are developing *PFCT Fluency Assessment Digests* for adults and for children (*FAD-A* and *FAD-C*), as well as revising the *PFCT Kit*.

I assume that most chronic stuttering is the result of multiple coexisting physiologic and psychological factors, a concept that is not new to speech-language pathology. McDonald used the concept of "multiple co-existing" factors in discussing the etiology of articulation disorders as early as 1964. The concept recognizes that a constellation of factors, each of which might be evaluated as normal when measured independently, must be present in a given time frame to produce a given speech disorder. Such a concept explains why we observe such variability in stuttering and why the causes of stuttering have eluded researchers. It also suggests why we should not be surprised that so many different therapeutic intervention procedures are successful with different segments of the stuttering population. Perhaps one day researchers and clinicians will be able to identify all of the significant etiologic factors and reconstruct the interaction of them graphically. At the moment, however, most of the multiple coexisting physiologic factors underlying stuttering remain to be definitively identified, and our understanding of the psychological factors is superficial at best.

During the late 1970s and early 1980s, undoubtedly motivated by the work of such researchers as Wingate (1966, 1969), Adams and Reis (1971, 1974), and Perkins and associates (1976), many clinicians viewed stuttering as a lack of coordination (resulting from multiple coexisting factors) of the basic speech processes of articulation, phonation, and respiration. Perkins (1979) later noted that any alteration in the coordination of these processes typically produced an alteration in the individual's fluency. While such an observation was not new to the field, its significance grew as the popularity of teaching stutterers "to stutter more fluently" decreased and the popularity of teaching stutterers to speak more fluently increased (Gregory, 1979). Applying these findings, which designate the relationship between the processes as the basis for eliciting fluency, I identified and described therapeutic techniques known as fluency-initiating gestures or FIGs (Cooper, 1976).

Assessment Procedures

If stuttering therapy should include procedures for dealing with the client's feelings and attitudes as well as with the disfluencies, then therapeutic success or failure should be judged on the basis of changes in the client's attitudes and feelings, as well as changes in fluency. Thus, any assessment of the stuttering problem should include procedures for evaluating not only fluency, but also feelings and attitudes. In addition, when young disfluent children are assessed, attempts should be made to predict the disorder's chronicity.

In previous articles (Cooper, 1977; Cooper, 1978) I discussed case selection procedures for school-aged disfluent children that involve a process beginning with the initial contact with the disfluent child and ending with the enrollment decision. Following is a brief review of those procedures.

INITIAL CONTACT

Teacher referral continues to be the major mechanism for identifying disfluent children in the schools. Investigating the ability of third-grade teachers to identify speech-handicapped children according to type and severity of speech problems, James and Cooper (1966) found that teachers most accurately identify children who stutter. They concluded that interruptions in speech fluency (hesitations, sound prolongations, and repetitions) and accompanying mannerisms interfere with communication to a greater extent than irregularities of vocal quality or pronunciation unless the disorders of the latter types are severe. As a result, teacher referrals are an effective means for establishing initial contact with disfluent children. Other means include parent referral, self-referral, clinician screening procedures, and referrals from other school and health care personnel.

APPROVAL FOR EVALUATION

The manner in which the speech clinician obtains parental approval to conduct a speech-language evaluation varies among school districts. Clinicians may need to obtain written approval; in some cases a simple verbal approval is sufficient.

SPEECH-LANGUAGE PATHOLOGIST'S EVALUATION

Initial evaluations of disfluent children involve (1) a review of health and education records, (2) an assessment of the problem through the use of formal test instruments, (3) observations of the client in varying communicative situations, and (4) preparation of a tentative description of the problem.

Prior to the scheduled initial diagnostic session, the clinician reviews the child's health and education records. This review helps the clinician decide which assessment instruments to use and provides insight into the child's background and current status. The first diagnostic session includes the following sequence of events.

The clinician reviews the events that resulted in the meeting and tells the child that in this initial session they will focus on a series of background questions, as well as complete several paper and pencil questionnaires. The clinician's questions elicit information from the child regarding the onset of the disfluent behavior and the child's perceptions of how the disfluent behavior has changed since he first became aware of it. The clinician also explains that, depending on the results of this meeting, the child may be observed in a few speaking situations outside of the testing room. Settings in the school environment would afford observation of the child's (1) participating in small-group activities in the classroom, (2) speaking before the entire class, (3) participating in organized and free-play activities, and (4) speaking to authority figures such as the teacher or the principal.

If the clinician decides to observe the child in a variety of speaking situations, she discusses the settings with the child to avoid any possibility that he might feel "spied-on."

After discussing these possibilities, the clinician and the child, working together, complete the following assessment instruments included in the *PFCT Kit* (Cooper and Cooper, 1976).

Stuttering Attitudes Checklist
The clinician asks the child if he agrees or does not agree with 25 statements about feelings and attitudes toward stuttering. The statements are worded to make them appropriate, in most instances, for use with both children and adults. The clinician reads the statements to the client if she believes that this would facilitate the client's responses. The wording of each statement is such that client agreement indicates an "undesirable" attitude on the part of the stutterer, independent of whether or not the attitude is justified. For example, the stutterer might agree that "My stuttering is my biggest problem." The child, by agreeing that stuttering is the major problem, indicates the stuttering is a significant, negative factor in his life. If the child, following therapy, no longer considers the stuttering to be a major problem, one might assume that the therapy has been beneficial.

The checklist is scored simply from the total number of statements with which the client has agreed. The greater the number of agreements, the less desirable are the client's attitudes and feelings. The scores have significance, however, only when compared with those from various other time intervals. While the checklist provides clues as to differences between stutterers with respect to attitudes and feelings, it really acts as a means of identifying a client's feelings and attitudes both for himself and for the clinician. The *Stuttering Attitudes Checklist,* then, not only assesses the client's attitudes toward stuttering before, during, and after therapy but also enables the clinician to initiate a discussion of these feelings and attitudes with the client.

Situation Avoidance Checklist

The client indicates which of 50 common speech situations he "avoids or would prefer to avoid" because of the stuttering. The clinician reads the list to any client who is unable to read, records the responses on the checklist, and determines the score by counting the number of speech situations the client avoids or prefers to avoid. The *Situation Avoidance Checklist,* then, provides information that is useful in assessing the stuttering problem, in determining changes with respect to the client's avoidances of speech situations, and in acquainting both the clinician and the client with the ramifications of the client's fluency disorder.

Concomitant Stuttering Behavior Checklist

The clinician observes the client's behavior during moments of stuttering to ascertain the presence of any of 32 concomitant behaviors falling into these five categories: posturing behaviors, respiratory behaviors, facial behaviors, syntactic and semantic behaviors (judged to be stuttering avoidance behaviors), and vocal behaviors. While these behaviors need not occur during every moment of stuttering, they should be in the current repertoire in order for the clinician to record their presence. The *Concomitant Stuttering Behavior Checklist,* then, helps both the client and clinician to assess stuttering, to determine necessary changes in the client's stuttering-related behaviors, and to develop an awareness of the client's stuttering behavior pattern.

Stuttering Frequency and Duration Estimate Record

The clinician records the client's stuttered responses in three activities: answering questions that typically elicit 1- or 2-word responses, reciting the alphabet, and reading a 200-syllable prose passage with second-grade level words. The questions, the alphabet, and the reading passage are included on the single page form for convenience. For the responses to questions, the clinician counts the number of stuttered syllables and estimates the average duration of the blocks. For the recitation and the reading, the clinician records (1) the time it took the client to complete the task, (2) the number of stuttered syllables, (3) the percentage of stuttering, and (4) the estimated average duration of the moments of stuttering. The *Stuttering Frequency and Duration Estimate Record,* then, provides the clinician with one more assessment instrument for estimating the stuttering severity, and should the clinician repeat the estimate during and following the therapy process, it serves also to indicate changes in the frequency and duration of the client's stuttering.

Client and Clinician Perceptions of Stuttering Severity Ratings
Global judgments of stuttering severity continue to be one of the most meaningful assessments of stuttering severity. Because of the variability in stuttering frequency within and between speech situations, judgments of stuttering severity are more meaningful when based on several observations of the client's speech performance in a variety of speech situations. For this reason, a summary of stuttering severity ratings by both the client and the clinician possesses face validity in assessing the stuttering severity. The *Client and Clinician Perceptions of Stuttering Severity Ratings* is a single page form completed by the clinician. In the first portion of the form, the clinician reads aloud three uncompleted sentences dealing with the client's perceptions of the severity of the stuttering problem. The client completes each sentence by choosing one to five possible conclusions which indicate how severe he perceives the problem to be. The client gives three indications on a one- to five-point scale of his perception of the severity of the problem.

The clinician's portion of the stuttering severity rating form contains a 1- to 5-point scale ranging from mild to very severe for each of four aspects of stuttering: frequency, duration, tension, and concomitant behaviors. On the basis of her observations of the client, the clinician selects the scale number that best describes her perceptions of that aspect of the client's stuttering. In this manner, she makes four such severity estimates, which provide not only further indications of the nature and severity of the client's stuttering problem but also useful comparisons of the client's and the clinician's perceptions of severity.

Upon completion of the five assessments noted above, the clinician prepares a list of tentative conclusions concerning (1) the frequency, duration, and type of disfluencies, (2) apparent situation-related variations in the disfluent behavior, (3) the child's perceptions of the disfluent behavior, (4) an impression of the child's feelings and attitudes regarding the stuttering, and (5) the child's apparent reactive behavior to the disfluencies. This list of tentative conclusions is used in the individualized education program meeting with the child's teacher and parents.

TEACHER INTERVIEW
The speech-language pathologist's primary purposes in interviewing the disfluent child's classroom teacher or teachers are to determine each teacher's perceptions of the child and the disfluent behaviors and to seek validation for the tentative conclusions concerning the nature of the problem made by the speech-language pathologist. Because teachers have more opportunities to observe children than any other professional

member of the educational team, they are able to add significantly to the clinician's list of observations. In addition, because classroom teachers frequently are the most significant individuals to children during their school days, the speech clinician should investigate not only the teachers' concepts of their roles in helping stuttering children but also the positive or negative attitudes that might influence the intervention activities ultimately recommended as part of the therapy. The speech clinician needs to understand how teachers view the problem and to evaluate how helpful teachers may be in carrying out a coordinated team-intervention effort.

Because the cooperation of classroom teachers is an essential element in successful treatment programs for school-aged disfluent children, the clinician wants to be certain that teachers are aware of her goals as therapy progresses. What is more, the clinician's position in discussing a client with his parents is strengthened when she and the teachers are in agreement regarding the children's attitudes and behaviors.

To increase the likelihood that classroom teachers share our clinical perceptions of stuttering, we instituted a program in the Tuscaloosa, Alabama, city schools. Classroom teachers were asked at one of their regularly scheduled meetings to complete a 25-item true-false test on knowledge of stuttering and an attitudinal inventory on their strength-of-agreement to 50 attitudinal statements regarding stuttering (Crowe and Cooper, 1977). At a subsequent teachers' meeting, we reviewed the teachers' responses and attempted to correct erroneous perceptions as well as to make teachers aware of attitudes about stuttering that are detrimental to progress in therapy.

PARENT INTERVIEW AND TESTING
The clinician's goals in the initial parent interview are to determine how the parents view their child's disfluent behavior and to identify parental attitudes that may facilitate or impede intervention activities. The clinician structures the interview by informing the parent that the first meeting will be devoted to seeking information, while subsequent meetings will deal with what should be done about the problem. If parents know that questions will not be answered during the first interview but that they will have opportunities to ask questions in future meetings, they are more informative in their responses and less likely to press the clinician for immediate answers. At the same time, knowing that a second interview is part of the procedure, the clinician is not pressured into premature conclusions.

The structure of the initial parent meeting derives from paper and pencil checklists and inventories such as the *Parent Attitudes Toward Stuttering Checklist* (Cooper and Cooper, 1976) which the parents complete just prior to the interview. This 25-item checklist contains statements of attitudes and feelings ordinarily expressed by parents of stutterers. The parents respond by indicating whether they agree or do not agree with each statement, and their responses of agreement pinpoint the feelings and attitudes that the clinician will explore. Thus, the greater the number of agreement responses, the greater the indication that the parent will benefit from instruction and counseling. The clinician uses the *Parent Attitudes Toward Stuttering Checklist* to (1) identify areas of parental concern and misperception, (2) structure parental therapy sessions by reviewing each item with the parents, and (3) assess changes in parental attitudes as therapy progresses.

Another inventory that is helpful in structuring the initial parent interview as well as providing critical information with respect to the child's stuttering, is the *Chronicity Prediction Checklist* (Cooper, 1973b; Cooper and Cooper, 1976). This checklist consists of 27 questions which the speech clinician answers with *yes* or *no* responses after observing and interacting with the stutterer and after consulting with the stutterer's parents. Responses to the questions provide historical data (such as onset, family history of stuttering) and information concerning the parent and child attitudes toward the stuttering (for example, "Do prolongations last longer than one second?"). *Yes* responses may be interpreted as predictors of stuttering chronicity, but we do not attempt to weigh individual questions for predictive value. Instead, we obtain information about variables that either relate to chronicity (for example, severity) or suggest a relationship (such as self-concept as a stutterer) though a cause-effect relationship *is not implied.* The observations recorded serve simply to assist the clinician in predicting recovery from stuttering and in identifying the variables with a cause-effect relationship to spontaneous recovery.

The *Prediction Checklist* is useful in introducing parents to potentially anxiety-producing topics (such as family history of stuttering and parental reaction to the child's disfluencies) in a straightforward and nonevaluative manner. Clinicians frequently report that parents who have completed the *Parent Attitudes Toward Stuttering Checklist* and reviewed each item on the *Chronicity Prediction Checklist* are more responsive and informative in discussions during the remainder of the initial interview.*

CHRONICITY ASSESSMENT

Assuming that as many as four out of every five stutterers recover without therapeutic intervention (Andrews and Harris, 1964) and that two out of every three stutterers whom speech clinicians meet in the school recover spontaneously (Cooper, 1972; Lankford and Cooper, 1974), the value in differentiating between the chronic and episodic stutterer is obvious. The *Chronicity Prediction Checklist* described previously assists the clinician in making the determination.

---

* Cooper's (1976) *Personalized Fluency Control Therapy* manual provides a review of the literature on recovery from stuttering as well as a discussion of probable clues to stuttering severity, articulatory patterns, concomitant extra-articulatory behaviors, and client affective-cognitive responses to stuttering that appear to relate to stuttering chronicity.

If we could measure precisely and then assign a weight to each of the variables that we have noted, we would be able to arrive at a score that would tell us which children need help; but unfortunately we do not have such a system. Consequently, each clinician must make the difficult enrollment or nonenrollment decision on the basis of imprecise measurements of variables whose significance to the chronicity of stuttering remains questionable. Assuming that the clinician has followed procedures such as those described previously, she will be as prepared as she can be to make enrollment recommendations.

IEP MEETING
Because disfluent children needing assistance with their speech most frequently are not placed in a special classroom situation, IEP meetings ordinarily do not require prior meetings to determine the placement of the child. Requirements vary among school districts as to who should be involved in IEP meetings for children whose primary handicap is a speech-language disorder that does not require special classroom placement. However, these meetings frequently involve the child's parents, the classroom teacher, the building principal, and the clinician. The disfluent child is also included when such attendance is judged by the committee members to be appropriate. Assuming that the child's handicap is limited to a problem in fluency, the speech clinician plays a leadership role in the IEP meeting. Her major responsibility at the meeting is to report conclusions and recommendations regarding the child's speech and, assuming that an intervention program is indicated, to obtain parental approval and active support for the program goals.

One approach to facilitating parental understanding of and support for the recommended intervention program involves a *Parent-Clinician Note of Agreement* (Cooper and Cooper, 1976) during the IEP meeting. At the conclusion of the meeting, the document is signed by all members of the IEP committee or at least by the parents and the clinician. The document has three major sections: a section for listing parent and clinician observations, a section for identifying long- and short-term goals, and a section for describing how the goals will be achieved.

The speech clinician arrives at the IEP meeting with a list of observations about the child on the apparent severity of stuttering, the child's reactions to the disfluencies, the need for therapy, and the number and duration of sessions being recommended. She presents these observations to the IEP committee for open discussion with the goal of arriving at an observation that each member of the committee perceives as being accurate. The agreed-upon observation then is written on the agreement form. If a consensus cannot be achieved on each observation, the conflicting observations are recorded with an indication of which committee members hold which observations.

Upon completion of the observations section of the agreement document, the IEP committee members begin to identify what changes, if any, in the child's attitude or behavior might be beneficial to him. At this time, the committee is not concerned with identifying who will be responsible for assisting the child in effecting these changes, but rather with arriving at an agreement among committee members as to the end goals of the therapy plan. Establishing target dates for the completion of each goal identified by the committee frequently assists committee members in keeping the goals realistic and in clarifying the roles that committee members might play in attaining them. The committee-approved long- and short-term goals then are written in the goals section of the *Parent-Clinician Note of Agreement.*

Following a discussion of the clinician's role, such issues as the frequency and time frame of the therapy program are addressed in the clinician's role section of the document. The committee then turns to the role of the parents, identifying response changes, attitudinal adjustments, and therapy duties as responsibilities to be written in the parent's role section of the *Parent-Clinician Note of Agreement.* When the agreement is complete, the individuals signing the agreement receive copies; and an appropriate number of copies are placed in the child's files. In some school districts, this signed agreement is acceptable either as the completed IEP, the therapy component of the IEP, a supplement to the IEP, or as a resource for completing the standardized IEP form. In any case, the completed *Parent-Clinician Note of Agreement* facilitates parental participation in the development of a stuttering therapy program by outlining goals that are acceptable to all parties concerned.

Cooper and Cooper (1980) developed a PFCT-IEP packet with a six-page IEP form to be used with the *Personalized Fluency Control Therapy Kit* (Cooper and Cooper, 1976). The first page is for recording client identification and fluency assessment data; and the four succeeding pages contain short-term instructional objectives, with recommended materials and techniques for each of the four stages of PFCT. The sixth page serves as a record-of-approval for the PFCT-IEP and enables the clinician to keep a record not only of when the long-term goals for each stage of therapy are completed, but also of the number, type, and duration of therapy sessions planned for the period of time covered by the program. A two-page *IEP Parent Guide* and a two-page *IEP Teacher Guide* are also available with the PFCT-IEP forms. Side one of the forms contains general introductory information, and side two provides a summary of the PFCT goals as well as ways in which the teacher or the parent may assist the child in achieving those goals.

Included in the PFCT Kit itself is a single page *Longitudinal Stuttering Assessment Summary,* attached to the front or back inside cover of the client's file, which enables the clinician to summarize changes in the client's and the parents' attitudes, feelings, and behaviors as therapy progresses. The form also provides space for the data obtained in each of the aforementioned inventories, checklists, and ratings as well as spaces for 24 different indicators of client change and 4 different indicators of parent change. By using all of the aforementioned assessment instruments, the clinician develops a "battery" of indicators which trace client changes with respect to both behavior and to feelings and attitudes. These checklists and forms indicate variables that should be evaluated in stuttering therapy. As noted previously, unidimensional approaches to evaluating pretherapy and posttherapy differences are misleading and provide little or no information to the clinician as to what aspects of the client's attitudes and behaviors need modification in the pursuit of increased fluency.

ENROLLMENT DECISION

The enrollment decision, of course, will have been made prior to the conclusion of the IEP meeting. By following a well-defined process of evaluation and consultation, the speech clinician assists all involved in arriving at an enrollment decision that will maximally benefit the child.

Description of the Therapy

THERAPY GOALS

Perhaps one of PFCT's unique features is its end goal of therapy: the feeling of fluency control. More specific long-term goals and short-term objectives for each of the four stages of PFCT are presented in Tables 1-1 and 1-2. As noted elsewhere (Cooper, 1979a), others have developed therapy programs in which the goals of therapy appear to be arbitrarily established stuttering frequency counts during predetermined speech activities in prescribed situations. Counting the frequency of disfluencies in controlled situations may be less difficult and demonstrably more precise than assessing a hypothetical construct such as "the feeling of fluency control." However, the latter is perhaps *the* key variable in determining if a stutterer will maintain an acceptable fluency level upon termination of formal therapy. Stuttering frequency counts in prescribed speech modes and situations simply are not valid indicators of an individual's general stuttering behavior in life situations. Clinicians know that such pretherapy and posttherapy assessments frequently have little validity in reflecting changes in the complexity of the stutterer's struggle behavior or in the stutterer's attitudes and feelings that facilitate or impede fluency. While the stutterer's feelings of fluency control are more difficult to define and to assess than stuttering frequency counts, the feeling of fluency control remains the most important single variable in determining how successful the client has been in obtaining a level of fluency acceptable to himself.

The term "feeling of control" refers to a response-specific, visceral re-

Table 1-1. Personalized Fluency Control Therapy Long-Term Goals and Short-Term Objectives for the First Two Stages of Therapy

Stage	Long-term Goals	Short-term Objectives
1. Identification and structuring	To help the client identify the feelings, attitudes, and behaviors that constitute the stuttering problem.	To enable the client to identify and describe the types of disfluencies experienced (prolongations, repetitions, hesitations).
		To enable the client to identify and describe the concomitant stuttering behaviors including: (a) posturing behaviors, (b) respiratory behaviors, (c) facial behaviors, (d) syntactic and semantic behaviors, (e) vocal behaviors.
		To enable the client to identify and describe situation-avoidance behaviors.
		To enable the client to identify and describe attitudes toward stuttering.
	To help the client understand the goals and the process of therapy.	To enable the client to describe the final long-term goals in therapy.
		To enable the client to describe the therapy process in general terms.
2. Examination and confrontation	To eliminate distracting body and facial movements occurring during stuttering moments.	To reduce and/or eliminate distracting and extraneous facial behaviors such as loss of eye contact, flaring nostrils, and excessive eyelid movements occurring during the moments of stuttering.

To establish a client-clinician relationship that will help the client explore feelings and make changes in speech behavior.

To assist the client in becoming aware of attitudes, feelings, and behavior patterns that impede or facilitate fluency changes.

To reduce and/or eliminate distracting and extraneous posturing behaviors such as hand, finger, trunk, or leg movements occurring during the moments of stuttering.

To reduce and/or eliminate distracting and extraneous respiratory, syntactic, semantic, and vocal behaviors occurring during the moments of stuttering.

To create a client-clinician relationship in which the client feels free to express positive and negative feelings about the stuttering, the therapy, and the clinician.

To identify and label the client's attitudes and feelings that facilitate or impede fluency changes, such as, "I don't think I have a speech problem," "I like therapy," and "I am dumb because I stutter."

To identify and label the client's behaviors that facilitate or impede fluency changes, such as appearing late for therapy, completing all speech assignments, and forgetting the speech notebook.

Source: Adapted from E. B. Cooper and C. S. Cooper, *Personalized Fluency Control Therapy: IEP Forms.* Hingham, Mass.: Teaching Resources, 1980.

Table 1-2. Personalized Fluency Control Therapy Long-Term Goals and Short-Term Objectives for the Last Two Stages of Therapy

Stage	Long-term Goals	Short-term Objectives
3. Cognition and behavior orientation	To help the client in adopting fluency-enhancing feelings and attitudes.	To shape and reinforce the client's accurate and fluency-enhancing perceptions as identified in Stage 2. To shape and reinforce fluency-enhancing behaviors as identified in Stage 2.
	To help the client in becoming an effective self-reinforcer.	To identify and develop the client's self-reinforcing activities such as expressions of positive feelings toward self.
	To help the client in the identification, development and use of fluency-initiating gestures (FIGs).	To identify the client's self-developed, fluency-initiating gestures, such as "slowing down," "changing words," and using "starter words." To identify fluency-related speech changes under various speech conditions, such as delayed auditory feedback (DAF).

4. Fluency control	To assist the client in developing the feeling of fluency control.	To develop the use of the "universal FIGs" in the clinical situations: slow speech, easy onset, deep breath, loudness control, smooth speech, syllable stress.
		To maintain and enhance the client's attitudes and behaviors that indicate: an accurate perception (as judged by the clinician) of the stuttering behavior and the interpersonal ramifications of that behavior; a realistic emotional and intellectual appreciation of self; a capability to self-reinforce; a knowledge, feeling, and belief in the capability to gain the feeling of fluency control.
	To generalize the client's use of FIGs in speech situations outside the therapy situation varying for the client from the least difficult (in terms of maintaining fluency) to the most difficult.	

Source: Adapted from E. B. Cooper and C. S. Cooper, *Personalized Fluency Control Therapy: IEP Forms.* Hingham, Mass.: Teaching Resources, 1980.

action which all have experienced in some aspect of their behavior such as in typing class, shooting baskets in basketball, or playing the guitar. It is the feeling of knowing that you are capable of controlling a complex motor act. Regardless of the procedures employed in the modification of the stuttering pattern, they are of value only if the stutterer *feels* he has changed the original stuttering pattern. Fluency-eliciting responses are of little value unless the stutterer is developing a feeling of control when using them. To prevent the stutterer from focusing on the modification technique rather than on the feeling of control, clinicians should refer to the fluency-facilitating behaviors descriptively, rather than attach labels to them. Unfortunately, once a label has been attached to a modification technique, stutterers focus on executing procedural aspects of the technique rather than on developing an ability to modify the speech act itself. For example, a stutterer might focus on doing a "good easy onset" rather than on being able to modify the speech act. To avoid this, clinicians might ask, "Do you *feel* you were able to change the speech pattern in any way?" rather than, "Did you do an easy onset or a deep breath?"

As clients continue to experiment with various fluency-initiating gestures (FIGs) in different speech situations, the feeling of control over the speech pattern is reinforced, and it is not unusual for them to announce dramatically that they have achieved the feeling of control. When asked to express this feeling, controlled stutterers frequently report, "No matter how tough a speaking situation I'm in, or no matter how much stuttering I might have initially, I *know* that I can use my FIGs until I feel in control."

Fluency is the by-product of the feeling of fluency control. The term *control* refers to the ability of the stutterer to use fluency-initiating gestures in any speaking situation. The terms *control* and *fluency* are not meant to be synonymous, for individuals may use fluency controls and continue to be disfluent. Individuals experiencing the feeling of fluency control and using fluency-facilitating behaviors in even the most difficult situations, however, are capable of decreasing the disruption in communication with fewer disfluencies.

THERAPY METHOD

Personalized Fluency Control Therapy has four stages labeled to indicate the primary nature of the therapeutic activity occurring within the state.

Identification and Structuring

During the initial stage of PFCT, the clinician assists the stutterer in identifying behaviors that occur during moments of disfluency and behaviors adopted as a result of the disfluencies. The clinician informs the stutterer of the procedures that will be followed in the therapeutic process and the rationale for focusing on the client-clinician relationship to facilitate removal of any disruptive cognitive processing. Through the resulting therapeutic involvement, the clinician facilitates the client's acquisition of fluency-initiating gestures.

The clinician's role in this stage is primarily instructional, and she assumes a teacher-student type of therapeutic relationship with her client. The clinician explains that a basic interest in therapy will be in how the therapeutic relationship develops, noting that many therapy discussions will center on how the client and the clinician "see" each other. The clinician also suggests that the client will feel uncomfortable at times and experience negative feelings toward her. Although the clinician's explanations may not be meaningful to the client at this time in the therapy process, they provide a structure to which the clinician refers as therapy progresses. Because she assists the stutterer in perceiving and defining his stuttering problem but has not yet sought modification of that behavior, the client typically is positive in his feelings toward her at this point. Also, the clinician describes the specific activities that will be undertaken to modify the stuttering behavior, and ordinarily the stutterer, feeling a sense of direction, is eager to begin.

The stutterer needs to experience positive feelings toward the clinician initially, because as the next stage commences and proceeds, there must be sufficient residual positive affect on the part of the client toward the clinician to sustain the relationship. If the client does not experience positive feelings towards the clinician at this stage, he may withdraw from therapy when the clinician begins pressing him for symptom modification in the next stage.

Examination and Confrontation
The second stage of therapy commences when the clinician directs the client to begin modifying the disfluency-related behaviors. For example, the clinician suggests that the client begin to change the "I look away when I stutter" behavior, asking the child to practice maintaining eye contact in front of a mirror in the therapy session. The client then is given a list of speaking situations outside of the therapy sessions in which to practice maintaining eye contact during moments of stuttering. Typically, clients make rapid changes in the more gross motor acts associated with the stuttering moments; the clinician also provides additional assignments on the most obvious and distracting extraneous hand, face, and body movements in the succeeding sessions of therapy with the primary goal of identifying attitudes, feelings, and behavior patterns that affect the client's ability to modify speech patterns.

Assignments typically evoke negative or resistive client reactions directed at the clinician and the therapy situation. The clinician utilizes these forms of resistance to develop an affectively meaningful interpersonal relationship with the client. Even as she becomes aware of the client's resistant behaviors, she continues to press for the behavior change, but the client, generally unaware of these resistive behavioral patterns, is typically less than totally successful in carrying out the assignments. Through observation of the client's behavior, however, the clinician perceives the client's resistive behavior, and, in effect, encourages him to express the resistances openly, using his entire repertoire of both therapy-impeding and therapy-facilitating behaviors. When the clinician feels that she is capable of identifying the client's basic patterns of interpersonal behavior, the confrontation phase of the second stage is initiated.

The term *confrontation* is defined as the clinician's verbalizations of client behavioral patterns which either facilitate or impede the client's modification of behavior. Confrontation is different from the act of identification in the first stage of therapy. There, the clinician assisted the client in describing and defining the symptoms of the speech problem. Here, through confrontation, the client is helped to perceive accurately his behavioral response patterns to the clinician's pressure for change.

The clinician cites behavior, free of value judgments (in terms of being either "bad" or "good") for, in fact, most of the client's patterns of adjustive behavior, identified as detrimental to behavior change during this period, are actually productive behavior patterns in many life situations (e.g., intellectualizing, which is a necessary skill for the college student). Such distinctions, however, generally are not made by the stutterer this early in therapy, and ordinarily he perceives the clinician's confrontations as indications of disapproval and rejection. Generally, it is only as the relationship continues that the stutterer is able to discern that even though the clinician calls attention to these behavior patterns, she really does understand and accept the feelings and attitudes underlying them.

As the clinician continues to direct attention to the observed resistive behaviors, the client typically responds in a defensive manner, either denying that the behavior is resistive or indicating a mere intellectual recognition of the clinician's perceptions. With continued confrontations, furthermore, the client begins to evidence a negativism (which is, perhaps, the first sign of involvement). The client may, for example, become nonverbal, appearing late for therapy or subtly indicating that he feels therapy is a waste of time. Such client behavior indicates that the clinician is successfully leading the client toward emotional involvement in the therapeutic relationship, and she confronts him with the resistive behavior to shape an emotional involvement for him, and thus create an affectively meaningful relationship.

Obviously the manner in which the confrontation is conducted is crucial to the success of therapy for this requires a sensitivity on the part of the clinician as to when and how to confront the client in order to provoke an emotional involvement in the situation. (For a more comprehensive discussion of clinician behaviors during this critical stage of therapy see the PFCT Kit's clinician's manual [Cooper, 1976].)

Involvement is evidenced by the stutterer's expression of feelings toward the clinician and the therapy process, and the clinician reinforces this expression of feelings (whether positive or negative) while not necessarily subscribing to the accuracy of the perceptions. With continued reinforcement of the verbal expressions of feelings, the clinician promotes a relationship in which the client expresses feelings honestly and freely. This establishes a therapeutic milieu that allows the client, primarily through the verbalization of feelings, to become aware of his feelings and evaluate them; and the emotionally honest relationship actually facilitates the client's adoption of the clinician's more accurate perceptions.

Cognition and Behavior Orientation
In the third stage, the clinician continues to reinforce client expressions of affect, facilitating client self-evaluation activities and maintaining client commitment to change. Assuming that the clinician is successful in reinforcing client self-evaluation activities with appropriate contingent responses, client introspection in the therapy sessions generally increases in frequency. Perhaps one of the most common problems encountered in shaping the client's behavior, however, is the tendency toward rumination rather than introspection, for clients frequently engage in nondirectional and nonproductive meditation rather than in goal-directed observations and analyses. Recognizing this as an obstacle, clinicians make the distinction for the client, reinforcing introspective activities while punishing ruminative responses in the therapy sessions.

Disruptive cognitive processing may take many other forms and are indicated by positive responses to any of the following questions: Does the client consistently evaluate himself from a negative point of view? Is he an unrealistic "negative" or "positive" thinker? Does he view people's reactions to his stuttering unrealistically? Does he intellectualize inappropriately? Does he consistently misinterpret affect-laden messages directed toward him? Does he misperceive the significance of his stuttering problem in relation to his total behavioral output?

Assuming that the clinician has been able to maintain the affectively honest therapeutic relationship throughout the client self-evaluative phase of therapy, clinician reinforcement of client appreciation results in an increased feeling of client self-worth and well-being (admittedly vague, but nevertheless very real, terms for individuals expressing these feelings).

As indicated in the goals for the third stage of therapy, the clinician introduces the concept of self-reinforcement as a significant factor in the modification of stuttering behavior (Cross and Cooper, 1976). The clinician instructs the client on administering self-reinforcers, identifying and defining disruptive cognitions just as she identifies the client's resistive behavior patterns. Thus, the client is taught to make appropriate, discrete, and contingent responses to reinforce both thoughts and acts.

Concomitantly with instruction in self-reinforcement, the clinician introduces the client to the concept of fluency control through the use of fluency-initiating gestures (FIGs). Elsewhere (Cooper, 1976, 1979a), I have discussed how my thinking with respect to "teaching stutterers to stutter more fluently" versus "teaching stutterers to speak more fluently" evolved. Perhaps my position at this time is best summed-up by the motto: "Don't fight it: FIG it!" Although clinicians are encouraged to assist older clients in developing their own "personal" FIGs, clinicians may introduce the following as "universal FIGs":

Slow speech: a reduction in the rate of speech typically involving the equalized prolongations of syllables

Easy onset: the initiation of phonation with as little laryngeal area tension as possible

Deep breath: a consciously controlled inhalation prior to the initiation of phonation and typically used in conjunction with the easy onset FIG

Loudness control: a conscious and sustained increase or decrease in the volume of the client's speech

Smooth speech (easy contact): a reduction in phonatory adjustments; also light articulatory contacts with plosive and affricate sounds, typically being modified to resemble fricative sounds

Syllable stress: a deliberate variation of volume and pitch

In working with young stutterers the clinician describes the concept of FIGs to both the parents and the child, noting that each FIG increases the coordination of the muscles for respiration, phonation, and articulation and thereby promotes increased fluency. The clinician instructs the child, generally in the presence of the parents, on the use of each of the FIGs, referring to a graphic representation of the FIG tree (see p. 29) to assist the parents and child in selecting the ones that appear most efficient and effective for the client's particular needs. The clinician, the parents, and the child then agree upon which FIG to begin working.

Neither the child nor the adult stutterer is asked to use FIGs immediately in situations outside of the clinic or the home because in the remainder of this third stage of therapy, the client must "over-learn" those FIGs that are found to be most effective in eliciting fluency primarily through drill. The third stage of therapy terminates when he demonstrates not only an ability to use FIGs successfully to elicit fluency in the clinic or home environment but also (to the extent possible) (1) perceives accurately (as must ultimately be determined by the clinician) the stuttering behavior and the interpersonal ramifications of the stuttering behavior; (2) possesses a realistic emotional and intellectual appreciation of self; (3) practices self-reinforcement; and (4) understands the feeling of control.

Fluency Control

The clinician assists the stutterer in planning and using FIGs in speech situations that previously resulted in fluency problems. The client strives to reinforce in life situations the feelings of fluency control that he has been developing in the clinical situation. As noted in the PFCT clinician's manual (Cooper, 1976), the clinician "psychs-up" the client to use FIGs in other environments and "going on controls" becomes a very real and highly desired goal for him. The clinician, knowing the client's feelings, attitudes, and skills in using FIGs, generally is the best judge of how and when the client should introduce them in the world outside. She, therefore, creates a hierarchy of speech situations based on the amount of fluency control which the client feels in a given situation; but as noted in the PFCT manual, most clients begin experimenting with their FIGs in a variety of life situations even before they are instructed to do so by the clinician. With older clients, the clinician does not have to develop elaborate guides to the utilization of fluency controls; however, with the younger client, she may want to continue assigning specific situations, using the *Assignment and Evaluation Worksheet* discussed in the materials section of this chapter. When the stutterer feels that no matter how difficult the speaking situation may be he is capable of employing FIGs to increase fluency, therapy is terminated.

PHYSICAL BEHAVIORS

Some clinicians (Perkins, 1979), using fluency-shaping methods rather than teaching the stutterer to stutter more fluently, conclude that there is no need to focus on concomitant behaviors (such as eye blinks) because they disappear when the client attains fluent speech. While such an assumption appears reasonable, my experience suggests that clients need to be taught to control their secondary behaviors, for even the most successful ones experience a few disfluencies with their new manner of speaking. These residual disfluencies are less distracting to the listener and less disturbing to the client if unaccompanied by extraneous mannerisms. What is more, as noted in the second stage of PFCT, the focus at the beginning of the therapy is on these secondary symptoms because they do not make premature demands on the client to learn to use FIGs.

ATTITUDINAL WORK

The extent to which the attitudes of stutterers have drawn attention in therapy has varied markedly during the past three decades. Clinicians in the 1950s maintained that developing objective attitudes in stutterers toward both their stuttering and themselves would lead to increased fluency. In the onrush of excitement with the new behaviorism of the 1960s and early 1970s, however, the focus on stutterers' attitudes all but disappeared. Then, although appreciative of the precision and obvious effectiveness of the behaviorally oriented therapy programs available to them, clinicians of the mid-1970s once again focused on the significance of stutterer attitudes.

The rebirth of interest in developing strategies that promote fluency-facilitating attitudes in stutterers pleases me, for any stuttering program is inadequate if it does not help the clients clarify and alter attitudes that impede fluency control. Others still believe that attention to attitudes and feelings are unnecessary (Ryan, 1974; Webster, 1975), however, for with the advent of detailed and systematic behavior modification programs based on a specific learning model, speech clinicians became aware of the vulnerability of the abstract hypothetical constructs that underlie insight approaches to stuttering therapy. As a result, clinicians adopted defensive attitudes when they discussed "self-actualization," "acceptance," "objectivity," or "self-concept"; for in comparison with the rigorously defined and experimentally manipulative behaviors described in behavior therapies, these terms appeared undefinable and irrelevant to the manipulation of behavior.

Unfortunately, behaviorally oriented therapy programs that do not attend to the stutterer's feelings and attitudes result in the belief that with the proper control of contingencies, fluency can be shaped and maintained without effort on the stutterer's part. While few doubt that stutterers can be conditioned to *temporary* fluency, we know, nevertheless, that stutterers wishing to maintain fluency must expend enormous effort to do so. Stutterers must possess energy which, in large part, is internally derived if they wish to maintain the fluency that is elicited with the clinician's conditioning strategies; in fact, for some, the amount of vigilance needed to sustain fluent speech requires such an outlay of energy that the stutterer is capable of accomplishing little else. The clinicians' duty, therefore, is to assist clients in assessing how much energy they wish to expend on maintaining fluency control, and by doing so, avoid imposing unrealistic fluency standards on them. If this variable is neglected, clinicians may force stutterers to feel even more incompetent because they are unable to maintain the fluency that was so easily elicited in the clinical situation. A therapy program that imposes externally derived criteria for success on its clients, then, runs the risk of belittling them.

For this reason alone, stuttering therapy programs should include activities attending to the client's feelings, beliefs, attitudes, goals, and dreams. These are real human responses that continue to evade the behaviorist's well-defined, measurable, and manipulative reinforcements.

The speech clinician's role with the preschool stutterer is critical, since at that age children are just beginning to acquire the language necessary for identifying feelings and attitudes. In her role as speech-language clinician, the therapist has the responsibility of helping her young client to identify, develop, and reinforce the attitudes and feelings that are fluency-enhancing as well as instructing him and his parents in how

FIGs are developed. The PFCT clinician, then, not only assists the child in developing a vocabulary for these but also guides the child in developing accurate perceptions of the stuttering problem itself.

In the case of older stutterers who have already identified and labeled feelings and attitudes, the speech-language clinician's role with respect to these varies markedly. In some instances, the stutterer accurately perceives the stuttering behavior and its ramifications but evidences fluency-enhancing attitudes and feelings as well, requiring only reinforcement by the clinician. In other instances, the stutterer's attitudes and feelings are based on inaccurate, therapy-impeding perceptions of the stuttering and its ramifications. In such situations, the clinician needs to attend not only to the feelings and attitudes of the client but also to the inaccurate perceptions on which they are based. Convinced that it is the speech clinician's responsibility to develop and maintain fluency-enhancing attitudes and feelings in stutterers of all ages, we designed PFCT to include procedures for the development, maintenance, and reinforcement of fluency-*enhancing* attitudes and feelings as well as for the modification of fluency-*impeding* ones. Clinicians need not alter client attitudes and feelings in all instances, but the clinician and the client must at least identify them if therapy is to proceed efficiently and effectively (Cooper, 1982b).

Effective therapy for stutterers focuses attention on attitudes and feelings when clients

1. Process significant misperceptions, not only about the problem itself, but also about the ramifications of the behavior
2. Process feelings about their problems or themselves that will significantly impede their successful utilization of speech and language modification procedures
3. Experience significant discrepancies between the way they think and the way they feel about their problem and about themselves.

If, at the beginning of PFCT, the clinician finds no problem in the areas noted above, she proceeds with the behavior modification procedures; but if she perceives problems in one or more of the three areas, she assumes that the client's feelings and attitudes need to be addressed in order for the client to obtain maximal benefit from therapy.

A recent national self-study project found that while speech clinicians recognize the frequent need for counseling-oriented activities in therapy, they have less confidence in their counseling skills than in the ones that address behavior modification. Clinicians know how to change behavior but are less certain as to how to change feelings and attitudes, for it is difficult, if not impossible, to develop or alter an individual's sense of emotional integrity or self-worth through simple instruction. Such attitudes and feelings evolve early in life through repeated emotion-laden interchanges with our parents and continue to develop later primarily through interchanges with others with whom we become emotionally involved. Obviously we adopt attitudes of individuals we love, respect or admire more readily than we adopt attitudes of those from whom we are emotionally detached. What is more, any abrupt or significant changes in our own self-concept typically are emotionally charged responses that result from an interaction or series of interactions with significant persons in our lives.

The clinician's task, then, is to establish with the client a helping relationship characterized by significant affect-laden verbal interchanges, providing her client with the opportunity to identify, evaluate, and adopt feelings and attitudes that facilitate therapy.

Unfortunately for our understanding of the clinical process, terms such as "warm," "personal," "supportive," "nurturing," and "friendly," are rather popular definitions of a helping relationship that facilitates attitudinal change. Clinical process studies indicate that while these terms are useful as an overall characterization of a relationship designed to alter feelings and attitudes, they are not helpful in describing the critical affective interchanges between client and clinician in such a relationship. We acknowledge the problems that terms such as "warm" and "friendly" have created when we review our therapy plans with the client, and the student then notes that the strategy is to establish rapport in the first 4 to 5 minutes of therapy before proceeding to the business at hand. One must assume that the student's attention to the clinical relationship will terminate after those 4 to 5 minutes. If we rely exclusively on terms such as "warm" and "nurturing" to describe the clinical relationship, we overlook the critical role affective interchanges play in changing attitudes in the therapy relationship process. In addition, such terms suggest that the ideal clinical relationship is static, for they fail to indicate that a helping relationship is not simply a state but also a process.

During the course of the helping relationship, the client's attitudes toward his clinician undergo a series of rather predictable changes that are independent of the type of therapy employed. Whether the clinician focuses the client's attention on feelings and attitudes or keeps the therapeutic activities focused on modifying behavior, the sequence of client feelings towards the clinician follows a fairly typical pattern. Research in our field (Cooper, 1966; Cooper and Cooper, 1969; and Manning and Cooper, 1969) as well as in clinical psychology (Snyder and Snyder, 1961) suggests the nature of that pattern. The client develops increasingly less positive feelings toward the clinician after the initiation of therapy, only to evolve even more positive ones later on in the process. Then, toward the end, the client's feelings, which tend now to be more positive, actually begin to stabilize in contrast with the shifts noted in earlier stages of therapy. Such a pattern of affect change is not surprising, for the client's initial positive feelings derive primarily from his expectations of symptom relief and from faith in the clinician's ability to effect it. The feelings decline, however, as the client comes to realize that the clinician has no instant cure and that improvement will come only after the expenditure of significant energies. Later, when the client reestablishes a sense of well-being as he experiences success in the therapy, the positive feelings return and begin to stabilize as the therapy process nears termination. By this time in the therapy process, the client has adjusted to the clinician; and the magnitude of behavioral and attitudinal changes decreases.

Because they are aware of these typical shifts in client feelings, clinicians, regardless of their therapeutic orientation, must avoid needless therapeutic failures. Those involved in instruction-oriented relationships, knowing that clients typically experience a down period following the initiation of therapy, must be more understanding of the client's apparent loss of enthusiasm and interest at this point. The clinician may actually need to make adjustments in therapy procedures in order to minimize the negativism and to hasten the client's sense of accomplishment.

These shifts in client feelings are of even greater significance for a clinician engaged in a counseling-oriented relationship. The clinician who focuses on assisting the client to identify and to adopt therapy-facilitating attitudes and feelings must capitalize on these universally observed changes in client feelings. By responding to these feelings, she initiates the kinds of affective interchanges between the client and herself that will facilitate changes in the client's feelings and attitudes.

TRANSFER AND MAINTENANCE
In my 20-odd years of experience with treatment programs for stutterers, I have been continually impressed with how easily even the most severe stutterer gains fluency in such an environment. My initial feelings of having solved the problem of stuttering through short-term intensive programs, however, were quickly abused by follow-up studies (Cooper, 1965a, 1968b) which showed that in the vast majority of cases, stutterers who gained total fluency in short-term intensive residential programs experienced significant relapses within 1 to 2 years following their enrollment. Aware, then, of the need to develop strategies that assist stutterers in maintaining their fluency once they leave therapy, I focused on the problem of transferring the stutterer's clinical fluency to his home environment and arrived at the following conclusions:

1. Fluency should not be the end goal of therapy.
2. Long-term, nonintensive stuttering programs are preferable to short-term intensive programs.
3. Training in self-reinforcement should be a basic element in every stuttering therapy program.

Earlier in this chapter, I identified the feeling of control, rather than the fluency itself, as the end goal of PFCT. That feeling of control is necessary if the stutterer is to successfully transfer the fluency gained in therapy to the home environment and maintain it. This observation is reinforced by the findings of others (Guitar and Bess, 1978), including Daly (1977), who in a follow-up study of stutterers enrolled in an intensive therapy program, makes the following observations about the feeling of control and the maintenance of fluency:

> It is our contention that stutterers must earn this "feeling of control." What happens when our clients acquire fluency too fast or when they experience "false fluency" very early in therapy? The change in speech fluency occurs so suddenly that the client is not aware of the monitoring he or she must do in order to maintain fluency in difficult situations. . . .
>
> These clients do not replace stuttering with normal speech—fluency just happens. Happy with their new speech pattern, many clients are not motivated to learn the speech components or targets necessary to retain fluent speech. These clients have not achieved the "feeling of control." Fluent speech and disfluent speech are still superstitious behaviors that just occur. It is with these "quick to fluency" clients that we have considerable difficulty.

Such observations support my opinion that one of the most important factors in the maintenance of fluency is the stutterer's feeling of control. For that reason, alone, it is more important for the stutterer to focus on the feeling of control than on an arbitrarily determined level of fluency.

My disenchantment with the results of short-term intensive residential treatment programs for stutterers continues. Although a combination of a short-term intensive program in which fluency skills are introduced and a long-term, nonintensive program of support might be ideal, such a situation rarely exists. Having observed my wife's work with stuttering therapy in public school settings for over 15 years, however, I now think the typical school situation provides the support that is necessary. In this setting, therapy is long-term, entailing one or two sessions per week for a period of 1 to 2 years, and, therefore, has the greatest potential for helping young stutterers acquire and maintain the feeling of control.

The fluency control stage of PFCT, as noted earlier in this chapter, focuses on guiding the stutterer to transfer the fluency skills learned in the clinic to life situations. Transfer activities are not simply an adjunct to PFCT but, in fact, are basic to the process that assists stutterers in developing an enduring feeling of fluency control in even the most difficult speech situations.

FOLLOW-UP PROCEDURES

Clients are not dismissed from PFCT simply because they have reached a predetermined level of fluency in a prescribed speaking situation or completed a predetermined number of therapy sessions within a prescribed time frame. Rather, clients begin to withdraw from therapy when they experience and maintain the feeling of control outside of the clinic situation without the clinician's assistance. For those who have attained this feeling, we alter the schedule of therapy appointments, gradually increasing the period of time between them until clients indicate they wish to terminate the formal therapeutic relationship altogether.

Follow-up procedures are relatively easy to complete in the school situation. We consider the initial phase of follow-up procedures, along with maintenance and transfer procedures, to be part of the therapeutic process. The clinician follows the children who have completed the program by conducting annual interviews throughout their school years; and, of course, we recommend re-enrollment in the therapy program for those children who evidence a need for "booster shots" (as several of the clients have referred to it).

EQUIPMENT AND MATERIALS NEEDED

A tape recorder and a stopwatch are the only equipment needed to use most of the PFCT materials described in this chapter. Although equipment such as delayed auditory feedback machines, devices to monitor the loudness of onset of phonation, metronomes, and noise generators effectively and efficiently assist clients in becoming aware of disfluencies and in identifying and adopting fluency-initiating gestures, they are not critical to effective therapy. Clients are able to develop a feeling for a slower rate of speech through the utilization of a delayed auditory feedback apparatus, but the feeling of rate control can be achieved simply with the use of a stopwatch. Similarly, an instrument indicating abrupt changes in phonatory activity may be an efficient means of assisting clients in developing the feeling of control over the easy onset of phonation, but a clinician can serve as a monitor of easy onsets without the benefit of such expensive instruments.

PFCT kit materials, some of which were described in the assessment section of this chapter, assist clinicians in assessing attitudes and behaviors and in structuring the therapy. Although these therapy materials are specific to the principles and procedures of PFCT, most of the instruments can be used effectively by clinicians with differing therapy orientations.

Three therapy guides are used in the second stage of therapy.

My Stuttering Apple

The stuttering apple therapy guide provides the young client with an easily grasped conceptualization of the stuttering problem. In order to promote his understanding of the things he does "when" and "because" he stutters, we use a graphic representation of an apple with a centrally placed circle, labeled "Core: getting stuck on words" and surrounded by several empty circles within the outline of the apple. Working together, the client and the clinician use the empty circles to write down the behaviors observed during the client's moments of stuttering as well as resulting behaviors that the client adopts because of the stuttering problem. The apple then constitutes the first page of a loose-leaf speech notebook into which the client and clinician insert additional pages concerned with the therapy schedule, assignment sheets, practice sheets, and other therapy-related items.

My Monkeys

To help both children and adults identify burdensome feelings and attitudes, we use a cartoon of a young man with three monkeys sitting on his back and waving blank flags. This particular therapy aid prompted one client to report that "all my life I have had the feeling that I must be odd because people say that stuttering is 'psychological.' " Another client who responded similarly wrote the comment, "stuttering is psychological" in one of the monkey's blank flags. Young stutterers frequently respond as well with the observation that "people think I'm dumb because I stutter." The act of not only verbalizing but writing down these kinds of observations seems to facilitate identification of stuttering-related feelings and attitudes that need attention.

Assignment and Evaluation Worksheet

A clinician uses this single page form both for giving assignments and for evaluating the client's response to them. After asking the client to alter a disfluency-related behavior (such as loss of eye contact, eye blinks, or facial grimaces), she observes his attitudinal and behavioral responses, recording these in the evaluation portion of the worksheet. Then at the beginning of each therapy session, she and the client review the responses which she identifies as either facilitating or impeding attainment of the goals of therapy. Typical therapy-impeding behaviors and attitudes are failing to complete the assignment, being late for therapy, forgetting the speech notebook, viewing therapy as a waste of time, and considering the assignment inappropriate.

The clinician completes the evaluation portion of the worksheet with the client's assistance, and the completed worksheet becomes a permanent part of the client's speech notebook. The first few minutes of each therapy session during the second stage of therapy are structured around this single worksheet, and the latter portion of the therapy session is spent preparing the assignment for the next time. Such assignments reduce extraneous disfluency-related behaviors and elicit client behaviors and attitudes to which the clinician can respond.

Several therapy guides exist for the third stage of PFCT.

Fluency Analysis Checklist

This single page checklist itemizes a number of fluency-eliciting conditions (for example, speaking in time to a metronome and speaking under delayed auditory feedback) and a number of speech situations (for example, conversational speech and reading aloud). The clinician monitors the fluency of her client's speech under the various conditions and identifies speech behaviors (changes in loudness, rate, and prosody) that typically characterize the fluent speech. After experimenting with the identified speech behaviors, the client determines whether or not the behavior elicits fluency, thereby heightening not only his awareness of speech motor acts but also his understanding of the feeling of fluency control.

My FIG Tree

To help young children identify fluency-initiating gestures, clinicians use a drawing of a fig tree with blank fig-shaped spaces scattered among the leaves. As these gestures are identified for the child, the clinician writes descriptions of them in the blank spaces of the fig tree. This activity serves to emphasize FIGs as significant to fluent speech and provides labels that facilitate communication between the child and the clinician in the same manner as the stuttering apple.

Fortunately for both the parents and the clinician, young children grasp the concept of FIGs easily. While the nonreading children represent FIGs in the empty figs with simple symbols, the older children actually write in the names of gestures which they, their parents, and clinicians have deemed effective and worthy of reinforcement.

Disfluency Descriptor Digest

This single page form (Cooper, 1982a) includes a list of 20 statements describing behaviors that are frequently observed in the disfluent speech of stutterers. When a behavior appears in the client's stuttering pattern, even if only occasionally, the clinician enters a check mark in the box preceding the statement. Following this list is a table indicating six universal FIGs and the number of described behaviors for which each FIG appears to predict success. Clinicians frequently observe that the behavioral checklist assists them not only in identifying the characteristics of individual disfluencies with greater precision, but also, and as a result, in developing client awareness of the vocal adjustments that are necessary to increase fluency.

As noted previously, the effectiveness of any one of the FIGs in eliciting fluency varies from client to client and appears related to the primary observable phonatory, respiratory, and articulatory posturings that occur during moments of disfluency. For example, the deep breath FIG is used effectively with stutterers whose disfluencies occur most frequently when they are "out of breath" and attempting phonation without an adequate air supply to sustain phonation. Stutterers with an abnormally rapid articulatory rate during both fluent and disfluent speech, on the other hand, find the slow speech FIG most useful in enhancing fluency. Thus, the *Disfluency Descriptor Digest* assists clinicians in determining which FIGs are most appropriate for the individual stutterer.

FIG Practice Sheets

The *Personalized Fluency Control Therapy Kit* (Cooper and Cooper, 1976) provides 26 different single page FIG practice sheets including sheets for each of the six "universal FIGs." The numbers in the lower right corner of each page indicate a recommended order in which to use the practice sheets although each sheet is used more than once. The directions on the sheets are simple and enable the clients to complete the practice with minimal assistance. Included in the kit are sample sheets which clinicians use to assist clients in developing a feeling of fluency control, but clinicians and clients develop additional, more individualized practice sheets as needed. Evaluations of the client's progress in mastering these FIGs ultimately include the question "are you beginning to feel or do you have a feeling of fluency control when you use the FIG?"

The order in which the FIG practice sheets are presented is not meant to mandate the order in which the client progresses through the FIGs. In the exploratory period when the concept of FIGs is introduced, clients may find that they feel more comfortable beginning with, for example, easy onset rather than the slow speech FIG. Clinicians use their own judgment in advising clients of an order in which to begin to master the motor acts of the various FIGs. In fact, they may find it helpful to have clients focus on more than one FIG at the same time; but again, these are judgments best left to the discretion of the clinician.

Client Readiness for Fluency Control Inventory

The PFCT kit includes a single page inventory used throughout the third stage of therapy to keep both client and clinician on track. The inventory consists of 25 statements describing client attitudes and feelings, self-reinforcement capabilities, and behavioral patterns to which the client and clinician respond during the last few minutes of each therapy session. After reading each statement together, the client and the clinician select a point on a 5-point scale (ranging from "substantial negative evidence" to "substantial positive evidence") which they agree most accurately reflects the client's behavior or attitude during the therapy session just completed.

The statements on the inventory describe behaviors and attitudes that are indicative of the client's readiness to initiate the final drive for a feeling of fluency control. Consequently, the more substantial positive evidence the clinician and client observe, the greater is the likelihood that the client is ready to undertake the final stage of therapy. The importance of utilizing the inventory consistently cannot be overemphasized. The clinician's attention to the attitudes and the behaviors that it assesses establishes and maintains a client perspective of the therapy process essential to the client's gaining and maintaining the feeling of control when therapy is terminated.

CLINICIAN SKILLS AND TRAINING REQUIRED
Recognizing the success of PFCT depends to a large extent upon the clinician's ability to be sensitive to and responsive in the client-clinician relationship (Cooper, 1965c, 1966; Cooper, Eggertson, and Galbraith, 1971; Crane and Cooper, 1983). In the PFCT kit clinician's manual, a chapter is devoted to reviewing the literature on clinician personality factors and to describing the attitudes and skills of the effective clinician (Cooper, 1976). As noted in that chapter, on the basis of research data available and over 20 years of observations of clinicians in training and professional practice with stutterers, I suggest that the following list of attributes are characteristic of the effective clinician:

Affectively verbal—Viscerally vocal
Affectively honest
Primarily positively and affectively verbal
Affectively reflective—Not affectively directive
Devoid of dogma
Noninterpretive
Persevering
Informative
Detail disciplined

In the PFCT clinician's manual (Cooper, 1976) and again in Gregory's (1979) *Controversies About Stuttering Therapy* I noted that the exclusively behavior-oriented stuttering programs proliferating on the market are inadvertently reinforcing the training of technicians without consideration of the skills necessary to assist clients in identifying and handling their feelings and attitudes. With the popularization of behavior modification principles and procedures, these training programs have been criticized for training amoeboid compassionates without technical skills; and emphasis has shifted to training the complete clinician; a humanist who is both a behaviorist and a phenomenologist.

CLIENT REQUIREMENTS
Personalized Fluency Control Therapy is designed for both children and adults. The rationale underlying the therapy process is as appropriate for very young children as it is for adults, so all of our materials are geared for use with clients of all ages.

One of the controversial issues in the treatment of stutterers concerns intervention procedures with the very young preschool disfluent child. Apparently many clinicians, clinging to the dubious notion that drawing attention to disfluencies causes stuttering, continue to advocate a hands-off policy with the young stutterer. On the basis of my own research in recovery from stuttering (Cooper, 1972; 1973b; Lankford and Cooper,

1974) and my research in parent, teacher, and clinician attitudes toward stuttering (Cooper, 1975; Crowe and Cooper, 1977; Fowlie and Cooper, 1978; McLelland and Cooper, 1977; and Cooper and Cooper, 1982), I disagree. Too many clinicians for too long have held parents responsible for stuttering on the theory that parents do wrong by reacting to their child's disfluencies. The evidence suggests that typical parental reactions, such as drawing attention to and suggesting means of altering disfluent behavior, actually facilitate the development of fluent speech. In fact, what little data we have in this area indicate that parents are a positive factor in the significant number of young children who spontaneously recover from stuttering. A review of the studies on recovery from stuttering indicates further that parents of recovered stutterers frequently advised their children to "slow down" or "take a deep breath before speaking," and variations of both these techniques obtain in many of the therapy programs currently available.

The recognition of the positive role parents play in recovery from stuttering led me to perceive early and active intervention by clinicians as facilitating recovery from stuttering as well. I am convinced that stuttering children, exhibiting either tension in the speech musculature or articulatory or phonatory struggle behavior during moments of disfluency, can be taught to use FIGs efficiently and effectively; and even very young children, with the aid of materials, are able to conceptualize their stuttering and what they can do to alter it.*

Evaluation of the Therapy

As noted in the Assessment and Evaluation Procedures sections earlier in this chapter, therapeutic success or failure should be judged on the basis of changes in the client's attitudes and feelings as well as changes in fluency. In keeping with that belief, the PFCT assessment instruments, which measure both attitudes and behaviors, are used to evaluate the therapy program. In addition, because of the universality of the relapse phenomenon following the termination of stuttering therapy, any evaluation of a therapy program must include follow-up evaluations for at least 3 years following the termination of therapy.

While we continue to develop new insights into the clinical process and new materials to facilitate the administration of PFCT, the basic PFCT process remains as it was when first published (Cooper and Cooper, 1976). Using this therapy system with its assessment instruments, my wife and I, over a 10-year period, have provided therapy for disfluent individuals ranging in age from 2½ to 58 years. We have watched as the preschool disfluent children with whom we worked matured and subsequently

---

*A more thorough discussion of the role of parents in early intervention programs for very young stutterers, written primarily for parents, is available in the National Easter Seal Society booklet *Understanding Stuttering: Information for Parents* (Cooper, 1979b).

completed their public school education; and we have followed for several years the careers of adults with whom we employed PFCT. On the basis of these observations and the data on these clients, and in the absence of vitally needed longitudinal studies on large populations of stutterers, the following evaluative comments appear justified.

1. As many as four out of every five abnormally disfluent preschool children can be helped to achieve normal fluency by the time they complete the primary school years.
2. The chance for complete recovery for an adult stutterer (over 18 years of age) is markedly less than for the preschool age stutterer. On the basis of my experience, the chance for complete recovery from stuttering in an adult stutterer appears to be about one in five.
3. Approximately 60 percent of the adult stutterers receiving PFCT experience prolonged periods of fluency once they have developed the feeling of control. At the end of a 3-year period, about 20 percent of those clients continue to experience normal fluency, giving little or no attention to the mechanics of fluency maintenance. Forty percent of the adults, although able to sustain periods of fluency through the use of FIGs, continue to experience periods of stuttering but consider themselves to be "controlled stutterers."
4. The remaining 40 percent of adult stutterers receiving PFCT, while being capable of maintaining a higher level of fluency than prior to therapy, continue to perceive themselves as stutterers and continue to be frustrated by their inability to maintain the feeling of fluency control in certain speech situations. Generally these stutterers perceive their therapy experience as having contributed significantly to a realistic view of their stuttering and to a positive self-image. Frequently, members of this group of adult stutterers seek supportive liaisons with clinicians on an infrequent but long-term basis.

In summary, PFCT has been helpful for both child and adult stutterers with young clients attaining normal fluency four times as frequently as older ones. Three out of five adult stutterers achieve fluency through PFCT while the remaining two, who continue to experience periods of uncontrolled disfluencies at a diminished rate, perceive the therapy experience positively in terms of their acceptance of the problem and themselves.

An editor for the PFCT kit publishing firm estimated in 1982 that at least 90,000 stutterers have been enrolled in treatment programs using concepts and materials from the PFCT kit. As we continue to develop new and improved therapy guidelines and materials to include in the PFCT process, we hope that the success rate, particularly with the adult stutterer, will improve. What is needed are longitudinal studies of large numbers of stutterers, but until then, we must rely on small samples of small populations with which to discuss our follow-up evaluations.

Reasons for Therapeutic Effectiveness

PFCT is effective because its therapy process efficiently and coherently integrates activities leading to the modification of attitudes and feelings as well as disfluent behaviors. Thus, in PFCT, as an individual learns to modify speech production behaviors for increased fluency, the individual's affective responses are modified to maintain the affective-cognitive congruity necessary for sustaining the feeling of fluency control.

Advantages of the Therapy

COMPREHENSIVENESS

PFCT's integration of behavior and attitude modification procedures is one major advantage of the therapy system, as well as the major reason for its effectiveness; and thus it offers a comprehensive approach to the modification of stuttering behavior.

COMMUNICABILITY

The therapeutic concepts used in PFCT are easily communicated to clinicians and clients of all ages. Very young children, for example, grasp the process of therapy through the use of the PFCT materials which indicate that therapy can be described simply as "moving from apples to FIGs." The four-stage PFCT process is easily grasped by clinicians, and the commercially available materials enable clinicians to communicate a sense of direction to the client.

ADAPTABILITY

PFCT is adaptable to a short-term, intensive therapy regime or to a long-term, nonintensive therapy situation, and the materials are adaptable either to children or adults, as well as to individuals of varying intellectual capacities.

AVAILABILITY

The commercially available PFCT kit, which includes instructional materials for both the clinician and clients, makes the therapy program easily accessible to therapists seeking a structured therapy program for stutterers.

References

Adams, M., and Reis, R. The influence of the onset of phonation on the frequency of stuttering. *J. Speech Hear. Res.* 14:639–644, 1971.

Adams, M., and Reis, R. The influence of the onset of phonation on the frequency of stuttering: A replication and evaluation. *J. Speech Hear. Res.* 17:752–754, 1974.

Andrews, G., and Harris, M. *The Syndrome of Stuttering.* London: Heineman, 1964.

Bloodstein, O. Stuttering as an Anticipatory Struggle Reaction. In J. Eisenson (ed.), *Stuttering: A Symposium.* New York: Harper, 1958.

Cooper, C. S., and Cooper, E. B. Variations in adult stutterer attitudes towards clinicians during therapy. *J. Commun. Dis.* 2(2):141–153, 1969.

Cooper, C. S., and Cooper, E. B. Clinician attitudes toward stuttering in the United States and Europe. *ASHA* 2:11–19, 1982.

Cooper, E. B. An evaluation of inter-personal communications therapy for stutterers. *ASHA* 7:401, 1965a.

Cooper, E. B. An Inquiry Into the use of Inter-personal Communication as a Source for Therapy with Stutterers. In D. Barbara (ed.), *New Directions in Stuttering.* Springfield, Ill.: Thomas, 1965b.

Cooper, E. B. Clinician personality factors and judged effectiveness in varying therapeutic relationships. *ASHA* 7:408, 1965c.

Cooper, E. B. Client-clinician relationships and concomitant factors in stuttering therapy. *J. Speech Hear. Res.* 9:194–207, 1966.

Cooper, E. B. An therapy process for the adult stutterer. *J. Speech Hear. Dis.* 33:246–260, 1968a.

Cooper, E. B. Effectiveness of an intensive rehabilitation program for adult stutterers: A follow-up study. Paper presented at the annual convention of the American Speech-Language-Hearing Association, Denver, 1968b.

Cooper, E. B. An integration of behavior therapy and traditional therapy procedures for stutterers. *Ill. Speech Hear. J.* 2(3):5–8, 1969a.

Cooper,E. B. An integration of behavior therapy and traditional therapy procedures for stutterers. *Speech Hear. Assoc. Ala. Letter* 6:4–7, 1969b.

Cooper, E. B. An integration of behavior therapy and traditional therapy procedures for stutterers. *Assoc. Adv.Behav. Ther. Newsletter* 4(2):10–11, 1969c.

Cooper, E. B. Integrating behavior therapy and traditional insight therapy procedures with stutterers. *J. Commun. Dis.* 4:40–43, 1971a.

Cooper, E. B. Reflections on conceptualizing the stuttering therapy process from a simple theoretical framework. *J. Speech Hear. Dis.* 36(4):471–475, 1971b.

Cooper, E. B. Recovery from stuttering in a junior and senior high school population. *J. Speech Hear. Res.* 15:632–638, 1972.

Cooper, E. B. Integrating Relationship and Behavior Therapy Procedures for Adult Stutterers. In L. Emerick, and S. Hood (eds.), *The Client-Clinician Relationship.* Springfield, Ill.: Thomas, 1973a.

Cooper, E. B. The development of a stuttering chronicity prediction checklist for school age stutterers: A research inventory for clinicians. *J. Speech Hear. Dis.* 38:215–223, 1973b.

Cooper, E. B. Clinician attitudes toward stutterers: A study of bigotry? Paper presented at the annual convention of the American Speech-Language-Hearing Association, Washington, D.C., 1975.

Cooper, E. B. *Personalized Fluency Control Therapy Clinician Manual.* Hingham, Mass.: Teaching Resources, 1976.

Cooper, E. B. Case-selection procedures for school-aged disfluent children. *Lang. Speech Hear. Services Schools* 8(4)264–269, 1977.

Cooper, E. B. Facilitating parental participation in preparing the therapy component of the stutterer's individualized education program. *J. Fluency Dis.* 3:221–228, 1978.

Cooper, E. B. Intervention Procedures for Young Children. In H. H. Gregory (ed.), *Controversies About Stuttering Therapy.* Baltimore: University Park Press, 1979a.

Cooper, E. B. *Understanding Stuttering: Information for Parents.* Chicago: National Easter Seal Society, 1979b.

Cooper, E. B. A disfluency descriptor digest for clinical use. *J. Fluency Dis.* 7:355–358, 1982a.

Cooper, E. B. Understanding the Process. In S. Ainsworth (ed.), *Counseling Stutterers.* Memphis: Speech Foundation of America, 1982b.

Cooper, E. B., Cady, B. B., and Robbins, C. J. The effect of the verbal stimulus words "wrong," "right," and "tree," on the disfluency rates of stutterers and nonstutterers. *J. Speech Hear. Res.* 13:239–244, 1970.

Cooper, E. B., and Cooper, C. S. *Personalized Fluency Control Therapy Kit.* Hingham, Mass. Teaching Resources, 1976.

Cooper, E. B., and Cooper, C. S. *Personalized Fluency Control Therapy: IEP Forms.* Hingham, Mass.: Teaching Resources, 1980.

Cooper, E. B., Eggertson, S. A., and Galbraith, S. A. Clinician personality factors and effectiveness: A three study report. *J. Commun. Dis.* 4:40–43, 1971.

Crane, S. L., and Cooper, E. B. Speech and language clinician personality variables and clinical effectiveness. *J. Speech Hear. Dis.* 48:140–145, 1983.

Cross, D., and Cooper, E. B. Self versus investigator-administered presumed fluency reinforcing stimuli. *J. Speech Hear. Res.* 19:241–246, 1976.

Crowe, T. A., and Cooper, E. B. Parental attitudes toward knowledge of stuttering. *J. Commun. Dis.* 10:343–357, 1977.

Daly, D. A. Intervention procedures for the young stuttering child. Paper presented at the annual meeting of the Council for Exceptional Children, Atlanta, 1977.

Daly, D. A., and Cooper, E. B. Rate of stuttering adaptation under two electroshock conditions. *Behav. Res. Ther.* 5:49–54, 1967.

Fowlie, G. M., and Cooper, E. B. Traits attributed to stuttering and nonstuttering children by their mothers. *J. Fluency Dis.* 3:233–246, 1978.

Gregory, H. H. *Controversies About Stuttering Therapy.* Baltimore: University Park Press, 1979.

Guitar, B., and Bass, C. Stuttering therapy: The relation between attitude change and long-term outcome. *J. Speech Hear. Dis.* 43:392–400, 1978.

James, H. P., and Cooper, E. B. Accuracy of teacher referrals of speech handicapped children. *Except. Child.* 33:29–34, 1966.

Lankford, S. D., and Cooper, E. B. Recovery from stuttering as viewed by parents of self-diagnosed recovered stutterers. *J. Commun. Dis.* 7:171–180, 1974.

Manning, W. H., and Cooper, E. B. Variations in attitudes of the adult stutterer toward his clinician related to progress in therapy. *J. Commun. Dis.* 2(2):154–162, 1969.

Martin, E. W. Client centered therapy as a theoretical orientation for speech therapy. *ASHA* 5:576–578, 1963.

Matthews, J. Communicology and individual responsibility. *ASHA* 6:3–7, 1964.

McDonald, E. T. *Articulation Testing and Treatment: A Sensory Motor Approach.* Pittsburgh: Stanwix House, 1964.

McLelland, J. K., and Cooper, E. B. Fluency-related behaviors and attitudes of 178 young stutterers. *J. Fluency Dis.* 3:253–263, 1978.

Murphy, A., and FitzSimons, R. *Stuttering and Personality Dynamics.* New York: Ronald Press, 1960.

Perkins, W. H. From psychoanalysis to discoordination. In H. H. Gregory (ed.), *Controversies About Stuttering Therapy.* Baltimore: University Park Press, 1979.

Perkins, W. et al. Stuttering: Discoordination of phonation with articulation and respiration. *J. Speech Hear. Res.* 19:509–522, 1976.

Ryan, B. *Programmed Therapy for Stuttering in Children and Adults.* Springfield, Ill.: Thomas, 1974.

Sheehan, J. G. Conflict theory of stuttering. In J. Eisenson (ed.), *Stuttering: A Symposium.* New York: Harper, 1958.

Snyder, W. U., and Snyder, B. J. *The Psychotherapy Relationship*. New York: Macmillan, 1961.

Van Riper, C. *Speech Correction: Principles and Methods* (4th ed.). Englewood Cliffs, N.J.: Prentice-Hall, 1963.

Webster, R. L. *The Precision Fluency Shaping Program: Speech Reconstruction for Stutterers*. Roanoke, Va.: Communication Development Corporation, 1975.

Wingate, M. E. Prosody in stuttering adaptation. *J. Speech Hear. Res.* 9:626–629, 1966.

Wingate, M. E. Sound and pattern in "artificial" fluency. *J. Speech Hear. Res.* 12:677–686, 1969.

2. The Preschool Fluency Development Program: Assessment and Treatment

Delva M. Culp

Overview

In the mid-1970s, a review of the literature indicated that clinicians were doing little direct work with fluency-disordered preschool children. In order for the Callier Center at the University of Texas at Dallas to meet the needs of such children more effectively, I designed the Preschool Fluency Development Program. The program stresses the importance of early intervention, and this intervention approach utilizes both assessment and therapy procedures. Through assessment procedures, a sample of the children's daily communicative activities is obtained which is then compared quantitatively and qualitatively to the fluency of normal and fluency-disordered preschool children. The therapy that follows includes direct programming for the children and training for their parents. Programming for the children focuses on the integration of hierarchies of fluency as well as their cognitive and linguistic development; the training for parents introduces the characteristics of fluency disorder and provides instruction on the management of fluency at home. Follow-up data collected on the program have shown that a high percentage of the children involved have achieved and maintained normal fluency.

History of the Therapy

During the last decade, several factors lent impetus to my formation of the Preschool Fluency Development Program. First, I discovered that researchers have noted that fluency disorder most commonly begins during the preschool years (Van Riper, 1982); in a review of seven reports on this subject, the mean age of the onset of "stuttering" ranged from 3 to 5 years (Bloodstein, 1976). From this research, I determined that fluency skills of the preschool age group obviously warranted increased professional attention. Second, I noted a limited data base regarding normal and disordered fluency which led me to believe that further study of fluency development in the young was essential to differential diagnosis. Third, I questioned the sparse documentation of traditional programs which managed preschool fluency disorder by parent training without systematic assessment or treatment of the child. Fourth, I noted that numerous clinicians viewed fluency disorder as mysterious and, as a result of Johnsonian training, feared management of the disorder, particularly in children; these clinicians, it seemed to me, needed systematic and well-documented procedures for use in a variety of professional settings. Finally, I decided that because early intervention with numerous other health and education problems had been documented as valuable, such an approach held potential in the management of fluency disorder.

These observations, along with insights from the Preschool Stuttering Group at Northwestern University, where I studied under Hugo Gregory and Diane Hill in 1973–1974, inspired the design of the Preschool Fluency Development Program. During 1975, I developed the program to treat children ages 2½ to 7 years; a year later, the first children were enrolled at the Callier Center for Communication Disorders, Dallas, Texas. From the outset, the objective of the program was clear: to establish and generalize a normally fluent speaking pattern in children who demonstrate fluency disorder.

RATIONALE FOR THERAPY

The rationale for the therapy program derived primarily from principles of child development and learning theory. I hypothesized that fluency behavior could be modified by a program aimed at the child's cognitive level, offering an alternate speech pattern, and systematically manipulating stimulus–response–reinforcement in a hierarchy of increasingly more difficult tasks.

A review of the Piagetian model of cognitive development provided me with insight into specific skill levels of the preschool child as they relate to fluency (Flavell, 1963). Onset of fluency disorder typically occurs in the preoperational representation period (approximately 2 to 7 years of age), the second of the four developmental stages proposed by Piaget. It is important to recognize that during this period the child has not developed the mental structures necessary for logical or abstract thought. Rather, he depends upon what he sees or touches and reasons without systematic logic.

Four specific characteristics of child behavior during the preoperational representation period seemed worthy of consideration in developing a fluency program: abstraction, centration, transformation, and replication—each relevant to fluency facilitation.

Abstraction develops substantially during the preoperational representation period so that early in the period the child remembers only the concrete (whatever he sees or touches), while later he begins to process more abstract stimuli. For example, if given an object, most 3-year-olds could describe how it felt (soft, scratchy, etc.); but if shown a picture of the same object, they would be unable to provide such a description, because the picture is more abstract. In contrast, 7-year-olds can easily describe numerous characteristics of picture stimuli. Because speech, particularly fluency, is a more abstract stimulus, not to be seen or touched and presented quickly, I concluded that fluency modification required therapy procedures evolving with the child's ability to manage abstraction.

Centration describes the ability to explore only those aspects of a stimulus made obvious. Piaget has noted that the early preoperational child typically singles out one aspect of a stimulus. For example, the child looks at an apple, a red, round, shiny, edible object, and reacts only to its roundness, saying "ball." Centration demands serious consideration as the speech stimulus has many aspects: vocal tone, semantic intent, syntactic content, and articulation, all of which are routinely much more obvious than fluency.

During the preoperational representation period, the child also has difficulty processing transformations, for he focuses on individual elements in a sequence, rather than one element's changing to another form. For example, the child sees no relationship between a balloon filled with air and the piece of rubber which remains after the balloon bursts. Accordingly, without special assistance, the young child would experience great difficulty understanding changes in his speaking pattern and evaluating his own speech production.

Finally, during this period replication develops, that is, the ability not only to imitate a modeled behavior, but also to remember that behavior and spontaneously reproduce it at a later date and in different situations. Parents have always noted that preschool children imitate and replicate both desirable and undesirable behaviors modeled at home. In fact, Piaget suggested that young children learn most effectively when someone models a behavior, which children can practice imitatively and with repetition learn to replicate it. So I concluded that modeling a desired speaking pattern would be a good strategy for establishing and for generalizing fluency.

Review of the literature on learning theory provided me with additional insight regarding the use of modeling procedures. Research has consistently found systematic modeling superior to no treatment controls in all areas of behavior modification (Rachman, 1972). What is more, Bandura (1969) has found that modeling with guided participation provides the most effective means of eliciting and generalizing a desired response.

Carefully considering principles of child development and learning theory, I identified and integrated hierarchies, outlines with increasingly more difficult target behaviors, for cognitive development, fluency production, and language stimulation. In regard to the cognitive hierarchy, I concluded that for the early preoperational representation period child who has not yet mastered abstractions, centration, and transformations, an exaggerated systematic modeling of a target behavior should facilitate vicarious learning and increase the frequency of the child's production of the target behavior. Still, as the child establishes the target and continues to develop cognitively, guided participation, during which a clinician labels and specifically reinforces the target behavior, would be needed to improve performance even more. Accordingly, the therapy program was designed to coincide with the child's varying states of cognitive development during the preoperational representation period.

In this program I invoke the term *fluency disorder* to refer to speech characterized by interruptions in sound initiations and transitions; these interruptions may be tense, frequent, and/or distracting to the speaker or listener. By using this term, I avoid the negative connotation of the word "stuttering." Furthermore, whereas "stuttering" suggests an unusual problem, even a mysterious one, the term *fluency disorder* remains consistent with professional terminology for other communicative disorders, such as language disorder, voice disorder, and articulation disorder. Clinicians need to recognize that fluency disorder is neither unusual nor mysterious. The etiology of and data on therapy effectiveness regarding, for example, language disorder are not significantly more developed than those that pertain to fluency disorder.

In developing the fluency hierarchy, I chose "easy speech," previously used to facilitate fluency (Adams, 1980; Johnson, 1980; Shames and Florence, 1980; Shine, 1980), as the target behavior. Easy speech is an exaggerated, soft, slow (approximately 80 to 90 words per minute) speech pattern in which vowels are slightly prolonged and normal stress, intonation and juncture are maintained. The emphasis on softness of easy speech derives from the concept that softness inhibits tension; similarly, slowness and vowel prolongation facilitate motor coordination of the respiratory, phonatory, and articulatory mechanisms and provide more time for linguistic organization. The fluency hierarchy requires the child to produce easy speech in speaking situations that are increasingly longer, more syntactically difficult, and more distracting.

The language stimulation hierarchy, included to facilitate the child's command of semantic and syntactic development, is based on literature concerning normal linguistic development. I believed that enhancement of the children's language abilities could only promote fluency and general performance while providing enjoyable developmentally appropriate activities for fluency practice. Thus, language stimulation progresses from basic vocabulary development to categorization, association, and sequencing.

To complete the program's design, I identified three factors: parental involvement, positive communication experiences, and desensitization to fluency disruption; I used all three to facilitate generalization and maintenance of fluency. Finally, I developed flexible procedures and materials to make the program workable in a variety of clinical settings.

To ensure that the program meets its objectives, I use a differential assessment procedure based on fluency abilities and communicative activities of young children, and I employ therapy procedures consistent with recognized principles of child development and learning theory. In view of the critical need for documentation of such programs, I have consistently attempted to maintain data on all aspects of the program, particularly the long-term fluency outcome.

Assessment Procedures

HISTORY OF ASSESSMENT

In order to treat fluency disorder in young children, clinicians first needed a systematic assessment procedure for distinguishing between fluency-disordered and normal children. I believed that data regarding the fluency and disfluency of these two groups in their usual communication activities were critical to the design of such procedures. In reviewing the literature, I found limited information on the perceptual, physiologic and quantitative variables of preschool fluency. We do know that the fluent speech of normal and "stuttering" young children is not perceptually different (Colcord and Gregory, 1981; MacIndoe and Runyan, 1981). The physiologic characteristics of speech in these two groups are under study, but they have not yet been reported in the literature. So far the primary quantitative variable on which researchers have focused is the number of disfluencies.

The data, although still sparse, on disfluencies of normal and fluency-disordered children are increasing. Researchers reinitiated study of normal children in the early 1970s (Silverman, 1972; Kowal et al., 1975; Culp, 1981; Wexler, 1982; Yairi, 1982). Although conclusions regarding disfluencies of normal preschool children are tenuous, some general trends have emerged in the data. Cross-sectional studies show few significant differences in quantity and quality of disfluency across age and sex groups; mean percentages of disfluency reported by the studies cited ranged from 3.46 to 14.6 percent. The types of disfluency that were noted as most frequent, however, varied from study to study; and one longitudinal study on normal 2-year-olds suggests some significant quantitative and qualitative differences in measurements taken at 4-month intervals (Yairi, 1982).

Only recently have researchers objectively examined disfluencies of disordered children (Wall et al., 1981a; Wall et al., 1981b; Bernstein, 1981; Culp, 1982). Whereas available data on mean quantity of disfluency in disordered children (range = 8.3 to 11.2%) seem to be in agreement, data on quality of disfluency remain inconclusive.

Although a review of the literature still reveals a lack of data on fluency and disfluency in normal and disordered children, it indicates an increasing number of fluency assessment procedures that address the preschool age group (Ryan, 1974; Adams, 1977; Riley, 1980; Shames and Florence, 1980; Costello, 1981; and Riley, 1981). Many of these procedures do not consider the spectrum of specific fluency abilities and/or communicative activities of the preschool children and therefore fail to compare fluency performance with that of normal and fluency-disordered young children. Further research was warranted, then, to obtain data on the fluency abilities of young children and to establish differential diagnostic procedures for the young fluency-disordered child.

RATIONALE FOR NEW ASSESSMENT PROCEDURES

In considering possible procedures for the assessment of fluency abilities of young children, I focused first on identifying the typical communicative activities of the young child and confirmed with a review of the available literature that the five basic speaking situations used at Northwestern University were, in fact, representative of the young child's daily communicative interactions. I then sought to standardize administration procedures and collect normative data on fluency abilities of young children during these situations and designed a procedure to emphasize objective analysis of quantity and quality of disfluencies. I also recognized a need to establish flexibility for clinical judgments and to form general guidelines for enrollment in treatn.ent.

NEW ASSESSMENT PROCEDURES

Assessment procedures for the Preschool Fluency Development Program include both parents and child. Before scheduling the first appointment, the parents complete a standard case history form which provides routine information regarding the child's prenatal, birth, developmental, medical, educational, and social histories. The evaluation begins with a clinician-parent interview which establishes the parents' concerns and goals in having their child's speech evaluated. Some time may be spent during the interview to clarify further the general case history, but for the most part attention focuses on information specifically concerned with fluency. Guidelines for attaining fluency information from parents have been previously outlined (Luper, 1964). Upon completion of the interview, the clinician has gained insight regarding the course of fluency disorder and is well prepared to evaluate the child's speech and language.

Preschool children referred to Callier Center with the presenting complaint of "stuttering" undergo a basic battery of testing which typically includes hearing screening, articulation and receptive-expressive language testing, oral peripheral examination, and visual motor and gross motor screening. The evaluation though, focuses on fluency; the clinician administers the *Fluency Baseline Record* (Culp, in press) which consists of five different speaking situations of 150 words each. To assure samples of adequate length in all speaking situations, the clinician during administration may wish to record by hand the number of words spoken. I have found, however, that with preschoolers a tape-recorded sample has greater reliability for calculating fluency; accordingly, the clinician tape-records all five speaking situations for later analysis.

The five speaking situations are:

1. Monologue. In this situation, the clinician shows the child a circus pop-up book and asks him to describe an imaginary trip to the circus. The clinician may at first find it necessary to model monologue behavior or to prompt a child by pointing to interesting pictures in the book.
2. Dialogue. The dialogue situations are self-explanatory; the clinician and child engage in a discussion typically on a topic most familiar to the child: pets, family, favorite toys, games, TV shows, and so forth.
3. Retelling a story. The clinician tells an unfamiliar story, most often using a six-picture sequence story. (Note: The clinician's version should be twice as long as the version desired from the child.) The pictures are then reintroduced in order, one at a time, to facilitate the child's retelling of the story. The clinician may use two or three such stories to obtain an adequate sample.
4. Play. A doll house is used with very young children in this situation. With 4- and 5-year-olds, building toys, such as blocks, are generally more effective. In this situation the child leads the activity, so the speech sample may reflect interaction with the toys and/or the clinician.
5. Pressure. This situation is generally a continuation of the play situation described above, but the clinician introduces daily communicative pressures, such as interrupting the child, hurrying the child, competing with the child, increasing the clinician's rate of speech and linguistic complexity, and failing to make eye contact with the child.

Following the evaluation, the clinician carefully analyzes the tape recording of the five speaking situations. Word-for-word transcription is usually helpful, but essential only for those children who demonstrate rapid rate, poor intelligibility, or severe disfluency. For analysis, the clinician chooses 150 consecutive intelligible words from each situation. In accordance with procedures described by Johnson (1959) and revised by Williams and associates (1968), the clinician counts the numbers and types of disfluencies which she then records on the *Fluency Baseline Record* summary sheet (see Appendix 2-A). Finally, the clinician calculates the percentage of disfluency in each speaking situation and for all five speaking situations and then compares these percentages to normative data.

I have collected normative data on the *Fluency Baseline Record* for 30 normal and 30 fluency-disordered Caucasian monolingual English-speaking children who were from middle-income families. Ten 3-year-olds, ten 4-year-olds, and ten 5-year-olds made up each group. In the normal group, there were five boys and five girls at each age level. All subjects in this group had passed a speech-language screening administered by or under the supervision of an examiner holding the Certificate of Clinical Competence—Speech-Language Pathology; and each child's parent and classroom teacher had described the child as exhibiting normal speech and language skills. The fluency-disordered group included nineteen boys and eleven girls. Some individual profiles included articulation and/or language deficits; however, a certified speech-language pathologist had diagnosed fluency as each child's primary deficit.

After I administered the *Fluency Baseline Record* to all subjects individually, I then transcribed and analyzed all 60 tape-recorded samples before submitting them to a second certified speech-language pathologist for an independent fluency analysis. From the results of the two analyses, I was able to determine interjudge reliability, obtaining Pearson product-moment correlation coefficients of .974 (normal subjects) and .962 (fluency-disordered subjects), both indications of high interjudge reliability.

The nature of the *Fluency Baseline Record* allowed me to obtain both quantitative and qualitative information on the disfluencies of normal and disordered children. Because an analysis of variance revealed no significant quantitative or qualitative differences between age or sex groups among either the normal or disordered subjects, I was able to compare the quantity and quality of disfluencies of the normal group as a whole with those of the disordered group.

From a quantitative standpoint, I used percentage of disfluency for all five speaking situations for comparison of the two groups. As would be expected, a t test revealed that the normal group demonstrated a significantly lower percentage of disfluency (3.46%; standard deviation = 1.66%) than the disordered group (11.2%; standard deviation = 5.8%). Comparison of these quantitative results with other studies indicate that while percentages of disfluency for normal subjects are somewhat lower than those previously reported for different speaking situations (Silverman, 1972; Wexler, 1982; Yairi, 1982), percentages for disordered subjects are consistent with previous reports.

From a qualitative standpoint, the mean numbers of part-word repetitions, whole-word repetitions, dysrhythmic phonations and tense pauses exhibited by the normal group were significantly lower than those of the disordered group. Data comparing the disfluency types of the two groups appears in Table 2-1. Among the normal children, interjections, whole-word repetitions, and phrase repetitions occurred most frequently; although some revisions and part-word repetitions were evident, dysrhythmic phonations, tense pauses, and multiple-unit repetitions of any sort were infrequent. Previous reports of clinical impressions have also recorded the preponderance of part-word repetitions, whole-word repetitions, dysrhythmic phonations, and tense pauses in the speech of fluency-disordered children; however, these findings are inconsistent with those of a recent study (Bernstein, 1982) which suggested that the types

Table 2-1. Comparison of Types of Disfluency
in Normal and Fluency-Disordered Subjects

	Mean total		
	Normal subjects	Fluency-disordered subjects	t Value
Part-word repetitions	3.80	39.03	5.80*
Whole-word repetitions	5.97	11.67	3.07*
Phrase repetitions	5.20	6.97	1.39
Revisions	4.40	3.53	0.80
Dysrhythmic phonations	0.23	7.00	3.59*
Interjections	6.23	11.73	2.50
Tense pauses	0.03	3.90	2.63*
Other	0.10	0.57	1.95

*$p < .01$.

of disfluency exhibited in sentences by slightly older normal and disordered children were not significantly different.

In addition to comparing fluency performance to normative data, the *Fluency Baseline Record* encourages other informal clinical observations, including judgments of tension, prosody, speaking rate, length (in seconds or syllables) of three longest disfluencies, associated behaviors, and the child's attitude toward communication. I find that these observations are helpful in planning therapy and monitoring a child's progress.

Once the clinician has administered the *Fluency Baseline Record*, she introduces the child to an easy speech model or, when appropriate, other fluency-facilitating techniques, taking base rates in increasingly longer and more spontaneous utterances. This activity yields information about the child's stimulability for easy speaking and thus determines the entry level of the child who enrolls in the treatment program.

Guidelines for enrolling a child in the therapy program are derived from *Fluency Baseline Record* data collected on normal and fluency-disordered children. I enroll in the program a child who demonstrates one or more of the following characteristics in the evaluation:

1. A high percentage of disfluency:
   a. Greater than or equal to 10 percent disfluency in one or more of the five speaking situations
   b. Greater than or equal to 7 percent disfluency in two or more of the five speaking situations
   c. Greater than or equal to 5 percent disfluency (one standard deviation above the mean) for all five speaking situations
2. Tension in association with speech and/or a significant number of dysrhythmic phonations, tense pauses, and/or multiple-unit part-word or whole-word repetitions

3. Discoordination of the speech mechanism and/or subtle language problems in conjunction with some evidence of either quantitative or qualitative significant disfluency
4. Poor concept of self as a speaker in conjunction with some evidence of either quantitative or qualitative significant disfluency
5. Family history of fluency disorder in conjunction with some evidence of either quantitative or qualitative significant disfluency
6. A parent and/or teacher who demonstrates significant concern about the child's fluency in conjunction with some evidence of either quantitative or qualitative significant disfluency.

The final portion of the evaluation consists of the reporting conference. After completing the child's assessment, the clinician schedules a conference as soon as possible with the parents to discuss the findings and recommendations. When a child's fluency appears to be within normal limits, the clinician reassures the parents by educating them about normal and disordered fluency. Although the clinician may recommend a follow-up phone call or visit to monitor fluency in 2 to 3 months, she encourages parents to feel free to contact the center anytime if they have additional concerns. When therapy is recommended, the clinician briefly explains the program and attempts to schedule the first day of therapy. I find that parents feel substantial relief when I can define a specific course of action in this manner. Throughout the conference, parents have the opportunity to voice any concerns and to ask questions.

For those children enrolled in the therapy program, assessment continues as an ongoing process, relying on periodic administration of the entire *Fluency Baseline Record* or one or more of the five speaking situations in conjunction with the progress notes to monitor fluency development. As children progress in therapy, the quality of disfluency gradually shifts from part-word repetitions, dysrhythmic phonations, and tense pauses to more normal word and phrase repetitions and interjections; gradually the quantity of disfluency decreases.

Numerous advantages result from the assessment portion of the program. The *Fluency Baseline Record* yields a comprehensive sample of the typical communicative activities of the preschool child in a brief 20- to 30-minute period. Furthermore, it provides for a reliable objective measure (percentage of disfluent words per total words) that can be compared quantitatively with the fluency abilities of normal 3- to 5-year-old children in the same speaking situations. The assessment procedure includes an analysis of the types of disfluencies exhibited which may be important to differential diagnosis as well as in monitoring the progress in therapy; and the information on the child's performance in different speaking situations assists the clinician in adapting the hierarchy to employ in therapy. Moreover, the *Fluency Baseline Record* allows flexibility for significant clinician observations and judgments that further promote differential diagnosis. Finally, the *Fluency Baseline Record* could be easily adapted to contemporary coding systems using the microcomputer.

Description of the Therapy

Therapy in the Preschool Fluency Development Program consists of two primary features, a direct therapy program for the children and training for the parents. While direct therapy is the essential component of the program, the parents contribute significant support outside the therapy session as role models, trained observers, and reinforcers. Both features, direct therapy and parent training, operate simultaneously and focus on offering the prolonged, slower speaking pattern labeled easy speech, which leads to fluency in an individualized hierarchy consisting of more difficult speaking situations.

THERAPY GOALS

The general goals of the therapy aspect of the Preschool Fluency Development Program are

1. To establish the abilities of the child, parents, and teachers to model an easy speech pattern
2. To improve the skills of the child, parents, and teachers as listeners
3. To provide information to parents and teachers regarding fluency development and disorders
4. To develop the skills of parents and teachers as objective observers at home and school
5. To identify factors that may disrupt or facilitate fluency
6. To provide guidelines for managing disfluent episodes
7. To provide increasingly more difficult speaking situations in which the child can maintain fluency and receive positive feedback regarding his communication skills
8. To desensitize the child to fluency disruptors
9. To extend basal fluency to spontaneous situations outside the clinic

THERAPY METHOD

The treatment design includes weekly 1-hour therapy sessions for small groups of two to four children or biweekly half-hour therapy sessions for individual children; a series of sessions (approximately 7 hours in all) that provide intensive group or individual parent/teacher training; and an ongoing parent observation and maintenance program. The group therapy has proved not only cost effective but also productive for both the child and parent training. For children, a group therapy setting serves to stimulate normal communicative activities and hence, expedites carryover of fluency. I group the children primarily according to age and development level and schedule availability. I also consider the severity of the fluency disorder. In the group setting, then, each child works at an individualized program. For the parents, the group setting ordinarily provides peer support, stimulates discussion, and encourages problem solving. Parent training groups may consist of two to three families, grouped according to educational level and schedule availability, but for those children and parents for whom there is no appropriate group I arrange individual sessions. In addition, if a parent or child has difficulty keeping up in the group or needs additional help, e.g., a child with articulation or language deficits, I introduce individual sessions to support the work in group therapy.

The therapy techniques, procedures, and activities of the children and parent programs require separate discussion; but in practice they require integrated and simultaneous execution.

THE CHILDREN'S PROGRAM
Specific Techniques, Procedures, Activities

The children's program may be described as a clinician-directed preschool play situation which focuses on hierarchies of fluency, cognitive development, and language stimulation. The primary purpose of the activities in the children's program is intrasession and intersession progression through increasingly more difficult fluency responses that are ordered according to length, linguistic complexity, and the presence or absence of disruptors. Disruptors often used include competition, physical activity, change of physical setting, and presence of family members or peers. Whereas use of easy speech in fluency responses is always the primary target behavior, the progression of therapy requires increasingly difficult cognitive and language responses. As a child's cognitive readiness develops, therapy becomes more direct; and the child's responsibility to self-monitor increases. Language responses, ordered developmentally, begin with simple categories and progress to association and sequencing tasks. Integration of the hierarchies of fluency, cognitive development, and language stimulation thus occurs continuously. Each of these hierarchies warrants specific consideration.

The fluency hierarchy (see Table 2-2) consists of two major phases: (1) establishing fluency; and (2) generalizing fluency in running speech.

The goal of phase 1 is to establish easy, fluent speech in spontaneous sentences; this phase works at three graduated levels of responses: (1) single words, (2) carrier phrases, i.e., a standard phrase in which only one original word is formulated, such as "I see _____"; and (3) formulated sentences. The clinician introduces seven steps for each of the three levels, slowly withdrawing modeling and introducing disruptors as the child progresses. The clinician may also insert intermediate steps by systematically varying linguistic complexity; for example, the clinician may introduce carrier phrase activities that are simple stereotypic utterances,

Table 2-2. Fluency Hierarchy

I. Establishing Fluency
  A. Single word
    1. Choral speaking
    2. Clinician provides immediate model
    3. Clinician provides immediate model in a disruptive situation
    4. Clinician provides a delayed model
    5. Clinician provides a delayed model in a disruptive situation
    6. Child produces spontaneously
    7. Child produces spontaneously in a disruptive situation
  B. Carrier phrases (1–7 above)
  C. Sentences (1–7 above)
II. Generalizing Fluency in Running Speech
  A. Story completion (gradually increasing mean length of response)
    1. Play setting
    2. Disruptive setting
    3. Home setting (optional)
  B. Monologue (1–3 above)
  C. Dialogue (1–3 above)

---

such as "I want a _____" or "I found a _____," but which later may employ varying tenses and interrogatives, such as "I will draw a _____" and "Do you have a _____?" The clinician may also use discretion in deleting steps.

When the child has developed the ability to spontaneously formulate fluent sentences, the clinician introduces the generalization phase of the program. The goal of phase 2 of the program is to generalize fluency in numerous speaking situations and focuses on three levels of response: story completion, monologue, and dialogue. A review of the *Fluency Baseline Records* of normal and fluency-disordered children has suggested that children are more fluent in a play situation. Accordingly, I offer two steps at each generalization level: the more fluency-facilitating play situation and a disruptive one. In addition, the clinician may include an optional step of home setting at each level, and again may add intermediate steps by varying the length and linguistic complexity of story completion, monologue, and dialogue.

The cognitive hierarchy is designed in accordance with the child's progression in the preoperational representation period. More specifically, it evolves with respect to the child's developing ability to deal with more abstract stimuli, to make transformations, to explore all aspects of a stimulus, and to internalize a model from an external source. I identify three primary cognitive phases. In the first phase, for the younger, less mature child, the clinician provides an exaggerated easy speech model as the target response. This technique directs the child's attention toward fluency by using positive nonspecific reinforcements such as "Good for you," and "Good story telling," "You can say the whole thing," for easy, fluent responses. At this point the clinician simply ignores disfluent responses and, accordingly, does not require the child to evaluate the abstract speech stimulus or to make transformations, thus allowing the child to learn easy speaking indirectly. In the second phase, as the child stabilizes the easy speech pattern in spontaneous sentences and demonstrates increasing cognitive maturity, the clinician introduces the label "easy speech" which she then specifically designates as the target response in both instructions and reinforcement. The clinician may either continue to ignore disfluent responses or request repetitions as she reminds the child to use easy speech. Finally, as the child begins to show attention to more than one aspect of the speech stimulus and to demonstrate ability to self-evaluate, the clinician moves to the third phase in which she introduces contrasting labels of "fast speech" and "hard speech" and identifies hard speech as the child's most typical disfluency, particularly in the form of part-word repetition. At this point, while sessions continue to focus on practicing easy speech, the clinician spends a portion of every session practicing *control* of the speaking pattern in words and sentences, having the children imitate and then spontaneously produce easy, hard, and fast speech on command. During control practice, the clinician reinforces the children, saying "Good. You can control the way you talk" or "Good. You can say that three ways." Although I cannot specify behavioral guidelines for progressing through the three cognitive phases of the program, clinical judgments ordinarily have proved successful, and have allowed the individualized fluency program to continue to evolve with the cognitive readiness of the children in the group.

The language hierarchy, the third and final hierarchy, has been designed to provide systematic developmental language stimulation. Accordingly, the therapy sessions begin initially with varying but familiar thematic categories such as body parts, household objects, foods, clothes, animals, toys, colors, shapes, transportation, textures, and community helpers. Later sessions require use of categories, opposites, parts of the whole, associations, and sequencing skills.

THE THERAPY SESSION

During the therapy session, each child works at an individualized level in the fluency hierarchy. The reinforcement is continuous verbal and/or verbal-tangible with the degree of specificity in the instructions and verbal reinforcement varying according to the child's level in the cognitive hierarchy. The clinician may choose from a variety of preschool activities, always keeping in mind the children's developmental level (see Appendix 2-B, Table 2-3). Early therapy sessions, highly structured by the clinician,

Table 2-3. Some Suggested Activities

I. Establishing Fluency
  A. Single word level
    1. Sentence completion
    2. Guessing games
    3. Grab bag games
    4. How many (animals) can we name?
    5. Hiding pictures for child to find
  B. Carrier phrase level
    1. Draw a man (children take turns drawing; "I can draw the _____ .")
    2. Grocery store
    3. Mr. Potatohead (children put him together; "Now, he has a _____ .")
    4. Fishing (with magnet pole; "I caught a _____ .")
    5. Go fish (card game; "Do you have a _____ ?")
    6. Twenty questions
    7. Language lotto
  C. Sentence level
    1. Interactive language stories
    2. Concentration
    3. Board games
    4. Hide and seek
    5. Grab bag games
II. Generalizing Fluency in Running Speech
  A. Story completion
    1. Flannel board stories
    2. Story picture books
    3. Poster stories
  B. Monologue
    1. Charades (of action pictures)
    2. "What's wrong?" pictures
    3. Commercials
    4. Position in space pictures (child describes his position)
    5. Restaurant (children order meals)
    6. Feelie meelie (child describes object he feels)
  C. Dialogue level
    1. Building a fort
    2. Dress-ups
    3. Making sundaes
    4. Making cookies
    5. Puzzles
    6. Crafts

rely upon enforcement of the "good listener rule," that is, talking only in turn. Therapy sessions begin typically with a review of the children who are present and reintroduction of a model of easy speech with a preschool song or fingerplay. In later sessions, once the children can maintain fluency in conversation, structure decreases. For all sessions, the clinician records responses and maintains response sheets for use in entering monthly progress notes in each child's file.

Standard criteria for moving through the fluency hierarchy are as follows:

1. A child must demonstrate easy, fluent speech on 95/100 words at one step before progressing to the next. If a dysrhythmic phonation, tense pause, or multiple unit repetition appears in the recorded disfluencies, the clinician retains the child at the same step.
2. In the event a child demonstrates easy fluent speech on fewer than 90/100 words, the child must return to the previous step and reestablish criteria.

Clinicians may find it useful to delete or insert intermediate steps depending on the child's progress, but must ensure, nevertheless, that therapy continually provides the child with as much practice in easy, fluent speaking as possible. In addition, the child must have positive communication experiences to reinforce his or her use of controlled speaking patterns.

PROBLEMS FREQUENTLY ENCOUNTERED: MANAGEMENT STRATEGIES
Resistance or Lack of Attention to Easy Speech
Occasionally, the clinician encounters a child who at the beginning of therapy appears to resist the model of easy speech. To counteract this problem, the clinician introduces appropriate tangible reinforcers which generally improve motivation and cooperation. Management for a child who does not seem to recognize the easiness of speech presents a different problem from the resisting child. In the later case, the clinician should further exaggerate the easiness of the model, relying heavily on choral speaking or more concrete visual cues, such as rolling a ball or drawing a line, to reflect the rate and rhythm of speech.

Resistance to or Dislike of Therapy
Children accustomed to unstructured environments often react negatively to the highly structured atmosphere of the initial therapy sessions. Because the clinician can often predict this reaction, I find it helpful to warn the parents of this possibility and assure them that after a month or so, once the child is happy and secure with the group structure and

has made friends with other group members, this reaction will subside. In most instances, the children begin to look forward to and enjoy the sessions.

Awareness of Disfluencies of Others

While a primary goal of the therapy session is to provide an opportunity for the children to practice easy, fluent speech as much as possible, a limited number of disfluencies will occur. Occasionally, one child will show excessive concern for another child's disfluencies; when this situation occurs, the clinician should handle it openly with a response such as, "That was a hard one. We all use hard speech sometimes, and it doesn't feel very good. That's why it's important to practice our easy speech."

Difficulty Making Transition

Children frequently have difficulty moving from the level of spontaneous sentence to that of monologue. For this reason, I designed story completion as an intermediate step, so the children can experience success in extending one sentence to two or three sentences when telling a familiar story. The rote nature of telling a familiar story assists most children in making the transition to monologue. For a number of children, however, that transition continues to be difficult. For some, expressive language deficits may interfere. Hence, extensive language work at the sentence level may make the fluency transition less difficult. In contrast, most children seem to have difficulty attending to the easiness of speech when they are sequencing sentences. The clinician should utilize appropriate tangible reinforcers at this point to help the child focus attention on easy speech as the target behavior. The clinician may also frequently introduce contrasting labels of easy, hard, and fast speech as well as the concept of speech control.

Articulation and/or Language Deficit

A child most often enrolls in a fluency group before enrolling in articulation or language therapy, but once fluency has stabilized in spontaneous sentences, he or she begins an additional half-hour weekly individual articulation/language therapy. In this manner, articulation and language deficits can be remediated at the sentence level without the interference of disfluency. Similarly, remediation of articulation and language deficits frequently aids in the development of fluency.

Inability to Reproduce Disfluencies Volitionally

In the final stage of the cognitive hierarchy, the clinician demonstrates hard speech to the children as their most frequent disfluency type. For most children, this will be the part-word repetition. Up until 5 or 5½ years of age, although children can imitate part-word repetitions, they very often have difficulty producing them deliberately. Attempts to produce hard speech may yield /b -b -b -dog/ and /b -b -b -cat/. This observation is consistent with knowledge of reading readiness and a child's developmental ability to isolate and identify the beginning sounds of words. Because attempts such as those noted do at least demonstrate the disruption of the smoothness of speech, the clinician accepts them as correct production of hard speech. As the children mature, true part-word repetitions emerge spontaneously.

THE PARENT PROGRAM

Specific Techniques, Procedures, Activities

The parent training program, like the children's program, must be individualized to meet educational and social-emotional needs of the parents. In establishing a procedure for the training, however, I considered three basic components fundamental: initial training, observation, and a parent maintenance group.

Initial training, which begins at the time of the child's enrollment in direct therapy, involves approximately 7 hours of direct contact that may be completed in several 2- to 3-hour blocks or in weekly 1-hour sessions. Accordingly, the parents complete this part of the training during the child's first 2 months in therapy. I have found initial training in groups of two to three families to be both economical and effective, resulting in increased family support and productive discussions. If group scheduling presents problems, I offer individual parent training. Whatever the case, I encourage all parents to attend and offer evening sessions as needed. The initial training program consists of seven basic units, which do not necessarily enforce behavioral objectives or specific criteria for moving through the units. With guidance from the clinician, each of the parents evaluates his or her own progress.

The second aspect of the parent program stresses monthly observation of the children in therapy. During observations, the clinician provides goals of each activity and frequently asks parents to record their child's responses. The parents have consistently reported that this part of the program is the most helpful in applying fluency techniques at home and recognizing their child's progress.

The final aspect of the parent program consists of the parent maintenance group, which parents are encouraged to attend throughout their child's enrollment. The group meets approximately every 2 months to help parents maintain interest, to review fluency facilitation skills, and to solve new problems as they arise. The meetings include activities such as discussing the parents' reactions during their child's fluent/disfluent episodes, reviewing current literature in preschool fluency, providing training for home program implementations, talking with parents of program graduates, and viewing the film *The Prevention of Stuttering*, Part II (Speech Foundation of America, 1975).

It may be argued that I have not objectively measured the contribution of the parent program and/or that in some settings, such as public schools, clinicians may not even have access to the parents. Although I consider the parent program vitally important to the child's progress, several school clinicians have informally reported success with primary grade children when only the classroom teacher participated in an abridged version of the parent program.

THE THERAPY SESSION
Although the clinician individualizes the initial parent training sessions, I have developed seven basic units from which to draw material for presentation.

Unit I: Introduction
The first unit provides a general introduction to fluency, fluency disorder, and the Preschool Fluency Development Program. The clinician defines fluency as the smoothness of speech sound initiation and transition, and describes disfluency as any interruption in this smoothness. The clinician then discusses normal disfluency and fluency disorder in the preschooler in terms of available quantitative and qualitative data. The clinician explains a preference for the term *fluency disorder* over the traditional term, *stuttering*, by showing the multiple connotations and associations of stuttering with adult behaviors. Further, she notes that the term is inconsistent with other scientific speech-language pathology terms, and suggests that fluency disorder describes the problem of the preschooler most specifically.

Possible causes of fluency disorder which the clinician discusses include physiologic predisposition, psychosocial factors, and environmental reinforcement. While the clinician cannot establish a single cause for an individual child, he or she can, and does, use examples of how such factors interrelate to assist parents in understanding. The clinician points out that even normal adults may have difficulty if they attempt a motor task that is physically difficult for them (e.g., threading a needle, swinging a golf club) when they are excited, fatigued, hungry, ill, or stressed. Thus, parents see that physiologic and psychosocial factors may interrelate as a child with poor motor coordination for speech experiences disfluency in an exciting or stressful situation.

The clinician spends most of this introductory session discussing fluency facilitation. He or she defines and demonstrates easy speech for the parents and explains that this new speech pattern allows the child to practice speech production and language skills more slowly, just as one would learn a golf swing or dance step through slow, exaggerated, and repeated practice. The clinician also presents general guidelines in terms of activities to avoid and those to encourage at home.

Activities to avoid include

1. Correcting, helping, calling attention to or showing concern about the child's speech.
2. Labeling disfluency as "stuttering."
3. Asking the child to display speech, such as reciting a verse or relating an event to relatives, company, classmates, and so forth.
4. Compelling the child to compete with others for a chance to talk.
5. Encouraging the child to speak when he is excited, upset, or tired.
6. Reinforcing disfluent speech; for example, the child comes to ask a question of a parent who is busy doing paperwork. If the parent does not respond, the child in all probability will ask again, this time disfluently; the parent, now concerned, will actually reinforce the disfluency as he or she attends and responds.

Activities to encourage include

1. Being good and patient listeners, reacting with interest to what the child says, rather than how he or she says it, and maintaining good eye contact. Situations in which the parent is unable to fill the function of a good listener should be handled by postponing the conversation. Parents should also encourage the child and others in the environment to employ good listening habits, and to take turns talking.
2. Using a soft, slow, exaggerated, easy relaxed speech pattern.
3. Identifying and modifying any circumstances that appear to increase the amount of disfluency.
4. Ensuring that peers do not tease the child about speech.
5. Encouraging the child to talk during more fluent periods or in situations that are more conducive to fluency; for example, the child comes in from outside excited and ready to tell a story. Before encouraging the child to speak, allow a minute for him to calm down. For instance, say "I can see you're anxious to tell me something. It must be really interesting, so why don't you go get a drink of water (or hang up your coat, or wash your face) and then we'll sit down and talk."
6. Encouraging short utterances by asking yes-no or short-answer questions. If the child has a long story to tell, make the task easier for him by asking him questions that require short answers, such as, "When was it?" "Who were you with?" and so on.

After outlining these negative and positive activities, the clinician discusses the general goals of the Preschool Fluency Development Program with the parents, provides data on children previously enrolled in the program, and describes the typical course of therapy which lasts from a year to a year and one-half. All information in Unit I appears in a handout given to the parents, but the clinician also allows sufficient time for questions and discussion.

It should also be noted that I frequently share this particular unit with the child's preschool teacher. Data from a questionnaire study of 10 classroom teachers, whom we surveyed both before and 3 months after training, suggest that the unit is effective in changing the teachers' strategies for managing fluency in the classroom.

Unit II: Analysis of Frequently Reported Disfluent Episodes
In this unit, the clinician provides parents with a handout that lists a variety of disfluent situations often reported, and parents, using easy speech, take turns reading descriptions of these situations to each other. The group then offers feedback regarding the reader's easy speech pattern and analyzes the disfluent situation in terms of possible fluency disruptors and management strategies. The following situation serves as an example:

> Mr. Smith is very fond of his daughter Jamie. First thing when he comes home, he grabs Jamie and playfully swings her through the air and affectionately tickles her. Then, as he reaches for the evening paper and begins to thumb through, he says, "Tell Daddy what you did today," Mr. Smith listens and corrects Jamie if she has trouble with a word. Soon, it is time for the news. Mrs. Smith notes that this experience is Jamie's most disfluent episode every day.

A discussion of possible fluency disruptors for this situation might include physical stimulation before the conversation, use of open-ended questions or statements, poor listening attention, and correction of disfluent words. In terms of management strategies, the clinician might then suggest a new routine in which Mr. Smith swings and tickles Jamie, but then retires to his room alone to relax and read the paper. Later he might come out for talking time with Jamie. During talking time, he would give Jamie his full attention, model easy speech, avoid correcting disfluent words, and direct the conversation with short-answer questions.

Unit III: Recording Fluency at Home
In parent training, the clinician stresses the importance of objective observers in the home throughout the course of therapy to monitor the child's fluency in a variety of speaking situations. The clinician teaches parents to record the number of disfluencies per minute and provides them with opportunity to practice this technique by using tape-recorded samples. The clinician asks the parents to record the disfluency for two 5- to 10-minute periods daily, and then, after they have actually counted the number of disfluencies, to consider the speaking situation they have recorded in terms of possible fluency facilitators and disruptors as discussed in Units I and II. This approach has frequently been helpful in identifying situations in which a child consistently experiences fluent or disfluent speech.

Unit IV: Child Development
I have observed that many parents question whether or not their expectations are appropriate for young children from a developmental standpoint. I have also noticed that when parents are unsure of their expectations they are more likely to be inconsistent in their discipline. The purpose of this unit then is to familiarize parents with normal child development so they will establish expectations that are appropriate for their child. The clinician discusses cognitive, social-emotional, fine motor, and gross motor areas, as well as common fears and behavioral problems, such as fear of the dark and thumb sucking. To present this material, the clinician uses a variety of resources (Fraiberg, 1959; Flavell, 1963).

Unit V: Discipline
In Unit V, the clinician presents three major principles of discipline (Ginott, 1969). First, the clinician considers the importance of setting limits on acts but not on feelings. Second, the clinician suggests that parents encourage their child to express feelings about the discipline situation, noting that such expression is often difficult for the disfluent child. Third, the clinician discusses the value of consistent discipline for the disfluent child and stresses that a child is more secure and relaxed when he understands what is expected of him. Finally, the clinician points out that consistent discipline should aid the child in learning a new mode of behavior such as easy speech.

Unit VI: Helping the Child Express Feelings
Portions of a filmstrip series, *The Development of Feelings in Children* (*Parents Magazine*, 1973), provide parents with information on children's emotional development and the expression of feelings, and again the clinician stresses the value of assisting the disfluent child to express emotion.

At the end of this session, parents receive a form for recording their own behaviors at home by charting the number of times each day that they consciously make use of each of the fluency-facilitating techniques previously discussed.

Unit VII: Review
In the last session, the parents discuss the charts they have kept and raise questions about specific techniques. The general discussion then revolves around overall changes that have been made in the home to date, problem situations that still persist, and individual family goals for the coming few months. This session concludes the initial training phase of the parent program.

PROBLEMS FREQUENTLY ENCOUNTERED IN THERAPY:
MANAGEMENT STRATEGIES

Discomfort with Modeling Easy Speech

At the beginning of parent training, parents are frequently inhibited about changing their speech pattern. Modeling by the clinician, choral practice in group session, single sentence activities, and reading aloud have been helpful in desensitizing parents in this regard. In addition, some parents have found it easier to slow down their speech gradually in increments of approximately 10 words per minute over a longer period of a month to 6 weeks.

Failure to Complete Home Assignments

Parents sometimes resist home assignments, and such an attitude poses a problem during their initial training and the generalization phase of their children's program. When the clinician notices resistance, she might talk with the parent or parents to determine its source. In some cases, parents are embarrassed to ask questions when they fail to understand an assignment so a quick review of the assignment will resolve that problem. More often, parents understand the importance of assignments, but feel they do not have time to complete them; in such instances, the clinician tries to compromise with the parents on the assignment in order to reduce the amount of time involved. I find that I can usually eliminate resistance and encourage parents to complete a task at least partially when I relate that task to the child's progress.

PHYSICAL BEHAVIORS

Few of the children enrolled in the Preschool Fluency Development Program have demonstrated physical behaviors in association with disfluency. When these behaviors have occurred, they have resolved themselves spontaneously as fluency develops, thus requiring no direct attention in either the children's or the parents' program.

ATTITUDINAL WORK

The children's program addresses attitudes by indirectly providing the child with positive feedback about his speech in a variety of age-appropriate activities. The parent program not only encourages parents to provide similar feedback at home but places emphasis as well on reducing the parent's anxiety about fluency disorder.

TRANSFER AND MAINTENANCE

Upon a child's enrollment, the Preschool Fluency Development Program addresses transfer and maintenance by incorporating hierarchies with fluency disruptors in the children's program; and it offers education on home fluency facilitation in the parent program. I have also established procedures for gradually phasing out therapy and discharging the child. When a child enters Phase 2 of his therapy, I provide weekly home activities. Once a child has maintained easy, fluent speech on 95/100 words in a variety of dialogues with disruptors for a 6- to 8-week period both in the therapy session and at home, therapy decreases to a single 1-hour session every 2 weeks. If criteria is maintained in therapy and at home for 6 to 8 additional weeks, then therapy decreases to a single 1-hour session per month. At the end of the second session of monthly therapy, if criteria are maintained, an unfamiliar clinician readministers the *Fluency Baseline Record* in an unfamiliar setting to evaluate formally the fluency performance in a variety of speaking situations. When performance on the *Fluency Baseline Record* falls within normal limits and reports from home, school, and therapy concur with this assessment, the clinician discharges the child.

FOLLOW-UP PROCEDURES
When the clinician discharges a child from therapy, she encourages parents to contact the center anytime they again become concerned about the child's fluency. The clinician should then see each child for reevaluation 3 months after his discharge. The reevaluation process involves both conferences with parents and teachers concerning the child's fluency and direct readministration of the *Fluency Baseline Record*. For research, as opposed to clinical purposes, I have also seen each child for a follow-up visit 2 years after discharge.

EQUIPMENT AND MATERIALS NEEDED
In designing the program, I allowed for substantial flexibility in equipment and necessary materials. Any standard collection of preschool materials provides adequate stimuli for the children's program (see Appendix 2-B), and although some specific media presentations enhance the parent program, they are not essential. A standard tape recorder will meet the needs of both programs.

CLINICIAN SKILLS AND TRAINING REQUIRED
Although I have not conducted a conclusive study to determine the effectiveness of clinicians from differing backgrounds in implementing this program, I do believe that the clinician's success depends upon basic training in fluency, knowledge of child development, a grasp of linguistic development and behavior modification, and ability in counseling.

CLIENT REQUIREMENTS
Client requirements for children's and parents' programs include regular attendance, cooperation within sessions, and completion of home assignments.

Evaluation of the Therapy

RESEARCH STUDIES

I do attempt to document carefully the effectiveness of the program by keeping records on active program enrollment, withdrawals, and discharges upon completion (see Table 2-4). Withdrawal typically occurs during the first 3 months of therapy with parents citing financial and transportation problems as reasons for withdrawing their children from the program. Phone interviews indicate that four of the six children who have withdrawn have received some additional fluency therapy and that fluency disorder persists in four of the six.

Procedures

Fourteen children (nine boys and five girls) who completed the program served as the subjects with a mean age upon enrollment in the program of 4 years and 1 month. Of these fourteen children, four demonstrated articulation and expressive language deficits, and two others presented with familial history of fluency disorder.

An unfamiliar clinician administered the *Fluency Baseline Record* to each child, then the mean percentage of disfluency for all five speaking situations was calculated. All children included in the study met the

Table 2-4. Fluency Development Program Statistics (March, 1983)

Number of children originally enrolled in program = 32
  12 Still enrolled
  6 Dropped out
  14 Discharged upon program completion
Mean percentage of disfluency on fluency baseline record for children who have completed the program:

Pretherapy % disfluency/ 5 situations	Posttherapy % disfluency/ 5 situations	3 Months posttherapy % disfluency/ 5 situations	2 Years posttherapy % disfluency/ 5 situations
N = 14	N = 14	N = 12	N = 7
Range = 5.5–29.3%	Range = 0.067–6.9%	Range = 0.07–6.9%	Range = 0.40–7.06%
Mean = 11.44%	Mean = 2.95%	Mean = 2.58%	Mean = 2.85%

Additional information (N = 14):
  Age of child upon enrollment
    Range = 2 years, 11 months–5 years, 10 months
    Mean = 4 years, 1 month
  Number of hours enrolled
    Range = 15–70
    Mean = 45

guidelines previously discussed for enrollment in the program, but I did not specifically describe disfluency as mild, moderate, or severe.

Results
The mean duration of the direct therapy program for the fourteen subjects was 45 hours. As demonstrated in Table 2-4, after therapy all fourteen children exhibited mean percentages of disfluency within the normal limits on the *Fluency Baseline Record*. Qualitative analysis of disfluencies and parent and teacher reports also confirmed fluency within the normal limits in each of the children. Further, all children had spontaneously progressed from exaggerated easy speech to perceptually normal rate and intonation patterns.

Follow-up Investigations
I collected follow-up data both 3 months and 2 years after discharge, readministering the *Fluency Baseline Record* during the 3-month follow-up visit of each child (N = 12). All twelve children continued to demonstrate fluency quantitatively and qualitatively within the normal limits on this measure. Reports of parents and teachers confirmed normal fluency. Two years after discharge, I again readministered the *Fluency Baseline Record* to each child (N = 7). Six of the seven children had continued to demonstrate fluency quantitatively and qualitatively within the normal limits on this measure, as well as by reports of parents and teachers. One girl exhibited disfluency that was quantitatively above normal expectations (7.06%) and qualitatively characterized for the most part by part-word repetitions and tense pauses. She had not presented with articulation/language deficits or a familial history of fluency disorder. Yet, it is noteworthy that upon enrollment in therapy, she had presented with the highest percentage of disfluency and the greatest chronologic age.

Finally, three children who have been discharged from therapy for as long as 4 years, continue, according to parent report, to exhibit normal fluency.

Reasons for Therapeutic Effectiveness
I propose that there are several reasons for the therapeutic effectiveness of the Preschool Fluency Development Program, the primary ones being the direct child therapy supported by parent training and focus on hierarchies of fluency, child, and linguistic development. The integration of child development principles in a program of speech remediation is unique and important. I also believe that both the child and the parent need a specific target speech behavior as an alternative, and I have found that easy speech helps the child to develop the ability to establish and generalize fluency. Another important contributor to the program's success is the consistent introduction of fluency disruptors in therapy to ensure

that fluent speech will be carried into real-world settings. Finally, the children's program provides positive feedback in enjoyable communication experiences that appear to enhance each child's fluency and general development.

Advantages of the Therapy

Three main advantages of the program are apparent. First, the program includes a reliable and objective assessment procedure which encourages fluency evaluation in the preschoolers' typical communicative activities and allows for fluency comparison with normal and fluency-disordered young children. Second, the flexibility of the program in terms of materials required and the option of individual or group therapy and parent or teacher training, makes it possible for the program to function in a variety of clinical settings. Finally, the program's documentation to date provides strong support for wider clinical use.

This program is posited to document more completely the effectiveness of early intervention with preschool fluency-disordered children and to offer clinicians an alternative to the more traditional indirect therapy programs. I encourage clinicians to utilize this and other preschool fluency programs and to maintain careful documentation regarding efficacy. The potential of differential diagnosis and therapy for the young fluency-disordered child is not encouraging. Yet, much research is still needed. Clinicians face a challenge to be active in data collection and to be involved in developing further fluency programs for the young child.

References

Adams, M. R. A clinical strategy for differentiating the normally nonfluent child and the incipient stutterer. *J. Fluency Dis.* 2:141–148. 1977.

Adams, M. R. The young stutterer: Diagnosis, treatment and assessment of progress. In W. Perkins (ed.), *Strategies in Stuttering Therapy.* New York: Thieme-Stratton, *Semin. Speech Lang. Hear.* 1:289–300, 1980.

Bandura, A. *Principles of Behavior Modification.* Chicago: Holt, Rinehart & Winston, 1969.

Bernstein, N. E. Are there constraints on childhood disfluency? *J. Fluency Dis.* 6:341–350, 1981.

Bloodstein, O. *A Handbook on Stuttering.* Chicago: National Easter Seal Society, 1976.

Colcord, R. D., and Gregory, H. A perceptual analysis of fluency in stuttering and nonstuttering children. Paper presented at the annual convention of the American Speech-Language and Hearing Association, Los Angeles, 1981.

Costello, J. M. Current Behavioral Treatments for Children. In D. Prins and R. J. Ingham (eds.), *Treatment of Stuttering in Early Childhood: Methods and Issues.* San Diego: College-Hill Press, 1983.

Costello, J. M. Pretreatment assessment of stuttering in young children. *Communicative Disorders.* New York: Grune & Stratton, 1981. *An Audio Journal for Continuing Education.* Cassette tape, no. 6.

Culp, D. M. The fluency baseline record—developing a preschool fluency assessment instrument. Paper presented at the annual convention of the American Speech-Language and Hearing Association, Los Angeles, 1981.

Culp, D. M. The preschool fluency baseline record—the young fluency disordered child. Paper presented at the annual convention of the American Speech-Language and Hearing Association, Toronto, 1982.

Culp, D. M. *The Preschool Fluency Baseline Record.* Dallas: University of Texas at Dallas, in press.

Curlee, R. F. A case selection strategy for young disfluent children. In W. Perkins (ed.), *Strategies in Stuttering Therapy. Semin. Speech Lang. Hear.* 1:277–288, 1980.

Flavell, J. H. *Developmental Psychology of Jean Piaget.* Princeton, N.J.: Van Nostrand, 1963.

Fraiberg, S. H. *The Magic Years.* New York: Scribner's, 1959.

Gregory, H., and Hill, D. G. Stuttering therapy for children. In W. Perkins (ed.), *Strategies in Stuttering Therapy. Semin. Speech Lang. Hear.* 1:351–364, 1980.

Johnson, L. J. Facilitating parental involvement in therapy of the disfluent child. In W. Perkins (ed.), *Strategies in Stuttering Therapy. Semin. Speech Lang. Hear.* 1:301–310, 1980.

Johnson, W. *The Onset of Stuttering.* Minneapolis: University of Minnesota Press, 1959.

Kowal, S., O'Connell, D. C., and Sabin, E. J. Development of temporal patterning and vocal hesitations in spontaneous narratives. *J. Psycholinguist. Res.* 4:195–207, 1975.

Luper, H., and Mulder, R. *Stuttering Therapy for Children.* Englewood Cliffs, N.J.: Prentice-Hall, 1964.

MacIndoe, C., and Runyan, C. M. Perceptual comparison of stuttering and non-stuttering children's nonstuttered speech. Paper presented at the annual convention of the American Speech-Language and Hearing Association, Los Angeles, 1981.

Martin, R. R., Kuhl, P., and Haroldsen, S. An experimental treatment with two preschool stuttering children. *J. Speech Hear. Res.* 15:743–751, 1972.

Myers, F. L., and Wall, M. J. Issues to consider in differential diagnosis of normal childhood nonfluencies and stuttering. *J. Fluency Dis.* 6:189–195, 1981.

Nelson, L. A. Language formulation related to disfluency and stuttering. Paper presented at the Speech Foundation of America conference, Northwestern University, Evanston, Ill. 1982.

Parents' Magazine. Child Development Sound and Color Filmstrips. *Understanding Early Childhood—The Development of Feelings in Children.* New York: Parents' Magazine Films, Inc., 1973.

Rachman, S. Clinical applications of observational learning, imitation and modeling. *Behav. Ther.* 3:379–397, 1972.

Reed, C. G., and Godden, A. L. An experimental treatment using verbal punishment with two preschool stutterers. *J. Fluency Dis.* 2:225–234, 1977.

Riley, G. *Stuttering Prediction Instrument for Young Children.* Tigard, Ore.: C. C. Publications, 1981.

Riley, G. *Stuttering Severity Instrument for Children and Adults.* Tigard, Ore.: C. C. Publications, 1980.

Riley, G., and Riley, J. Evaluation as a Basis for Intervention. In D. Prins and R. J. Ingham (ed.), *Treatment of Stuttering in Early Childhood: Methods and Issues.* San Diego: College-Hill Press, 1983.

Ryan, B. *Programmed Therapy for Stuttering Children and Adults.* Springfield, Ill.: Thomas, 1974.

Shames, G., and Florence, C. *Stutter-Free Speech: A Goal for Therapy.* Columbus, Ohio: Merrill, 1980.

Shine, R. E. *Systematic Fluency Training for Children.* Tigard, Ore.: C. C. Publications, 1980.

Silverman, E. M. Generality of Disfluency Data Collected from Preschoolers. *J. Speech Hear. Res.* 15:84–92, 1972.

Speech Foundation of America. *The Prevention of Stuttering II—Family Counseling and Elimination of the Problem.* Silver Springs, Md.: Seven Oaks Productions, 1975.

Van Riper, C. The Nature of Stuttering (2nd ed.). Englewood Cliffs, N.J.: Prentice-Hall, 1982.

Wall, M. J., Starkweather, C. W., and Cairns, H. S. Syntactic influences on stuttering in young children. *J. Fluency Dis.* 6:283–295, 1981.

Wall, M. J., Starkweather, C. W., and Harris, K. The influence of voicing adjustments on the location of stuttering in the spontaneous speech of young child stutterers. *J. Fluency Dis.* 6:299–310, 1981.

Wexler, K. B. Developmental disfluency in 2-, 4-, and 6-year-old boys in neutral and stress situations. *J. Speech Hear. Res.* 25:229–234, 1982.

Williams, D. E., Silverman, F. H., and Kools, J. A. Disfluency behavior of elementary school stutterers and non-stutterers: The adaptation effect. *J. Speech Hear. Res.* 11:622–630, 1968.

Yairi, E. Longitudinal Studies of Disfluencies in 2 Year Old Children. *J. Speech Hear. Res.* 25:115–160, 1982.

Zwitman, D. H. *The Disfluent Child: A Management Program.* Baltimore: University Park Press, 1978.

Appendix 2-A. Fluency Baseline Record

Fluency Baseline Record Summary Sheet
Delva M. Culp

Name: A.G.
Date: 9-1-82
Examiner: D. Culp

Type of Disfluency	Monologue	Dialogue	Retelling Story	Play	Pressure	Total
Part-word repetition	5	8	4	8	7	32
Word repetition	1	1	1	0	2	5
Phrase repetition	0	0	0	3	1	4
Revision	0	0	0	0	0	0
Dysrhythmic phonation	0	2	2	2	1	7
Interjection	2	9	3	3	0	17
Tense Pause	0	0	2	0	0	2
Other	0	0	0	0	0	0
Total no. disfluencies	8	20	12	16	11	67
Percent of disfluency	5.33	13.33	8.00	10.67	7.33	8.93%

Additional observations
  Tension: intermittent on bilabials
  Prosody: unremarkable

Summary and recommendations
  Significant fluency disorder
  Enroll in Fluency Development Program

Speaking rate: 110 words/min
              with disfluencies
Length of three longest disfluency
(in sec or syllables): 5 syllables
                       4 syllables
                       4 syllables
Associated behaviors: none noted
Child's attitude about communication: No overt awareness or concern.
  A. was observed to talk with hand over mouth frequently.
Other:

Appendix 2-B. Sample Therapy Plans

Sample Therapy Plans

1. Beginning Therapy Session
    Theme—Foods
    Clinician presents good listener rule and makes introductory remarks to establish easy speech model.

    Target 1
    Name 10 out of 10 foods with no model using easy, fluent speech.
    Materials   30 imitation foods in a box.
    Procedures   Child reaches in box and chooses and names food.
    Reinforcement   Continuous verbal for cooperation.

    Target 2
    Name 10 out of 10 foods with no model in a competitive situation using easy, fluent speech.
    Materials   30 food pictures, board game, and die.
    Procedures   Child draws card and names food, then rolls die and takes turn on board.
    Reinforcement   Continuous verbal for good naming.

    Target 3
    95/100 easy, fluent words in carrier phrase "I want to buy (food)" following an immediate model.
    Materials   30 pictures of foods, pennies, or play money.
    Procedures   Clinician plays storekeeper and directs child to point to the object he wishes to purchase. Clinician then provides the model, e.g., "I want to buy a banana." Child imitates. Clinician tells child how much. Child pays. Next child . . . .
    Reinforcement   Intermittent verbal for being able to say the "whole thing."

    Target 4
    95/100 easy, fluent words in carrier phrase "I need a _____ " with no model.
    Materials   Art project (paper plate mobiles): 15 food pictures, paper plates, string, scissors, and glue.
    Procedures   Clinician explains art project to children, lays pictures on table and children take turns choosing foods each time using the phrase "I need a _____ ."
    Reinforcement   Continuous verbal for saying the whole thing.

2. Intermediate Therapy Session
   Theme—Community Helpers
   Clinician makes introductory remarks to establish and label easy speech
     model. The good listener rule is presented.

Target 1
95/100 easy, fluent words in sentences in response to a delayed model.

Materials	Interactive language story, "Going to the Fire Station," flannel board, illustrations.
Procedures	Clinician tells story requiring participation from each child following a delayed model.
Reinforcement	Intermittent verbal for easy speech.

Target 2
95/100 easy, fluent words in sentences in response to delayed model in
competitive situation.

Materials	30 pictures of community helpers.
Procedures	Clinician hides pictures around room. Children compete to see who can find the most pictures, bringing them back one at a time to the clinician who provides a delayed model of a sentence about the picture, e.g., "A librarian helps us find the books we need. Now you tell me."
Reinforcement	Intermittent verbal for easy speech.

Target 3
95/100 easy, fluent words in spontaneous sentences.

Materials	Community helper spinner.
Procedures	Children take turns spinning the spinner and making up a sentence about the community helper.
Reinforcement	Intermittent verbal for easy speech.

Target 4
95/100 easy, fluent words in spontaneous sentences in a distracting
situation.

Materials	Sugar cookies, ready-made frosting, cake decorator.
Procedures	Each child is given a baker's hat and told "We are going to work like bakers." Each child decorates a cookie step-by-step taking turns making a sentence about what he will do next.
Reinforcement	Intermittent verbal for easy speech.

3. Advanced Therapy Session

   Target 1

   Control easy-fast-hard speech on command in 10 out of 10 spontaneous single word production.

Materials	Spinner and list of opposites.
Procedures	Child spins and gets easy, hard, or fast. Clinician gives adjective from opposite list. Child produces opposite pair using speaking pattern designated by spinner.
Reinforcement	Intermittent verbal for controlled speaking.

   Target 2

   95/100 easy, fluent words in monologue in a play situation.

Materials	Flannel board sequence stories.
Procedures	Clinician gives sequence cards to child. Child places cards on flannel board in order and spontaneously tells story.
Reinforcement	Intermittent verbal for easy speech.

   Target 3

   95/100 easy, fluent words in monologue in a disruptive situation.

Materials	What's wrong or missing pictures and ball.
Procedures	Child looks at picture and tells what's wrong while playing catch.
Reinforcement	Intermittent verbal for easy speech.

   Target 4

   95/100 easy, fluent speech in dialogue in a play situation.

Materials	Butcher paper, scissors, crayons.
Procedures	Clinician traces each child's body and leads discussion regarding body parts, hair and eye color, types of clothing, etc., while children discuss and color their pictures.
Reinforcement	Intermittent for easy speech.

3. Double Tape Recorder Therapy for Stutterers

Maryann Peins
W. Edward McGough
Bernard S. Lee

Overview

Double Tape Recorder Therapy for stutterers, which requires the use of two tape recorders, has as its goal, speech that is similar to the speech heard in normally fluent individuals. The method, utilizing twelve 30-minute lessons recorded on cassette tapes, provides the stutterer with one tape-recorded lesson and a half-hour therapy session from a speech clinician every 2 weeks for 6 months. The taped lessons focus on teaching speech skills that will enable stutterers to produce more effective, expressive communication that emerges in continuous, forward-flowing, connected legato speech. At home the client listens daily to the taped lesson in one tape recorder and responds onto another tape in a second recorder. The client listens, learns legato speech, responds, and listens to the tape again. The taped lessons provide encouragement to self-monitor as well as a variety of oral reading and realistic speaking exercises designed to give incentive to the clients to transfer their improved speech habits from the practice room to the real world. Based on data from a follow-up study and on our clinical experience in working with stutterers for more than 20 years, we know that Double Tape Recorder Therapy is an effective method of speech improvement for stutterers.

History of the Therapy

EARLY RESEARCH: HOW THE THERAPY EVOLVED

Double Tape Recorder Therapy for stutterers is the outgrowth of research begun in 1966 by Maryann Peins, a speech-language pathologist; W. Edward McGough, a psychiatrist; and Bernard S. Lee, a biomedical engineer. In spite of our diverse backgrounds, we joined efforts to develop and evaluate a new method for the treatment of stuttering because we recognized certain problems with current stuttering therapy: the time and energy it took to administer conventional therapy; the narrow range of effectiveness; the delayed emergence of speech improvement; and the lack of maintenance of speech improvement after termination of therapy. We

The investigators wish to acknowledge with grateful appreciation the support received from the Department of Health, Education, and Welfare, Social and Rehabilitation Administration Research Grant 2932-S, a Rutgers University Research Council Grant, and a Rutgers Medical School General Research Support Grant (PSPHS, NIH).

perceived a need for a therapy that would shorten the clinician's preparation time; reduce the amount of actual client-clinician contact; reduce the cost (in time and money) for the client; increase the amount of home practice time for the client; insure rapid improvement for all degrees of stuttering severity—the mild, moderate, and severe stutterer; and facilitate maintenance of the speech improvement.

A fortuitous coincidence caused us to meet and eventually collaborate. Our professional venture began in 1966 when Peins and Lee met to discuss problems associated with an acoustical chamber in a rehabilitation hospital speech and hearing clinic where Peins served as clinic director. After solving the acoustical chamber problem, Lee discussed the possibility of employing some of the successful therapy techniques, such as white noise masking and shadowing (Cherry and Sayers, 1956), with stutterers. Instead of replicating their work, Lee speculated that these techniques might be programmed onto tapes with oral reading and speaking exercises and that tape recorders could be used for the primary delivery of the stuttering therapy program. No one had ever done this before with stutterers.

The suggestion that a stutterer spend a considerable amount of time with a tape recorder and minimal time with a speech clinician was a radical departure from conventional ideas on therapy procedures in 1966. Peins was by training a client-centered conventional clinician, that is, she had trained to administer a stuttering modification therapy (Van Riper, 1963). Nevertheless, she was intrigued by the possibilities of Lee's innovative therapy idea for she had not achieved a success rate greater than 50 percent when using a conventional therapy with stutterers. What is more, even though cassette tape recorders were not yet available in the late 1960s and the existing recorders were large, cumbersome reel-to-reel machines, the use of tape recorders in therapy was increasing; and Peins recognized several advantages of them, both for the clinician's delivery of a stuttering therapy and for the reinforcement and maintenance of the client's speech through home use of tape recorders. She promised Lee, then, that she would try the tape recorder therapy on a pilot basis with the next stutterer in the clinic program who requested that therapy be terminated before achieving adequate speech improvement.

In 1967 Peins and Lee administered the first tape-recorded therapy program to a 15-year-old severe stutterer who had received 1 year of conventional speech therapy (Van Riper, 1963). Despite substantial gains made in the conventional therapy program, improving from a severe stuttering rating of 7 on the seven-point Scale for Rating Severity of Stuttering to a moderate rating of 4 (Darley and Spriestersbach, 1978), the adolescent's motivation decreased and he wished to stop therapy. In a final attempt to avoid a clinical dropout or clinical failure, Peins decided to take a chance with the new tape-recorded therapy being developed by Lee. When she suggested the alternative to the stutterer, he was receptive to the change because of the reduced number and length of the client-clinician therapy sessions, and he warmed to the idea of having a tape recorder for his home use since tape recorders were a rarity in homes in 1967.

The 5-month therapy program consisted of a 30-minute lesson with a clinician every 2 weeks and daily practice with a 40-minute tape used on a two-track tape recorder similar to ones used in language learning laboratories. Over the 5-month period, the client worked with three different 40-minute tapes.

The material on these three early tapes had the following components: (1) shadowing, (2) oral reading without shadowing, (3) reading and speaking with gradual attenuation in masking the auditory feedback, (4) impromptu speaking without masking the auditory feedback, (5) passages of real-life questions, (6) oral reading with and without masking of the auditory feedback, and (7) motivational comments.

One of the therapy tracks was permanent (the teacher track) and one was erasable (the student track). The client listened to the teacher track through headphones and recorded on the student track. Then, every 2 weeks throughout the 5-month period, Lee spent 30 minutes with the client during which time both client and clinician listened to the most recent taped practice session and discussed the client's progress.

Peins made serial evaluations of the client with oral reading and speaking tasks (Darley and Spriestersbach, 1978) prior to the tape-recorded therapy, at the end of the 5-month therapy period, and 5 months after termination. Prior to Double Tape Recorder Therapy, the client received a rating of 4, indicating a moderate degree of stuttering severity on the Scale for Rating Severity of Stuttering; after 5 months of the therapy, the young man received a rating of 2, which indicates a mild degree of stuttering; and 5 months after the termination, he received a rating of 1, a very mild degree of stuttering severity. Observable physical behaviors such as movements of the body, arms, legs, or head which accompanied the client's stuttering before the taped therapy program had disappeared by the termination of therapy, and audible noisy breathing, the most persistent and obvious physical behavior, was no longer evident even though we had given no attention to the elimination of any physical behaviors during the program period. Reading aloud and reciting in classes were no longer problems for the client, nor was answering the telephone a feared situation. The client was enthusiastic about the tape-recorded program and said he felt confident and able to cope with any real-life situations. (Peins, Lee, and McGough, 1970).

Peins and Lee realized at this initial stage of the research that the tape recorder therapy had possibilities both as an independent therapy and as an adjunct to others. Encouraged by the results of this pilot study, Peins and Lee discussed their findings with W. Edward McGough, M.D., a colleague with whom Lee had collaborated on several research projects. McGough, impressed with the results of the pilot study, urged the authors to publish their findings and to evaluate the tape-recorded therapy in a more elaborate research experiment. Thus it was that we three diverse professionals began to collaborate. At first we thought we could design a modest study using a few tape recorders with only a few stutterers. However, we soon recognized through our clinical impressions that something in this tape-recorded program contributed to improvement in the client's communicative behavior and should be studied in greater depth. Thus we designed a series of controlled experiments to validate our clinical impressions and to evaluate the new tape recorder therapy.

Assessment Procedures

An integral part of any speech therapy program should be an assessment of the client prior to and periodically throughout the therapy program. To determine whether the clients who receive Double Tape Recorder Therapy achieve speech improvement, we assess the client's speech behavior during both oral reading and spontaneous speaking tasks before our program begins and every 3 months thereafter until termination of therapy. Our assessment battery and procedures can be used with other assessment instruments.

DISFLUENCY CLASSIFICATION

Before beginning an assessment of a stutterer's speech, the clinician should identify in the client's case folder the disfluency classification system used to assess the client's speech or the clinician's definition of a stuttering behavior, a disfluency, or an instance of stuttering. Anyone referring to the client's case folder in the future then knows exactly what the clinician identified as a stuttering behavior and how the examiner determined whether the therapy program altered the client's speech.

In our research and therapy programs we use Wendell Johnson's revised disfluency classification which divides an instance of stuttering or a disfluency into the following categories: part-word repetitions *(b-b-boy)*; whole-word repetitions *(boy-boy-boy)*; phrase repetitions *(I have the . . . I have the book)*; interjections of sounds and syllables *(I feel . . . uh, uh, uh, sick)*; revisions (correcting or changing the content of a phrase or utterance such as *"I'll have a duggle . . . I mean a double burger"* or *"He'll finish it now . . . no, change that to tomorrow"* or *"We should . . . we will . . . we can't go)*; tense pauses or tension existing between words, part-words, or before initiation of a word such as audible breathing or perceptions of muscular tension; also, dysrhythmic phonations, which are events that occur within words and may not involve tension, such as the prolongation of a sound, an unusual accent or timing, a break within a word, improper stress, or some other speech behavior that is incompatible with fluent speech (Williams, Silverman, and Kools, 1968).

PROTOCOL

In Double Tape Recorder Therapy, every speech assessment session is tape-recorded with only the examiner and the client present. The materials needed for each speech assessment include

1. A cassette tape recorder with external microphone
2. Audio-cassette tapes: one 60-minute tape for the case history initial interview session and one 30-minute tape for each evaluation session
3. An interview or case history form (see Appendix 3-A), administered at the initial evaluation session
4. Two copies of an oral reading passage, 200 to 300 words in length and appropriate to the reading level of the client*
5. A copy of a picture with sufficient details to elicit a 3-minute sample of conversational speech†
6. A check list of instances of disfluencies‡
7. A check list of physical behaviors accompanying stuttering (see Appendix 3-A)
8. A severity scale§
9. A stopwatch
10. A clipboard with note pad

Elaborate equipment is not required for our assessment procedure, only a good high-fidelity tape recorder and a clinician with attentive listening ability and acute visual observational skills. In addition to tape-recording the assessment session, the clinician may wish to simultaneously videotape the session if videotape equipment is available. Researchers have indicated the value of studying videotapes for identifying physical behaviors that accompany stuttering and for comparing the client's speech behavior in pretherapy and posttherapy tapes.

We find it useful to tape-record the entire initial evaluation session, rather than relying only on memory or on note taking, which may intrude on the listening process or distract the client. To put the client at ease, however, we explain the confidentiality of the recording.

*We use the 300-word oral reading selection entitled, "Your Rate of Oral Reading." This selection appears in two books: Voice and Articulation Drillbook, by Grant Fairbanks (New York: Harper & Row, 1940), p. 144, and Diagnostic Methods in Speech Pathology (2nd ed.), by Frederick L. Darley and D. C. Spriestersbach (New York: Harper & Row, 1978), p. 276.
†We use Card No. 2 from the Thematic Apperception Test by H. A. Murray (Cambridge, Mass: Harvard University Press, 1943).
‡We use Johnson's Revised Disfluency Classification System which appears in D. Williams et al. Disfluency behavior of elementary school stutterers and nonstutterers: The adaptation effect. J. Speech Hear. Res. 11: 622-630, 1968.
§We used the Scale for Rating Severity of Stuttering in our original research. This scale appears in F. L. Darley and D. C. Spriestersbach, Diagnostic Methods in Speech Pathology (2nd ed.) (New York: Harper & Row, 1978), p. 313. Currently, we are exploring other instruments described in Darley and Spriestersbach (pp. 309–313) as well as unpublished instruments.

As a result of our research, Peins developed a comprehensive interview form *(Rutgers Interview Form for Stutterers)* (see Appendix 3-A) which we use to elicit information from the client. The *Rutgers Interview Form* serves as a guide, stimulating the flow of information about the onset and development of the speech problem; family, education, social, and vocational history; previous therapy; the client's description of the stuttering problem; and the client's attitudes toward previous and present therapy. In addition to our interview form, the clinician may wish to use additional commercial case history forms and alternate questionnaires or to develop an original form for obtaining background information from the client. Although we use the interview form at the initial assessment session only, we believe the clinician should continue to elicit background information and to note changes in the client at every therapy and assessment session. The more thorough the knowledge of the client's behavior and attitude toward stuttering, the better able the clinician will be to make appropriate clinical decisions regarding therapy for the client. If the clinician finds that her client needs counseling, for example, and she is not academically or professionally qualified to offer this, then she must refer the client to a qualified counselor on the basis of information she has gleaned subsequent to the initial assessment session. In our own group, we tend to explore current problems as they may arise, if the stutterer wants to talk about them, rather than to ignore them for we believe that assessment or diagnosis is an ongoing, dynamic, and continuous process. There is great truth in the maxim, "Diagnosis is therapy, and therapy is diagnosis," which was frequently expressed by Eugene T. McDonald to his students at Pennsylvania State University.

In Double Tape Recorder Therapy, our basic speech assessment is based on a 3-minute tape-recorded sample of an oral reading task and a 3-minute tape-recorded sample of spontaneous conversation which we obtain from each client every 3 months following standard procedures.

Using Johnson's revised disfluency classification system to assess the speech, our clinicians listen to the tape-recorded samples, mark the disfluencies on a check sheet, count and tabulate the types and instances of these, and make judgments as to the client's severity of stuttering during both the oral reading and spontaneous speech. In the past, we have used the seven-point Scale for Rating Severity of Stuttering, but now we are exploring other severity scales.

To obtain information about the client's overt or physical behaviors, we use the *Checklist of Physical Behaviors Accompanying Stuttering* developed by Peins (see Appendix 3-A) and observe the client's behavior during the oral reading and spontaneous speech tasks. We note any extraneous or distracting bodily movements, irregularities of breathing, facial grimaces, or changes in vocal patterns.

Description of the Therapy

THERAPY GOALS

We recognize that it is difficult for stutterers to become absolutely free of stuttering; however, it is possible for them to speak more fluently and effectively. Our therapy goal is not stutter-free speech, but rather speech that is similar to the speech heard in normally fluent individuals. We teach stutterers certain speech skills which enable them to produce speech that emerges in a continuous, forward-flowing manner, thereby promoting the speakers' fluency.

Although there is no consensus on a definition of "fluency," Martin Adams' description seems closest to the one we use in our therapy program:

Fluency is an attribute of utterances that start *promptly* and *easily*, and are characterized throughout by the *coordination* of respiratory, phonatory and articulatory activity as the speaker moves sequentially from sound to sound and syllable to syllable in a *continuous, forward-flowing* manner [emphasis in original] (1982, p. 174).

Because we believe that fluency is central to the stutterer's social and emotional improvement as well as to improved communication skills, we focus on this characteristic. This emphasis on forward-flowing speech is the cornerstone of our method; and the techniques we employ reinforce fluency and enable the client to achieve the goal of effective speech.

THERAPY METHOD

Double Tape Recorder Therapy consists of twelve taped 30-minute lessons which the stutterer uses over a 6-month period. He receives one tape-recorded lesson every 2 weeks from a speech clinician who asks him to listen to the taped lesson daily on one cassette tape recorder and to respond onto another tape placed in a second tape recorder. In this way, the stutterer uses the tape recorder much as a student uses a language-learning tape recorder: for listening, learning, responding, and listening again at the conclusion of each daily session at home. Each time the stutterer re-records, he erases his previous performance, while the instruction tape remains intact and unharmed.

The taped lessons instruct the stutterer to speak in a slower, smoother *legato speech,* a name that derives from the musical term meaning "smooth, flowing, and connected." The clinician's voice on the instruction tape serves as a model or pacesetter for the stutterer who listens to the voice and learns to speak in a slower, smoother manner that will not call attention to itself or to the stutterer.

Double Tape Recorder Therapy does not utilize delayed auditory feedback (DAF), the metronome, or computer-assisted instruction (CAD) to assist the stutterer in establishing a slower rate of speaking. Instead, the human voice on the taped lessons is the sole model for the stutterer's daily practice with the instructor's rate of speech on the twelve tapes ranging from 102 words per minute to 123.

The beneficial effect of slowing down is consistent with the finding of several researchers. Shearer and Williams (1965), who investigated self-recovery from stuttering in 58 ex-stutterers, found that 69 percent of their sample felt the factor that helped or would help most in the recovery from stuttering was speaking more slowly. Sheehan and Martyn (1966) also reported that the technique of slowing down was one of the reasons given by spontaneously recovered stutterers for their speech improvement. Wingate (1964, 1976) reported similar findings.

Every 2 weeks, the client meets with a speech clinician in a half-hour therapy session and together they listen to the stutterer's most recent tape recording. The two then analyze the stutterer's disfluent and fluent speech and discuss speech progress, with the clinician offering additional suggestions to assist the client in attaining forward-moving, smoother speech. The clinician may demonstrate, for example, how to link uttered words to achieve greater fluency. Also, by emphasizing the importance of self-monitoring through all sensory channels, the clinician can help the stutterer to become more aware of how to produce fluent ongoing speech. Kinesthetic awareness (muscle sense feedback) of phonemes uttered in the overlapping movements of conversational speech can be enhanced when the stutterer uses a slower speech rate. Kinesthetic and auditory awareness can provide the stutterer with feedback on his speech so he can determine when he is using fluent speech with the components described by Adams (1982).

Therapy instructions and complete transcriptions of the taped lessons appear in the *Double Tape Recorder Therapy Clinician's Manual* that accompanies the set of tapes. The time allotted for client response is indicated in the right-hand margin of each lesson's transcripts. The taped lessons incorporate therapy suggestions, procedures, techniques and activities which we and other speech-language pathologists (Van Riper, 1973; Wingate, 1976) have found effective in working with stutterers; these include encouragements to self-monitor while speaking to people daily; exercises to enhance expressive speech; oral reading assignments; practice of difficult words and phrases; stressful and nonstressful role-playing activities; telephone conversations; impromptu and extemporaneous speaking; and self-assignments. Excerpts from these tapes appear later in this chapter. There are no novel therapy techniques on the tapes; their particular outstanding contribution is simply that they deliver a major portion of the therapy; this method is unique and has not been reported prior to our research.

SPECIFIC TECHNIQUES, PROCEDURES, ACTIVITIES
Legato Speech
To achieve our therapy goal, we use certain techniques to develop the characteristics of forward-flowing speech. One of the techniques is legato speech which incorporates the use of a slower rate of speaking.

Legato speech has certain requirements: (1) Begin every speech utterance with air flow (breath) or voice (phonation) a fraction of a second before initiating articulatory movements. (2) Initiate speech without tension of the oral speech structures (easy initiation of articulatory movements). (3) Link each speech syllable or phoneme to the next in overlapping, connected articulatory movements, and link one word to the next word in each breath unit (with the goal of forward-moving, ongoing speech). (4) Use a slower rate of speaking.

The stutterer learns to initiate legato speech by emitting either air or voice phonation (depending on whether the first phoneme is voiced or voiceless) a slight fraction of a second before articulating a word or syllable. Stutterers often do the reverse: (1) start to preform a word (and often incorrectly) without any air flow or voice (phonation); (2) start to speak by making a hard articulatory contact (for example, pressing the lips hard together or pressing the tongue to the alveolar ridge or velum) and thus prevent any air flow or voice from being emitted; or (3) hold the breath and not allow any sound to emerge. In the first lesson, however, the speech clinician demonstrates legato speech so the stutterer will understand that starting an utterance with air flow (breath) or voice (phonation) leads directly into an easy initiation of speech. The speech clinician then guides the stutterer as he begins to learn it, refusing to accept schwas or extraneous sounds such as "uh" or "umm" as the client's "starters." In addition, the clinician should also help the stutterer to learn to monitor his feedback systems as he is speaking.

For too long, the stutterer has been speaking in a staccato style of speech which has broken, jerky, or uneven delivery; now, he will learn to speak using legato style. He will be reminded to strive for gentle, easy, relaxed onset of speech, to link words together, and to aim for a continuity of vocalization or the "ongoingness of speech." The script for lesson one of Double Tape Recorder Therapy in which we teach legato speech to the stutterer appears in its entirety in an earlier publication (Lee, McGough, and Peins, 1973).

The following is an excerpt from an instructional tape used for training students and clinicians in legato speech prior to their use of Double Tape Recorder Therapy:

> *Instructor:* I will say my name now in legato speech: Maryann Peins. Maryann Peins. Did you notice that I started with vocalization a slight fraction of a second before uttering "m" and

linked it to the next phoneme? If that sounds complicated, let me demonstrate again: Maryann Peins, Maryann Peins.

I said a slightly prolonged voiced sound (not a schwa vowel) as I said the "m" of my first name, and then I connected the "m" phoneme to the next phoneme. I also connected the "n" phoneme at the end of my first name, Marya*nn*, to the first phoneme of my last name, the "p." Listen again: MaryannPeins (repeat the name several times). There was no break between the two words.

Will you say your name? Remember, start with air or voice, depending on the first phoneme of your first name; then initiate articulatory movements; link your first name to the last name; and use a slower rate of speaking your name, please. Begin.

Student: (Student says his name.)

Instructor: Were you successful? I will demonstrate saying my name again: Maryann Peins, Maryann Peins. Will you say your name? Begin.

Student: (Student says his name.)

Instructor: Were you more successful this time? Let's try saying a sentence: My name is Maryann Peins, and I am speaking in legato style. (Use hand gestures to indicate the "ongoingness"of speech and a blackboard to show the links between the words in the sentence.)

Now, please say that same sentence in legato style, and substitute your name. Link each word to the next word. Say the sentence smoothly and slowly. I'll repeat the sentence again; and then when I say, "Begin," will you please say your sentence. My name is Maryann Peins and I am speaking in legato style. Begin.

Student: (Student says sentence.)

Instructor: Will you practice saying it again? "My name is . . . " and then say your name. Then add, "And I am speaking in legato style." Remember, link each word. Say the sentence smoothly, slowly, using overlapping connected speech movements. Begin.

Student: (Student says sentence.)

Instructor: Once you have learned legato speech, you will be able to teach it to your clients. You should be able to demonstrate legato speech before you begin to administer Double Tape Recorder Therapy. It will take practice to learn legato speech, so have patience with your clients who are learning this new way of speaking slowly and smoothly. Strive to become a good model of the legato style of speaking for your clients to imitate. By your example, you will help motivate them to learn legato speech.

Self-Monitoring

We encourage the stutterer to listen consciously or to become more auditorially aware of his slower rate of utterance and his more fluent speech. We also encourage the stutterer to become aware of proprioceptive feedback or the movement of his speech muscles during daily communication. We want the client to feel or be aware of the articulators moving easily in the overlapping movements of fluent, forward-moving, conversational speech. We believe that improvement in this self-monitoring ability will help him recognize what he is doing when he is speaking fluently, effectively, and expressively, and what he is doing when he is disfluent or stuttering.

The following excerpt from our therapy tapes is an example of encouragement to the client to self-monitor.

Encouragements to Self-Monitor (From Lesson 10)
Are you remembering to slow down? I'll often remind you on the practice tapes, but you must carry your own responsibility for your speech with you wherever you go. You must understand that stuttering is not a "thing" that happens to you. Stuttering is something that you do. Think of stuttering as a habit—a habit that you must exchange for a new, smooth style of speaking that you are learning. We know that you are learning this new, smooth style because you read and speak so well on the tape recorder. Are you remembering and succeeding in your daily, real-life speech? I hope so.

Enhancing Expressive Speech

Early in the therapy program the speech clinician explains and demonstrates what is meant by expressive speech. The clinician stresses the importance of developing good speech habits and of using expressive speech that maintains optimum pitch but which is varied in intonation, loudness, emphasis, and rate. We coach the client in vocal variety techniques so that when he practices daily at home with the tape recorder, he will use and reinforce fluent and expressive speech. We encourage the client to vary his speech at timed intervals on the tape for we do not want him to adopt an unnatural, unusual, or artificial speech pattern such as speaking lifelessly, devoid of any vocal expressiveness.

Exercise Focusing on Vocal Variety (From Lesson 5)
Here is an illustration to show how speech can be slow, but without expression. You can imitate me in stretching out legato style with no inflection in your speech.

This is an imitation of a mechanical man named, "Robot." Imitate this: "My name is Robot. I operate by means of transistors." Robot has no expression in his voice. He speaks monotonously. Let's give him expressive speech. Imitate me now, with melody or inflection in your speech: "My name is Robot. I operate by means of transistors." You can make your speech slow, yet bright and lively. Try to speak slowly, using vocal inflections and emphasis. Now I would like you to talk about something pleasant that you plan for the future. It may be a trip, a vacation, a party, anything at all. Just talk for three minutes, and remember to use expressive legato speech.

Instructor's Voice	*Time Allotted for Client Response*
Please begin to talk for 3 minutes.	1 minute
Continue talking about your plans.	1 minute
Let me hear some more, please.	
Use expressive legato speech.	1 minute
Okay, that's enough about the plans. Now what is your name, please?	5 seconds
And, what is the day?	5 seconds
And, what is the date?	5 seconds
Thank you. Listen to your own recording now.	

Oral Reading Activities

Each taped instructional lesson includes oral reading practice; so, we suggest that the client select reading materials for daily practice that not only interest him but that have practical application to his schoolwork, to his job, or to social activities.

The following are representative excerpts from this segment of the tapes:

Oral Reading Exercise (From Lesson 3)

We will now have an oral reading exercise. Get a book, magazine, or newspaper, something interesting that you would like to read aloud. Read it aloud slowly, in legato style and with expression. Look at the first paragraph. With a pencil or pen, underline the words you consider important as you read. Emphasize these words with your voice. You can learn which words to emphasize properly if you read ahead or scan to plan your vocal expression before reading aloud.

	Time Allotted for Client Response
Go ahead and read aloud.	1 minute
Continue reading slowly. Slow is better.	1 minute
Read with expression, emphasize the important words, and use inflections.	1 minute
Continue for another minute.	1 minute
Okay, that's enough reading.	

Oral Reading Exercise (From Lesson 11)

For the next exercise, choose some pleasant reading. I hope you have practiced reading aloud to someone who enjoys listening. Read as you have been taught, with expression, slowly, and smoothly. Start with air or voice first and let the word follow with no break. Go ahead and read, slowly, smoothly, and with vocal variety. Slowly, please.

	Time Allotted for Client Response
Slow is better.	1 minute
With expression, please, in your voice.	1 minute
Don't read in a monotone.	1 minute
Continue in long, connected phrases, please.	1 minute
Use emphasis on the important words.	1 minute
That's sufficient reading.	
Listen now to portions of your readings—were they as slow as you felt them to be while you were reading?	3 seconds

Practice of Difficult Words and Phrases (From Lesson 4)

Okay, now let us drill, with vocal variations, for one minute each, over and over, four words or phrases of your own choice that you use in real life.

	Time Allotted for Client Response
The first word, please.	1 minute
And now a second word or phrase with vocal variety.	1 minute

	Time Allotted for Client Response
And now a third word or phrase with vocal expressiveness.	1 minute
And now a fourth word or phrase that you may be called upon to use tomorrow. Use an expressive voice.	1 minute
Okay, that's enough drill. That's the end of the first part of Lesson 4.	

Realistic Speech Experiences

The speech experiences, activities, and assignments on our tapes simulate the real speaking world and daily living communication activities so that the clients will quickly attempt to transfer the fluent speech used in the practice sessions to conversational speech in daily speaking situations. To facilitate this transfer and reinforcement of fluent speech we include role playing activities, telephone conversations, impromptu and extemporaneous speaking, and encouragements to use a slower rate of speech.

Representative segments extracted from the taped lessons follow:

Role-Playing Activity (From Lesson 5)

Here is some threatening conversation with a store clerk. Try to retain your composure and answer in a slow, legato style of speech. This is a typical situation with a clerk in a store.

You are returning a device or gadget because it is not satisfactory. The clerk is not too pleasant. Answer calmly, in slow, legato style.

	Time Allotted for Client Response
Let's go. What's the trouble?	10 seconds
Speak up, I can't hear you!	5 seconds
When did you buy it?	5 seconds
Have you got a receipt?	5 seconds
This doesn't look like our receipt at all! Are you sure you bought it here?	3 seconds
Did you read the instructions carefully?	3 seconds
What happened?	7 seconds
What do you expect us to do about it?	7 seconds
A refund or a replacement? Which do you prefer?	5 seconds

	Time Allotted for Client Response
Okay, I have to fill out this form. It'll take a while. What's your name, please?	5 seconds
How do you spell that last name?	7 seconds
What's your address?	7 seconds
Spell the street, please.	7 seconds
What town is that? Say it again!	5 seconds
Okay, we'll take care of it.	

Role-Playing Activity (From Lesson 9)
Some introductions:

	Time Allotted for Client Response
Introduce yourself to the receptionist at the front office and state why you are there	15 seconds
Introduce yourself at the dentist's office. What time is your appointment?	10 seconds
Inquire at a hospital desk for the room number of some person who is ill.	8 seconds
That person is in Room 522. Are you a relative?	3 seconds
How are you related?	7 seconds
Introduce a friend to your family.	7 seconds
Introduce a person to someone in authority, for instance, a principal, a teacher, or your employer.	7 seconds
Do that again.	7 seconds
Introduce a friend of yours to another friend.	7 seconds

Speaking on the Telephone (From Lesson 3)
Now, the telephone is going to ring. Each time, answer in words you would ordinarily use at home or at work. It helps to have a telephone instrument handy. Disconnect it and take it off the phone cradle while you simulate real answering.

	Time Allotted for Client Response
Ring	6 seconds
Ring.	6 seconds

	Time Allotted for Client Response
Ring.	6 seconds
Ring.	6 seconds
Ring.	6 seconds
Ring.	6 seconds
Ring.	6 seconds

Your speech clinician will help to desensitize you to the problems that you have with the telephone. It is a matter of practicing with a disconnected telephone instrument when you are relaxed. First, you will learn to pick up the telephone, put it in place, and sound your voice. Then, continuing to speak in a relaxed manner, learn to pick up the telephone and say, "Hello," or whatever it is that you wish to use when answering. This exercise may require many hours of patient practice. You can attempt to answer a *real* ringing telephone, after you have practiced enough with this taped lesson to feel confident to answer the telephone.

And now, here is some threatening telephone conversation. Even though I shout at you and urge you to answer quickly, do not do so. You are the one who decides at what rate you speak. The telephone rings.

	Time Allotted for Client Response
(Ring, ring.) Hello. Who is this?	5 seconds
Is Frank there? Frank. Frank. What number is this?	5 seconds
Where are you?	5 seconds
What's your area code?	5 seconds
Okay, thanks, I'll tell the operator not to charge it.	

Impromptu and Extemporaneous Speaking (From Lesson 3)
Now we shall have some exercise in ad lib or extemporaneous speaking. Simply open your eyes and describe everything you see before you. Describe what is on the desk, on the shelves, the furniture, the painting on the walls, the fixtures, or doors. If you can open the window and look out, describe what you see.

	Time Allotted for Client Response
Go ahead for 1 minute.	1 minute
Okay, that's enough description of the room. Now I would like you to hold before you a picture, one	1 minute

| | *Time Allotted* |
| | *for Client Response* |

with a lot of detail, and describe
the picture for one minute.
Begin.
Okay, that's enough about the
picture.

Now, what is your name, please?	1 minute
And where do you live?	5 seconds
In what town?	5 seconds
What is your telephone number?	5 seconds
Where do you work or go to	5 seconds
school?	
How many members in your	5 seconds
family? Give their names,	
please.	
What day is this?	5 seconds
And, what is the date?	5 seconds

Thank you. That's all for Lesson 3.

Encouragements to Use Slow Rate (From Lesson 1)
Okay, that's enough reading. When you listen to your reading, take note
of your improvement in slower rate. You may have felt you were going as
slow as cold molasses, but your reading was probably smoother, pleasant
to listen to, and more fluent. Speech rate is one of the hardest concepts
to grasp—the speed of one's own speech. Let's talk about that a bit. Remember, you are the one who decides at what rate you speak. Perhaps
you feel pressured to answer quickly when your friends engage in rapid
conversation—too rapid for you. The typist, the musician, and the steno-
grapher all have their top speed, beyond which they may get into trouble.
You have a top speed also—probably slower than others around you. Do
not be concerned about this. Almost all of the greatest speakers such as
Franklin Delano Roosevelt, Winston Churchill, and Martin Luther King
have been slow and deliberate in their style of speaking, and people listened to them.

| | *Time Allotted* |
| | *for Client Response* |

Say, "I am the one who decides at	8 seconds
what rate I speak. Slower speech	
is better speech."	
Say that again, please.	8 seconds

Self-Assignments
The more the stutterer deliberately uses and reinforces legato speech, the more stable his fluent speech will become. In therapy sessions and on the taped lessons, we motivate the stutterer to talk more, to use legato style speech, and to remember successful speaking experiences. For example, we suggest to the client that after he concludes his daily speech practice session he should speak to his family or to a friend, using legato speech, or make a telephone call to get immediate transfer and reinforcement of legato speech. We introduce self-assignments beginning with Tape 3. A segment of this taped lesson follows:

> *Self-Assignments* (From Lesson 3)
> You should, about now, be ready to do a speech self-assignment in real life. This is somewhat equivalent to going on stage for the first time. You should be well-rehearsed, confident, and prepared to attempt rather simple things at first. For example, rehearse asking for a brand-name product from a store clerk; or ask for a newspaper, candy bar, ice cream, or food at a store. Plan to do one assignment today. Then, with a feeling of confidence, go ahead. If you have the feeling of confidence, you are very likely to succeed. Rehearse, plan, and do at least one speaking self-assignment in real life each day. Let us rehearse right now some practical self-assignments you can do today.

	Time Allotted for Client Response
Go ahead, talk for one minute.	1 minute
Continue talking about an assignment you will do tomorrow. Talk for one more minute.	1 minute

THE THERAPY SESSION
The goals of every therapy session are to (1) assist the stutterer in attaining more effective, expressive, fluent speech; (2) encourage self-monitoring to develop the stutterer's awareness of the production of fluent speech; (3) encourage daily practice with the tapes; and (4) foster the use of good speech habits in all communicative experiences to reinforce and maintain fluent speech.

At the beginning of every therapy session, the speech clinician and the stutterer listen to portions of the stutterer's most recent tape recording and analyze the speech progress. By listening to the client's tape recording and comparing it with the client's spontaneous speech in the session, the clinician can quickly determine whether the client is using legato speech consistently. If the client does not demonstrate use of legato speech, then the clinician can review the essentials of legato speech and provide practice for it until the client uses legato speech spontaneously, speaking more slowly, more smoothly, and with greater fluency. The speech clinician should focus on the client's fluency and help the client analyze what he does as he speaks and reads fluently. How does this effective way of speaking and reading differ from the stutterer's moments of stuttering?

During each therapy session, we remind the client to listen consciously to his fluent, slower rate of utterance. We also encourage the stutterer to become aware of proprioceptive feedback, that is, to become more conscious of the speech muscles and their movements during daily communication. We want the stutterer to feel the articulators moving easily in the overlapping movements of fluent, forward-moving, conversational speech. As the stutterer learns the importance of self-monitoring and the roles of auditory and proprioceptive feedback, one or both of these feedback systems may help him to become more cognizant of his new controlled, slower rate of utterance and his use of legato speech.

Early in the therapy program, the clinician explains and demonstrates what is meant by vocal variety or expressive speech. The clinician stresses the importance of using expressive speech that is varied in intonation, pitch, loudness, stress, and rate, and coaches the client in vocal variety techniques. The client should practice these techniques daily at home with the tape recorder and avoid artificial speech patterns devoid of expressiveness. In the therapy sessions and on the taped lessons, we encourage the stutterer to talk more, to use legato speech, and to remember the successful speaking experiences.

Toward the conclusion of each therapy session, the clinician discusses the goals, the speech activities, and the rationale for each segment of the next taped lesson. The client must have a clear understanding of the speech objectives of each taped lesson so that his daily practice of the taped speech experiences will be meaningful. As the client listens to each tape, he is reminded to practice with materials that are interesting and have practical value in his daily activities.

Double Tape Recorder Therapy can be used successfully with stutterers as the sole therapy or as an adjunct or auxiliary therapy. The speech clinician should feel free to make therapeutic suggestions based on other therapies rather than following our therapy program rigidly. Stutterers have different symptoms, backgrounds, personalities, attitudes, and interests; and the speech clinician may wish, therefore, to individualize the therapy sessions according to the needs of the client.

PHYSICAL BEHAVIORS

Although conventional stuttering modification therapy places considerable emphasis on changing physical behaviors which often accompany the stuttering, Double Tape Recorder Therapy does not stress the elimination or modification of these behaviors. We base this decision on findings from our research (Peins, Lee, McGough, 1970; Peins, McGough, Lee, 1971b; McGough, Peins, Lee, 1971). In those studies, although we did not attempt to modify the physical behaviors of the stutterers during therapy, there was a very significant reduction of observable physical characteristics accompanying stuttering.

Why do the stuttering behaviors decline without direct intervention? We hypothesize that these physical behaviors decrease or disappear as the stutterer becomes more fluent because he no longer has a need to use them to assist him when speaking. Ryan reached a similar conclusion regarding the physical behaviors that accompany stuttering.

> . . . we have noticed that the need for these behaviors declines as the stutterer becomes more fluent—an observation we have made of most of the behaviors that have traditionally been defined as secondary symptoms. Presumably, the original reason for the acquisition of all these behaviors was stuttering (1970, p. 60).

ATTITUDINAL WORK

We do not recommend attempts to foster acceptance of stuttering in Double Tape Recorder Therapy. To instill in the stutterer acceptance of his stuttering or a more tolerant attitude toward his speech problem, we believe, is unrealistic and incongruous with our goals of speech improvement. Instead, we focus on motivation to help the stutterer become a more fluent speaker and improve his speech, utilizing motivational techniques such as encouragements and positive statements. We tell the stutterer that he can improve his speech through daily home practice of the taped lessons, the use of slower rate of legato speech in daily speech experiences, and attendance at therapy sessions every 2 weeks. We do not wish the stutterer to take a passive attitude toward the therapy program or toward his speech problem; instead, we encourage him to take control.

Based on our personal and clinical observations of the clients in our therapy program over the past 15 years as well as our research, we find that the stutterers' feelings and attitudes toward themselves and their speech do change in the course of therapy (Peins, McGough, Lee, 1971b). Ryan also corroborates our observations of a change in feelings and attitudes when stutterers become more fluent:

> Feelings, important as they may be, are not easily observed and measured, so that it is difficult to deal with them systematically. Furthermore, we have observed that many of our clients change their feelings and attitudes when they become more fluent. We all know that one's self-concept can change as one becomes better able to perform certain tasks, such as speaking (1970, p. 59).

TRANSFER AND MAINTENANCE

A constant concern of clinicians during the course of a therapy program is whether a client will be able to maintain speech improvement after termination of therapy. Will the reduction in stuttering continue after termination of therapy? What can the clinician and the stutterer do to insure maintenance of speech improvement?

At our laboratory, we are satisfied that Double Tape Recorder Therapy can help the stutterer maintain speech improvement. How is this accomplished?

First, the convenience and portability of this method makes it easy for the stutterer to practice daily at home. We believe that fluency must be continuously practiced. Speech is a skill, and our clients learn a new speech skill: how to speak in a more fluent manner.

Second, the pragmatic, communicative role-playing experiences incorporated in every taped lesson encourage carry-over or transfer as well as greater generalization of good speech habits into real-life situations. The taped speaking exercises simulate real-life speaking experiences which the stutterer will encounter daily. Thus, the stutterer practices speech exercises at home that he can transfer to life situations immediately after his daily practice session.

In many forms of therapy, there is no assurance that when the stutterer leaves the therapy session he will practice his speech assignments daily or transfer newly-learned speech fluency to various communicative situations. The therapy program with the format of daily speech practice and listening sessions at home, daily reinforcements of speech fluency, plus encouragements to instill confidence, however, provides clients with incentive to transfer their improved speech habits from the practice room to the real-life world and, thus, to maintain speech improvement.

FOLLOW-UP PROCEDURES

Completion of 6 months of Double Tape Recorder Therapy does not necessarily mean termination of therapy. We tell our clients that the door is always open to them to return for additional therapy, if necessary, and we provide them with a 30-minute posttherapy tape for use at home to help them maintain speech improvement. The tape reviews the main ideas presented in the program and serves to remind the client of techniques that he has learned in therapy. We encourage him to listen to the tape and practice as often as possible if he notices any increase in stuttering. In addition, we urge our clients to return once a month for a half-hour lesson for 6 months following conclusion of the therapy program, which gives us the opportunity to assess and monitor the clients' speech patterns and to offer suggestions if we notice any changes in speech behavior.

Follow-up of subjects is not an easy task; there is always subject attrition and for the predictable reasons: some clients move away from the area, some change jobs or employment hours, and some are unavailable at evaluation times. In spite of these and other reasons, we are gratified with the number of clients who returned for follow-up evaluations (Peins, McGough, and Lee, 1974). We continue to contact our clients and request that they return for follow-up evaluations every 3 months for 1 year and then every 6 months thereafter.

The follow-up speech evaluations consist of a 3-minute reading task and a 3-minute speaking task. Procedures for conducting the speech evaluations are discussed in this chapter in the section on Assessment Procedures.

EQUIPMENT AND MATERIALS NEEDED

At every therapy session, the speech clinician must have the following equipment to administer Double Tape Recorder Therapy:

1. A set of twelve instructional tapes*
2. A clinician's guide book, containing a complete transcript of the 12 instructional tapes
3. Two cassette tape recorders
4. Cassette tapes for recording speech evaluations

CLINICIAN SKILLS AND TRAINING REQUIRED

Any speech-language pathologist, speech clinician, or student under the supervision of a speech-language pathologist should receive training† in the use of Double Tape Recorder Therapy which includes learning legato speech prior to administering therapy.

In any therapy program, success rate probably cannot be based on the therapy method alone. Success also depends on many variables, some nonspecific and some unmeasurable, such as the client-clinician relationship, the clinician's personality and teaching style, and those skills involved in motivating a client to improve. Every clinician should see each client as a unique individual with special needs and respond empathetically to those needs.

We recognize that personal styles of teaching vary and influence the way therapy is delivered. All clinicians must have the freedom to choose a teaching style that they find effective in establishing and maintaining rapport as well as in developing a therapeutic relationship that will facilitate change in the client and assist him to achieve and maintain optimum speech improvement.

Also, unless a clinician has confidence in a therapy method and believes firmly that the method *will* work and will help the client, improvement probably will not occur. This confidence in the method will serve to strengthen the client's motivation and desire to improve his speech.

Double Tape Recorder Therapy for Stutterers is available from The Speech Therapy Group, Department of Psychiatry, University of Medicine and Dentistry of New Jersey–Rutgers Medical School, Piscataway, NJ 08854.
†Training workshops on Double Tape Recorder Therapy are given frequently at Rutgers, The State University of New Jersey, at the University of Medicine and Dentistry of New Jersey–Rutgers Medical School, and at various professional meetings throughout the country. Inquiries regarding training workshops may be addressed to the authors.

CLIENT REQUIREMENTS

Initially, we accepted stutterers 13 years and older into our research program. We set this minimum age limit of 13 years because we wanted to use a particular reading selection, "Your Rate of Oral Reading" (see Assessment Procedures), used by numerous researchers to measure the amount and severity of stuttering. The passage is at the eighth to ninth grade reading level, and this was the determining factor in setting the minimum age limit at 13 years. Thus, we evaluated our therapy method on a population of stutterers with a minimum age of 13 years. Since then we have administered the therapy to younger stutterers who could read at eighth or ninth grade levels and carry out daily home practice assignments. We have also begun to develop materials for younger children who stutter, and believe our therapy program is applicable to them if they have sufficient intelligence and maturity to operate a tape recorder. We are gradually accumulating data on the effectiveness of our therapy program with young children who stutter.

In addition, the client must practice daily for 1 hour at home with the instructional tapes. He is told to (1) listen to the instructional tape daily, (2) learn the training material, (3) respond and record his answers, and (4) replay the tape and listen to his recording at the conclusion of every daily practice session.

The client must also remember to transfer the therapy ideas continually into daily communicative situations whether at home, on the job, or in school.

Evaluation of the Therapy

To evaluate the Double Tape Recorder Therapy, the authors designed several controlled studies (Peins, McGough, Lee, 1970; 1972a; 1973; 1974; McGough, Peins, Lee, 1971) which included (1) a comparative study of 36 stutterers' improvement in speaking and oral reading tasks, reduction in physical behaviors, and attitude changes when assigned to one of two therapy conditions or no therapy for 6 months; (2) a study of the effectiveness of Double Tape Recorder Therapy as an adjunct therapy to eight stutterers formerly treated with a conventional form of stuttering modification therapy; and (3) a follow-up study of 25 stutterers who received Double Tape Recorder Therapy either as the sole treatment for 6 months or as an adjunct therapy to 6 months of a conventional therapy.

THE COMPARATIVE STUDY

The initial evaluation of Double Tape Recorder Therapy was a comparative study of 36 stutterers' improvement in speaking and oral reading tasks, reduction in physical behaviors, and attitude changes.

The 36 stutterers, between the ages of 13 to 43 and with stuttering severity that ranged from mild to severe, were randomly assigned to one of three groups for 6 months: (1) Double Tape Recorder Therapy, (2) a conventional (Van Riper) stuttering modification therapy, and (3) a control group (no therapy).

A speech pathologist administered an assessment battery (see p. 77) which included speaking and reading tasks, the Iowa Scale of Attitude Toward Stuttering, and the *Checklist of Physical Behaviors* (Darley and Spriestersbach, 1978) (utilized during the TAT task) prior to the subjects' group assignments and at the end of 3 and 6 months.

Using the TAT speaking task and a standard reading passage, a speech pathologist, who administered neither the assessment battery nor the therapy to any of the stutterers, made severity rating judgments on the subjects in each group prior to therapy, at 3-month intervals during the 6 months of therapy, and also at several points in the adjunct therapy and follow-up of the subjects. She used the seven-point Scale for Rating Severity of Stuttering (see footnote, p. 77) to evaluate the first minute of the tape-recorded 3-minute TAT speech samples and the first minute of the tape-recorded reading samples in random order without knowledge of either the time or nature of the treatment condition.

Before making a statistical assessment of the ratings, we determined the reliability of the speech pathologist's judgments, comparing the two ratings she had given to each of the 38 one-minute speech samples of 29 stutterers. An interval of 3 months separated the two ratings for each sample, and our comparison of the two yielded a Pearson correlation coefficient of 0.96 ($p = 0.01$).

Results

Improvement in a speaking task. Table 3-1 presents the severity ratings of speech samples (TAT Task) in the conventional (Van Riper) stuttering modification therapy group (N = 12), in the double tape recorder group (N = 12), and in the control (no therapy) group (N = 12).

Among the subjects in the group receiving the conventional (Van Riper) stuttering modification therapy, eight of the 12 stutterers, or 67 percent, showed a reduction in the severity of their stuttering after 6 months of therapy. Application of the sign test, one-tailed (Siegel, 1956), to the data indicated that the speech improvement was statistically significant ($p = 0.02$). The rate of improvement for more severe stutterers conformed to those reported by other researchers, with little speech improvement during the first 3 months of therapy and most speech progress between 3 and 6 months of therapy.

In the Double Tape Recorder Therapy group, 11 of the 12 subjects, or 92 percent of the stutterers showed a reduction in severity of stuttering after 6 months of therapy. Using the sign test, one-tailed, with this data indicated that the improvement observed in this group was significant (sign test, $p = .003$). An important finding is that at the end of the therapy

Table 3-1. Serial Severity Ratings of Spoken Samples (TAT Task) in the Conventional Therapy Group, the Double Tape Recorder Therapy (DTR) Group, and the Control Group

Subjects	Conventional Therapy[a]			DTR Therapy[a]			Control Group[a]		
	Initial Assessment	3 Months	6 Months	Initial Assessment	3 Months	6 Months	Initial Assessment	3 Months	6 Months
1	5	5	4	5	4	4	6	6	6
2	7	7	6	7	6	5	7	5	6
3	5	4	3	6	6	5	4	4	3
4	3	3	3	3	2	2	7	7	7
5	5	5	5	7	7	5	4	4	4
6	6	6	4	3	3	2	4	3	4
7	4	4	3	7	6	6	6	6	6
8	4	4	4	6	5	3	7	7	6
9	4	4	4	6	6	3	6	1	2
10	6	5	5	4	3	5	3	5	6
11	5	4	4	6	5	5	4	4	5
12	5	6	6	3	4	4	5	4	5
$\bar{X}^{b}$	4.92	4.75	4.17	5.25	4.75	4.08	5.25	4.92	5.08

[a] N = 12.
[b] $\bar{X}$ = weighted mean.

period, the degree of improvement did not seem related to the initial severity of stuttering as it did with the conventional therapy group. In comparison to conventional therapy, Double Tape Recorder Therapy is not only effective with mild, moderate, and severe stutterers, but also yields improvement in the first 3 months of therapy (seven of the 12 subjects showed some speech improvement).

In the control group (no therapy for 6 months), four of the 12 stutterers showed some improvement, one stutterer lost ground and seven stayed at the same severity level. Application of the sign test to these data indicated that any significant speech improvement seemed to relate to initial severity of stuttering.

Analysis of the data indicated that stutterers who received either therapy method improved markedly while stutterers who did not receive therapy did not, and the difference between the two therapy groups and the control group was highly significant (Fisher Exact Probability Test, $p = .01$ [Siegel, 1956]).

Even though more stutterers improved with Double Tape Recorder Therapy than with the conventional therapy, the difference in the effect of the therapies was not significantly different (Fisher Exact Probability Test). However, Double Tape Recorder Therapy is effective with mild, moderate, and severe stutterers; whereas only the more severe stutterers showed improvement in the conventional therapy group. Moreover, improvement also seemed to occur more quickly with Double Tape Recorder Therapy, often within the first 3 months.

Physical Behaviors

The two therapies, Double Tape Recorder Therapy and conventional stuttering modification therapy, differ in their treatments of physical behavior. Conventional stuttering modification therapy places considerable emphasis on the elimination or modification of observable physical behaviors that often accompany stuttered speech, such as conspicuous or inappropriate movements and postures of parts of the body. Double Tape Recorder Therapy does not focus on any physical behaviors.

In our pilot study we observed that as stuttering severity decreased, the observable physical behaviors that accompanied the stuttered speech similarly decreased without any direct intervention by the clinician. Although reduction of physical behaviors had not been a goal of the therapy program, upon review of our data we found a dramatic reduction in physical behaviors. Based on this incidental finding, Peins developed a checklist for observable physical behaviors accompanying stuttered speech (see Appendix 3-A) for use during the oral reading and speaking tasks.

This checklist requires making separate judgments for specific anatomic areas: the head, eyes, nose, mouth, torso, arms, hands, legs, and feet as well as many of the observable concomitants which accompany stuttering that are commonly accepted in the field.

In the conventional therapy group, eight of the 12 stutterers showed a reduction in observable physical behaviors accompanying stuttered speech after 6 months of therapy. Application of the sign test showed this to be significant ($p = .05$).

After 6 months of Double Tape Recorder Therapy, 10 of the 12 subjects showed a reduction in physical behaviors accompanying stuttered speech. Using the sign test, the change is significant ($p = .01$).

In the control (no therapy) group, there was no significant reduction in physical behaviors.

To summarize, there was significant reduction of physical behaviors accompanying stuttered speech in the conventional therapy group and even more significant reduction of physical behaviors in the Double Tape Recorder Therapy group, even though no direct emphasis is given to physical behaviors in the therapy program (Peins, McGough, Lee, 1971b).

Attitude
What happens to stutterers in regard to their attitude toward stuttering in the different therapy groups? Does a reduction in stuttering severity result in a positive change in attitude?

In 1968 when we were doing our research, one of the most widely used instruments for measuring attitude was the Iowa Scale of Attitude Toward Stuttering. This scale indicates the respondent's attitude toward stuttering, specifically, his tolerance or intolerance of stuttering.

The Iowa Scale of Attitude Toward Stuttering was administered as part of the total stuttering test battery to all the subjects in all groups prior to their group assignment, and at 3-month intervals.

In Double Tape Recorder Therapy, encouragements to the stutterer were interspersed throughout the taped lessons, but we did not place direct emphasis on the stutterer's need to accept or tolerate his stuttering. In contrast, in the conventional therapy group, the speech pathologist placed considerable emphasis in therapy on the concept of acceptance or tolerance of stuttering.

The conventional (Van Riper) stuttering modification therapy group evidenced a small but significant reduction of the mean score from 1.987 to 1.664 for the attitude scale at the end of 6 months of therapy. Application of the sign test indicates that the change is significant ($p = .01$).

The Double Tape Recorder Therapy group attitude scores did not decrease over 6 months, but rather experienced a slight increase in group mean scores from 1.833 prior to therapy to 1.885 at the end of 6 months of therapy. However, this change over 6 months was not significant (sign test).

In the control group, the change in mean scores from 1.71 to 1.76 over 6 months was not significant (sign test).

Thus, all the subjects in all three groups had "average" attitudes toward stuttering prior to assignment to their groups and at the conclusion of the 6 months' study. Only in the conventional group was the change in mean scores significant.

It is conceivable that the stutterers in the conventional therapy group learned their lessons well regarding tolerance toward, or acceptance of, their stuttering; whereas, the Double Tape Recorder Therapy group which was instructed not to accept their stuttering also learned their lessons well. Although attitude did not change among stutterers in the Double Tape Recorder Therapy group according to the Iowa scale, their attitudes did appear to change from our personal and clinical observations and conversations with them. Perhaps we did not have a sensitive tool to measure or quantify the attitudes that we were observing in our subjects and this accounts for the disparity between the ratings and our observations.

Improvement in Reading Tasks
Table 3-2 presents the severity ratings of reading samples in the conventional (Van Riper) therapy group (N = 12), in the Double Tape Recorder Therapy group (N = 12), and in the control group (no therapy) group (N = 12).

Four of the 12, or 33 percent of the stutterers who received the conventional stuttering modification therapy showed a reduction in the severity of stuttering during oral reading tasks after 6 months of therapy. Using the sign test, one-tailed, with this data indicated that the improvement observed in this group was not significant.

Comparing these findings with those for the speaking task (Table 3-1), we found that only four stutterers improved in the reading task, whereas, eight had improved in the speaking task. Interestingly, although two stutterers who registered gains in reading also improved in the speaking task, two others improved in the speaking task, but not in the reading.

In the group receiving Double Tape Recorder Therapy, 10 of the 12 stutterers, or 83 percent, improved on the reading task. Improvement seen in the reading tasks is almost identical to that seen in the speaking task and greater than the amount of improvement seen in the conventional therapy group. Application of the sign test, one-tailed, to this data indicated that the improvement observed was statistically significant (p = .006).

In the control group (no therapy), the findings are almost identical with the speaking task data: four subjects improved, six stayed at the same severity level, and two stutterers increased in stuttering severity. Application of the sign test, two-tailed, indicated that there was no statistically significant improvement in oral reading tasks in the control group.

In summary, analysis of the data indicates that the 12 stutterers who received the Double Tape Recorder Therapy improved significantly more in the reading task than the stutterers who received no therapy and more

Table 3-2. Serial Severity Ratings of Spoken Samples (reading task) in the Conventional Therapy Group, in the Double Tape Recorder Therapy Group, and in the Control Group

Subjects	Conventional Therapy[a]			DTR Therapy[a]			Control Group[a]		
	Initial Assess.	3 Months	6 Months	Initial Assess.	3 Months	6 Months	Initial Assess.	3 Months	6 Months
1	5	5	5	3	3	2	6	6	6
2	4	6	4	6	6	3	7	7	7
3	5	5	4	7	6	6	6	6	5
4	1	1	1	5	5	7	7	7	7
5	5	5	5	7	4	4	6	5	6
6	7	7	7	4	1	2	5	5	6
7	4	5	4	7	5	6	7	6	6
8	5	5	5	4	4	3	3	3	4
9	5	5	4	7	7	6	6	6	3
10	6	6	6	5	4	3	4	3	3
11	7	7	6	4	3	4	6	6	6
12	4	3	1	5	5	4	5	4	4
$\overline{X}$[b]	4.83	5	4.33	5.33	4.42	4.17	5.7	5.3	5.5

[a] $N = 12$.
[b] $\overline{X}$ = weighted mean.

than the stutterers who received the conventional stuttering modification therapy.

Double Tape Recorder Therapy and the conventional stuttering modification therapy are in some ways similar and in many ways quite different. One of the differences is the emphasis on reading exercises. Most of the daily taped therapy sessions include a reading exercise; whereas, the conventional therapy does not emphasize oral reading nor require daily oral reading exercises. It is not surprising, then, to see differences in the degree of improvement in the oral reading task in our groups.

ADJUNCT THERAPY

Can Double Tape Recorder Therapy be used after administration of other therapies? Based on clinical observations made during our pilot work and early research, we believed that our therapy program might have value as an adjunct or auxiliary therapy to more conventional forms of therapy. We also believed that the daily structured home practice time required would assist the stutterer to maintain his speech improvement after he had received a conventional form of speech therapy.

In order to determine whether Double Tape Recorder Therapy might be an effective maintenance therapy, we offered 6 months of the therapy program to the 12 stutterers who received the conventional (Van Riper) therapy for 6 months in our research program. As previously reported, eight of these stutterers, or 67 percent, showed a reduction in the severity of their stuttering after 6 months of therapy. Application of the sign test to the data indicated the improvement observed was significant ($p = .02$). Ten of the 12 stutterers elected subsequently to receive Double Tape Recorder Therapy and were placed on a 6-month no-therapy schedule to rule out the possibility that the effects of the previous therapy would carry over to the new therapy. After that 6-month period, a speech pathologist conducted speech assessments in the same manner as in our original research program.

Application of the sign test, one-tailed, to the data indicated that the changes after 6 months without therapy were not significant and, interestingly, that the changes did not occur in any one particular direction (Table 3-3). Four of the 10 subjects showed speech improvement, four of the 10 subjects' speech increased in stuttering severity, and two of the 10 subjects remained at the same severity level. This variability in speech performance seems to indicate that some stutterers may need adjunctive or maintenance therapy following 6 months of conventional therapy in order to maintain speech improvement.

Ten stutterers were available to receive Double Tape Recorder Therapy after 6 months of no therapy. Of the 10 stutterers receiving this adjunct therapy, we have data on eight of them after 3 months of therapy and on eight after 6 months of therapy. Significant improvement is seen at both points in therapy. Application of the sign test, one-tailed, to the

Table 3-3. Serial Severity Ratings of Spoken Samples
(TAT Task) in the Conventional Therapy Group and
After 6 Months of an Adjunct (Double Tape Recorder) Therapy

Subjects	Conventional Therapy Group[a]			Adjunct Therapy Group (Double Tape Recorder)[b]		
	Initial Assessment	3 Months	6 Months	Initial Assessment	3 Months	6 Months
1	5	5	4	4	3	4
2	7	7	6	7	4	4
3	5	4	3	2	2	1
4	3	3	3	4	—	3
5	5	5	3	4	4	3
6	6	6	5	—	—	—
7	4	4	4	4	3	3
8	4	4	3	5	4	3
9	4	4	4	3	—	—
10	6	5	5	—	—	—
11	5	4	4	3	2	1
12	5	6	6	5	1	—
$\overline{X}$[c]	4.92	4.75	4.17	4.10	2.87	2.75

[a]$N = 12$.
[b]$\underline{N} = 8$.
[c]$\overline{X}$ = weighted mean.

data indicates that the speech improvement is significant at both 3
months ($p = .016$) and at 6 months ($p = .008$), which indicates that
Double Tape Recorder Therapy in conjunction with a conventional form
of stuttering modification therapy is effective in further reducing stuttering severity (Peins, McGough, and Lee, 1973).

FOLLOW-UP INVESTIGATIONS
Reports of successful short-term therapy methods often meet with skepticism. Thus, we initiated a long-term follow-up investigation of the 31
subjects who had received Double Tape Recorder Therapy either as the
sole treatment or as an adjunct therapy. We wanted to determine whether
speech improvement attained by subjects who received our therapy for
6 months was maintained over a long period of time without further
therapy, or whether a relapse in speaking performance occurred following
termination of Double Tape Recorder Therapy.

We sent written inquiries to all who had received the Double Tape Recorder Therapy, but as is true in most longitudinal studies, we lost contact
with some subjects. Of the 31 subjects who had received Double Tape
Recorder Therapy, 6 subjects never returned for the first follow-up evaluation after completion of the program. Some subjects moved away, and
others did not respond to our request although some continued to write

reports on their speech improvement. Twenty-three subjects were seen 6 months after completion of the therapy program; twelve subjects were seen at 1 year; nine were seen at 1½ years; six were seen 2 years later; and seven were seen 2½ years after therapy.

At each interval a speech pathologist measured speech progress by readministering the entire assessment battery explained earlier in this section. Severity ratings were determined by using 1-minute tape-recorded speech and oral reading samples. To guard against researcher bias, the speech pathologist who conducted the speech assessments did not administer therapy to any of the subjects.

Results

Table 3-4 presents the serial severity ratings of spoken samples (TAT Task) for 31 stutterers seen for evaluations after Double Tape Recorder Therapy.

Table 3-5 presents the statistical data on the overall speech improvement (reduction in stuttering severity) for subjects who received follow-up evaluations after Double Tape Recorder Therapy. Twenty-three subjects were available for follow-up evaluations after they had last received Double Tape Recorder Therapy. Twenty-two subjects had maintained or increased speech improvement from their pretreatment severity level with an average improvement of 1.7 of an interval on the stuttering severity scale. This finding is significant (non-parametric sign test, one-tailed) (p = .001).

Twelve stutterers were seen 1 year after receiving Double Tape Recorder Therapy with an average improvement of 1.2 of an interval on the stuttering severity scale. Nine subjects maintained or showed increased improvement from their pretreatment severity level. This finding is significant (sign test, one-tailed, p = .01).

One and one-half years later, nine subjects were evaluated, showing an average improvement of 2.3 of an interval on the stuttering severity scale. All nine subjects had maintained or increased in speech improvement from their pretreatment severity level. This finding is significant (sign test, one-tailed, p = .002).

Two years after having received Double Tape Recorder Therapy, six subjects were seen for evaluation, and showed an average improvement of 2.2 of an interval on the stuttering severity scale. All six subjects had maintained or increased in speech improvement from their pretreatment severity level (sign test, one-tailed, p = .016).

Two and one-half years after receiving Double Tape Recorder Therapy, seven subjects showed an average speech improvement of 2.1 of an interval on the stuttering severity scale; and of these seven subjects, all but one had maintained or shown an increase in speech improvement from the original severity rating (sign test, one-tailed, p = .016).

Statistical analysis of the data on the mean change in stuttering severity for 18 stutterers evaluated 1½ years to two and a half years after Double Tape Recorder Therapy indicates that their average speech improvement

Table 3-4. Serial Severity Ratings of Spoken Samples (TAT Task) at Follow-up Evaluations After Double Tape Recorder Therapy

Subjects	Initial Assessment	After DTR Therapy	Months After Double Tape Recorder Therapy				
			6	12	18	24	30
1	7	5	5	4			
2	6	5	3	4	3		4
3	7	5	6				3
4	3	2	1	5	1		1
5	7	6	6				
6	6	3			4		4
7	4	3	1	2	1		1
8	6	5	5	6			6
9	3	4	3	3			1
10	4	4	3				
11	2	1	1		1		
12	4	3	3		1		
13	4	3	2		1		
14	4	3	2		2		
15	5	3	3				
16	3	1			1		
17	6	6	5	5		5	
18	6	4	4	5		5	
19	4	2	2				
20	4	3	2	2		2	
21	6	6	4				
22	6	5	4	5		4	
23	6	6	4				
24	6	6	4	5		2	
25	5	2	3	2		2	
26	5	4					
27	3	2					
28	6	5					
29	4	5					
30	3	1					
31	7	4					

was 2.2 of an interval on the stuttering severity scale for which the finding is significant (sign test, one-tailed, p = .001).

In summary, statistical analyses (see Table 3-5) of our follow-up data indicate that speech improvement achieved as a result of Double Tape Recorder Therapy was maintained up to 2½ years without further formal therapy (Peins, McGough and Lee, 1974).

In addition to analyzing speech improvement, we were curious about whether our subjects continued to practice and apply the ideas inculcated in the therapy program. So, in our follow-up procedures we asked a number of questions at the 2½-year evaluation stage, such as, "Did Double

Table 3-5. Reduction in Stuttering Severity for
Subjects Evaluated after Double Tape Recorder Therapy

Length of Time After Double Tape Recorder Therapy	Number of Subjects	Mean Change in Stuttering Severity	p*
6 months	23	1.7	.001
1 year	12	1.2	.01
1½ years	9	2.3	.002
2 years	6	2.2	.016
2½ years	7	2.1	.016

*Sign test, one-tailed.

Tape Recorder Therapy help you to improve your speech?" "Do you continue to practice daily with or without a tape recorder?" "Do you continue to use legato speech?" We sent written inquiries to all who had received Double Tape Recorder Therapy.

Twenty clients who returned and received follow-up evaluations responded to our inquiry. The clients reported that they no longer avoided speaking and reading situations, that they were enjoying speaking situations more, and that they felt more confident in communicative situations.

Eleven clients wrote that they did continue to practice at home by speaking into a tape recorder. Some wrote that they mentally referred to the principles taught in the therapy program: using legato speech, speaking more slowly, and self-monitoring. The clients' posttherapy regimes ranged from the daily half-hour practice sessions reported by one subject to "a few times a month" as reported by another subject. Other clients claimed that they did not practice formally, but rather, "practiced as they spoke" by speaking more slowly and fluently. Two subjects reported that they never practiced. Twelve subjects did not write comments about their practice regime, but their continued maintenance or improvement in speech after termination of therapy suggests that they did practice principles of Double Tape Recorder Therapy. However, we should not discount factors such as subjects' motivation, their desire to continue to self-improve, or the follow-up study itself which may have contributed to our subjects' continuing speech improvement over the 2½-year period.

Three of the subjects who did not return after the 6-month evaluation did reply at the time of the 2½-year evaluation stage, and all three reported their speech improved as a result of Double Tape Recorder Therapy. One client wrote, "My speech has improved so much that I am no longer worried about speaking anywhere or anytime." Another client wrote, "I am less self-conscious, more confident in my personal relationships with others. I still use legato speech when I think I will have trouble speaking."

Unfortunately, these subjective, personal speech assessments could not be confirmed with an objective evaluation since these clients had not returned for the 2½-year evaluation.

Reasons for Therapeutic Effectiveness

We cannot point with certainty to any single feature that contributes to the effectiveness of Double Tape Recorder Therapy. Instead, the therapeutic effects are probably based on a combination of factors. These include emphasis on slower rate of utterance, control of vocalization, improvement in self-monitoring ability, and daily practice using the tape recorder (Peins, McGough, and Lee, 1972a; McGough, Peins, and Lee, 1971).

SLOWER RATE

The use of techniques such as modeling the slow speech rate of the instructor's voice on the taped lessons and directives to establish a volitional, slower, controlled rate of utterance when speaking and reading aloud is one factor that may have contributed to the reduction in stuttering severity in our clients.

Work by other investigators in the field seems to support this conclusion. In his discussion of conditions that ameliorate stuttering, Wingate (1976) called attention to the slowing down of speech as a beneficial therapy method. If, as Van Riper asserts, stuttering may be a disorder of disrupted timing (1982), then slower speech might aid stutterers to use their speech muscles or speech mechanism in a more coordinated manner and thus synchronize their speech movements, that is, their timing for speech, so that more fluent speech would be the end result.

CONTROL OF VOCALIZATION

Double Tape Recorder Therapy emphasizes control of vocalization through modulation and modification of phonatory patterns, major factors that may contribute to the improved fluency noted in our clients. Our method stresses use of legato speech for which the stutterer learns to initiate every utterance with an easy onset of air flow or with glottal vibration a slight fraction of a second before articulating any phoneme. The stutterer learns to speak in unbroken, connected, expressive utterances in order to achieve continuity of vocalization and more fluent speech; and he reinforces this continuity of vocalization through daily practice.

Several other investigators have identified control of vocalization as an important contributor to fluent speech. Wingate (1969) was the first to point to the importance of control and continuity of vocalization and fluency in stutterers. Adams (1972) reported that the success of many contemporary stuttering therapy programs might be attributed to the fact that they include steps that help the stutterer adjust his respiratory and laryngeal activities so that air flow and glottal vibration can be readily started and sustained. Freeman (1982) wrote that a number of treatment programs (Wingate, 1976; Weiner, 1978) emphasize modifying phonatory components in stuttered speech and remarks that she has used this approach effectively with stutterers.

IMPROVEMENT IN SELF-MONITORING ABILITY
Because of the possible link between stuttering and a disturbed feedback or monitoring system, we believe it is important for the stutterer to improve his proprioceptive and auditory awareness whenever reading aloud or speaking. Van Riper (1973), too, writes about the importance of increasing the stutterer's proprioceptive awareness of his speech. If we assume that speech production involves a closed feedback system, that is, if a speaker can monitor his own speech production (Cherry and Sayers, 1956; Lee, 1950a, 1950b, 1951; Mysak, 1966; Peins, Lee, McGough, 1970; Van Riper, 1982), then another factor that may contribute to our clients' speech improvement is increasing auditory and proprioceptive awareness or self-monitoring ability.

Early in the therapy program the terms *proprioceptive* and *auditory feedback* are explained to the client. Then the taped lessons lead the stutterer through exercises to make him more proprioceptively aware of what is involved in speaking fluently. We ask the client to concentrate on the "feel of fluency" in order to enhance this awareness and strengthen feedback. We also encourage the stutterer to really listen to his speech when practicing and when conversing with others in order to increase his auditory awareness. It may well be that the daily use of legato speech and the utilization of tape recorders aid the stutterer to concentrate upon his feedback systems and thus in time improve his speaking ability.

DAILY PRACTICE USING TAPE RECORDERS
A fourth factor that may contribute to the reduction of stuttering severity in our clients is daily practice of reading and speaking tasks using the tape recorder.

Speech is a skill which, like other motor skills, should be practiced with consistency for greatest effectiveness. The daily use of tape recorders when practicing reading and speech exercises may expedite speech improvement for stutterers by reinforcing and stabilizing the newly-acquired slower, more fluent speech, as well as assisting the stutterer to improve his self-monitoring ability.

Although several investigators recently have incorporated tape recorders into therapy programs for voice, articulation, and language disorders, as well as for stuttering, our study was the first to cite the effectiveness of tape recorders as a delivery system for stuttering therapy.

At the present time, we do not know which of these four factors—establishing a slower rate of utterance, control of vocalization, improvement in self-monitoring ability, or daily practice using the tape recorder—plays a more dominant role in the attainment of speech improvement in our clients. Possibly the interplay among these contributes to the speech improvement achieved by the stutterers who receive Double Tape Recorder Therapy.

Advantages of the Therapy

Double Tape Recorder Therapy offers definite advantages for both the speech clinician working with stutterers and for the stutterer: economy and convenience; improvement with mild, moderate, and severe stutterers; effectiveness as an independent therapy or as an adjunct therapy; and maintenance of speech improvement.

ECONOMY AND CONVENIENCE
Double Tape Recorder Therapy is time-efficient. The client attends therapy sessions administered by a speech clinician once every 2 weeks for one-half hour, reducing the number of therapy sessions for the stutterer and permitting the clinician to schedule additional clients who otherwise might remain on waiting lists for therapy.

Double Tape Recorder Therapy is also cost-efficient. The stutterer attends therapy every other week which reduces the number of therapy sessions and results in a reduction in the cost of therapy for the stutterer.

With the increased emphasis today on accountability in many school and clinic programs, the application of Double Tape Recorder Therapy can be justified in terms of its efficient and economical results which show a high number of clients treated in low number of therapy sessions and presenting a high rate of speech improvement. Moreover, the therapy does not require as much time, preparation, effort, or client contact from the clinician in order to obtain measurable results.

Another advantage is the convenience of Double Tape Recorder Therapy which allows clients to work at home daily with the taped lessons and make biweekly visits to the speech clinician. This greater convenience tends to motivate the clients and leads to a positive attitude toward therapy.

IMPROVEMENT WITH MILD, MODERATE, AND SEVERE STUTTERERS
In our therapy experiences and in our research with stutterers, we have found that speech improvement occurs within the first 3 months of therapy and continues even after termination of therapy. This rapid rate of improvement serves to increase the client's motivation toward redoubled practice efforts and serves as an incentive to transfer the improved speech pattern into real-life communicative situations.

Moreover, based on our research program and our clinical therapy experiences, we have concluded that Double Tape Recorder Therapy is effective and efficient in reducing mild, moderate, and severe degrees of stuttering severity. This is in contrast to some therapies which are more effective with severe stutterers than with less severe stutterers.

INDEPENDENT OR ADJUNCT THERAPY

Our research findings indicate that Double Tape Recorder Therapy is effective as the only method of treatment or as an adjunct or auxiliary therapy to conventional forms of stuttering therapy. It can also be used effectively as a maintenance therapy.

MAINTENANCE OF SPEECH IMPROVEMENT

Our research findings indicate that speech improvement attained by clients who received Double Tape Recorder Therapy can be maintained over a long period of time. Although our follow-up studies have been limited to 2½ years, the high maintenance rate at that point suggests that it has an enduring effect.

CONCLUSIONS

We view Double Tape Recorder Therapy as a promising therapeutic alternative to conventional methods for speech clinicians who want to provide therapy to stutterers, but do not have time in their schedules to work individually with them. However, we wish to emphasize that our method is not rigidly programmed. There is more to the therapy than dispensing a taped lesson every 2 weeks to evoke a change in speech behavior, for a dialogue, arising from a dynamic client-clinician relationship, must exist for the client to attain speech progress.

The clinician must have the ability to motivate the client to maintain a consistent daily practice schedule and to transfer his fluent speech into all communicative situations, to encourage the client to self-monitor his speech so that he can recognize his speech improvement as well as his speech regressions, and to guide the client in setting attainable speech goals. This requires a clinician who not only has patience, flexibility, and understanding of stuttering and of client needs but can inspire clients to reach desired goals. Although the therapy requires the same hard work and motivation from the stutterer as other therapy methods, the client can observe tangible changes more rapidly while working continually on his speech at home with fewer clinical visits.

Based on our research and on our clinical experience in working with stutterers for more than 20 years, we know that Double Tape Recorder Therapy is an effective method of inducing speech improvement in stutterers.

References

Adams, M. R. Fluency, nonfluency, and stuttering in children. *J. Fluency Disord.* 7: 171–185, 1982.

Adams, M. R. Some motor determinates of fluency and stuttering. Paper presented at the annual convention of the American Speech-Language and Hearing Association, San Francisco, 1972.

Cherry, C., and Sayers, B. McA. Experiments upon the total inhibition of stammering by external control and some clinical results. *J. Psychosom. Res.* 1:233–246, 1956.

Darley, F. L., and Spriestersbach, D. C. *Diagnostic Methods in Speech Pathology.* New York: Harper & Row, 1978.

Fairbanks, G. *Voice and Articulation Drillbook.* New York: Harper & Row, 1940.

Freeman, F. J. Stuttering. In N. J. Lass, et al. (eds.), *Speech, Language and Hearing,* Vol. 2. *Pathologies of Speech and Language.* Philadelphia: Saunders, 1982. Pp. 673–691.

Guitar, B., and Peters, T. J. *Stuttering: An Integration of Contemporary Therapies.* Memphis: Speech Foundation of America, 1980.

Lee, B. S. Effects of delayed speech feedback. *J. Acoust. Soc. Am.* 22:824-826, 1950a.

Lee, B. S. Some effects of sidetone delay. *J. Acoust. Soc. Am.* 22:639–640, 1950b.

Lee, B. S. Artificial stutter. *J. Speech Hear. Disord.* 16:53–55, 1951.

Lee, B. S., McGough, W. E., and Peins, M. A new method for stutter therapy. *Folia Phoniatr.* 25:186–195, 1973.

Lee, B. S., McGough, W. E., and Peins, M. Automated desensitization of stutterers to use of the telephone. *Behav. Ther.* 7:110–112, 1976.

McGough, W. E., Peins, M., and Lee, B. S. A home-based tape recorder approach to rehabilitating the stutterer: Evaluation of an economic treatment. Final report, Research and Demonstration Project 2932-S. New Brunswick, N.J.: Rutgers Medical School, Department of Psychology, 1971.

Murray, H. A. *Thematic Apperception Test.* Cambridge: Harvard University Press, 1943.

Mysak, E. D. *Speech Pathology and Feedback Theory.* Springfield, Ill.: Thomas, 1966.

Peins, M. Innovative therapy methods and accountability. *J. Speech Hear. Assoc. N.J.* 4:7–11, 1973.

Peins, M., Lee, B. S., and McGough, W. E. A tape recorded therapy method for stutterers: A case report. *J. Speech Hear. Disord.* 35: 188–193, 1970.

Peins, M., McGough, W. E., and Lee, B. S. The evaluation of a home-based method of stuttering therapy using tape recorders. Paper presented at the annual convention of the American Speech-Language and Hearing Association, New York, 1970.

Peins, M., McGough, W. E., and Lee, B. S. Tape recorder therapy for the rehabilitation of the stuttering handicapped. *N.J. Speech Hear. Assoc. J.* 9:2–4; 22, 1971a.

Peins, M., McGough, W. E., and Lee, B. S. Effects of therapies on stuttering and attitude. Paper presented at the annual convention of the American Speech-Language and Hearing Association, Chicago, 1971b.

Peins, M., McGough, W. E., and Lee, B. S. Evaluation of a tape-recorded method of stuttering therapy: Improvement in a speaking task. *J. Speech Hear. Res.* 15:364–371, 1972a.

Peins, M., McGough, W. E. and Lee, B. S. Tape recorder therapy for the rehabilitation of the stuttering handicapped. *Lang. Speech Hear. Serv. Schs.* 6:30–35, 1972b.

Peins, M., McGough, W. E., and Lee, B. S. Tape recorder therapy as an adjunct to standard therapy for stutterers. Paper presented at the annual convention of the American Speech-Language and Hearing Association, Detroit, 1973.

Peins, M., McGough, W. E., and Lee, B. S. Long term follow-up of stutterers after tape recorder therapy. Paper presented at the annual convention of the American Speech-Language and Hearing Association, Las Vegas, 1974.

Ryan, B. An Illustration of Operant Conditioning Therapy for Stuttering. In *Conditioning in Stuttering Therapy*. Memphis: Speech Foundation of America, 1970.

Shearer, W. M., and Williams, J. D. Self-recovery from stuttering. *J. Speech Hear. Res.* 30:288–290, 1965.

Sheehan, J. G., and Martyn, M. Spontaneous recovery from stuttering. *J. Speech Hear. Res.* 9:121–135, 1966.

Siegel, S. *Nonparametric Statistics*. New York: McGraw-Hill, 1956.

Van Riper, C. *Speech Correction: Principles and Methods* (4th ed.). Englewood Cliffs, N.J.: Prentice-Hall, 1963.

Van Riper, C. *The Nature of Stuttering*. Englewood Cliffs, N.J.: Prentice-Hall, 1982.

Van Riper, C. *The Treatment of Stuttering*. Englewood Cliffs, N.J.: Prentice-Hall, 1973.

Weiner, A. E. Vocal control therapy for stutterers: A trial program. *J. Fluency Disord.* 3:115–126, 1978.

Williams, D., Silverman, E., and Kools, J. Disfluency behavior of elementary school stutterers and nonstutterers: The adaptation effect. *J. Speech Hear. Res.* 11: 622–630, 1968.

Wingate, M. E. Recovery from stuttering. *J. Speech Hear. Disord.* 29: 312–321, 1964.

Wingate, M. E. Sound and pattern in "artificial fluency." *J. Speech Hear. Res.* 12: 677–686, 1969.

Wingate, M. E. The fear of stuttering. *ASHA* 13: 3–5, 1971.

Wingate, M. E. *Stuttering: Theory and Treatment*. New York: Halsted Press, 1976.

Appendix 3-A. Assessment Materials

Rutgers Interview Form for Stutterers (RIFFS)
Maryann Peins, Ph.D.

Instructions to the Clinician
This interview form is part of the assessment battery for stutterers. The speech clinician administers this interview form orally to the stutterer during the intake interview and before the client's assignment to therapy. You may add questions as warranted to obtain additional information. Please read aloud the *Instructions to the Client* before asking any of the questions.

Instructions to the Client
"I am going to ask you some questions which will help me to understand your speech problem. The information you give me will be kept completely confidential. What you discuss with me today and in the future will not be told to your family, to your employer, to your teachers, or to school officials."

Copyright 1968 by Maryann Peins, Ph.D.

Name _____ Age _____ Birth date _____
Interviewer _____ Date _____

History of Problem
1. When were you first aware that you had a speech problem or difficulty speaking? _____
2. Were you ever told that as a young child you had difficulty learning to talk? _____
3. When you were a child did you talk a great deal _____
   Very little _____ Average amount _____?
4. At what age did you begin to "stutter" (3–5, 5–7, 7–10, 11–14, 15–17, 18 and over? _____.
5. Who first noticed your stuttering or told you that you were "stuttering"? Self _____ Speech Therapist _____ Relative _____
   Father _____ Mother _____ Teacher _____ Friend _____
   Other _____.
6. Did you know you were "stuttering" or having speech difficulty when the "stuttering"was called to your attention? Yes _____ No _____
7. How did you react when you were told you were stuttering? Were you surprised _____ Shocked _____ Scared _____ Puzzled _____
   Knew you were stuttering before being told _____ Other _____.
8. Did your parents correct your speech when you stuttered? Yes _____
   No _____ Sometimes _____ All the time _____.

9. How did they try to correct your speech? By criticizing _____
   Tell you to slow down _____ Taking a deep breath _____
   Thinking before you speak _____ Relax _____
   Take it easy _____.
10. Do you think this was helpful? Yes _____ No _____.
11. Do you recall receiving any penalties for the way you talked at home,
    for example: Punishment _____ Ridicule _____ Annoyance
    from parents _____ Laughter _____ Anger _____
    Criticism _____ Other _____.
12. When you were growing up, were there any important incidents or
    events that were related to your speech problem or seemed to affect it—
    to make it *better* or *worse* (an accident, illness, death in family, parents
    divorced, a new job, moving to another town, new school, receiving
    speech therapy, etc.)? _____
    _____
    _____
13. What do you think caused your stuttering? Nervousness _____
    Home atmosphere _____ Thinking too fast _____ Lack of
    confidence _____ Labeling _____ Physical _____
    Emotional _____ Mental _____ Illness _____ Shock _____
    Fright _____ Don't know _____ Talking too fast _____
    Getting excited _____ Other _____.

Family Background
14. What is your father's present occupation? _____.
15. What is your mother's present occupation? _____.
16. Educational background of father? Grade school _____
    Jr. H.S. _____ H.S. _____ College _____.
17. Educational background of mother? Grade school _____
    Jr. H.S. _____ H.S. _____ College _____.
18. Do you have any sisters (list ages)? _____
    Any brothers (list ages)? _____
19. Are there other stutterers in your family? Father _____
    Mother _____ Sister _____ Brother _____
    Grandmother _____ Grandfather _____ Uncle _____
    Aunt _____ More than one _____ None _____.
20. Which is your preferred hand? Right _____ Left _____
    Ambidextrous _____ Changed _____ Do you write with the
    right _____ Left _____ Do other tasks with the right _____
    Left _____ Both _____.
21. Are there left-handed persons in your family? Father _____
    Mother _____ Sister _____ Brother _____
    Grandmother _____ Grandfather _____ Uncle _____
    Aunt _____ More than one _____ Other _____
    No one in family _____.

Previous Therapy

22. Have you received any formal speech therapy? _____ Age you started therapy _____.

23. Length of time you have received speech therapy? _____

24. Where did you receive speech therapy? _____

25. Did the therapy help you? Yes _____ No _____. In what specific ways did the therapy help you? _____

26. How much has your speech improved through the years? Very little _____ A great deal _____ Became worse _____ Remained the same _____.

27. At what age did your speech improve the most (3–5, 5–7, 7–10, 11–14, 15–18, 18–23, 23–26, 27 or over)? _____.

28. What do you think brought about this speech improvement? Relaxing _____ Slowing down _____ Talking more _____ Thinking before speaking _____ Speech therapy _____ Don't know _____ Other _____.

29. Was this speech improvement sudden _____ Gradual _____ No speech improvement _____.

30. Have you received any other type of therapy (psychotherapy, counseling, medical treatment for stuttering, hypnosis, etc.)? _____ Was the treatment helpful? In what way? _____

The Problem Now

31. How would you rate your stuttering? Severe _____ Moderate _____ Mild _____ Don't know _____.

32. Is your stuttering *much worse* at some times than others? Yes _____ No _____.

33. Are there any times or situations in which you *do not* stutter at all? _____

34. At what times or in what situations do you stutter *very little*? _____

35. Do you have particular *difficulty* speaking in certain *situations* or *places* (school, home, certain classes, in store, on telephone, at work, etc.)? Tell me about them. _____

36. Do you tend to *avoid* certain *speaking situations* because of your stuttering? Yes _____ No _____ Sometimes _____ Tell me about them. _____

37. Do you have any particular difficulty saying certain *sounds* or *words*? Which? _____

38. Do you have particular difficulty talking to certain *people?* Who (mother, father, teachers, boss, etc.)? _____
_____

39. Is your speech better or worse when speaking with your mother _____ With your father _____ With your brothers _____ With your sisters _____.

40. Does your stuttering increase or decrease in severity:
    a. At home _____
    b. In school _____
    c. With strangers _____
    d. On the telephone _____
    e. In social situations _____
    f. Speaking or answering questions in the classroom _____
    g. At your place of employment _____

41. Does your stuttering become more severe or less severe when you are:
    a. Very happy or pleased _____
    b. Tired _____
    c. Nervous _____
    d. Angry _____
    e. Talking to good friends _____
    f. Talking before a group _____
    g. Talking to teachers _____
    h. Talking to parents _____

42. Do you stutter when reading aloud? Yes _____ No _____
    Sometimes _____.

43. Are you able to predict the words on which you will stutter in a reading passage if you were going to read the selection aloud? Yes _____
    No _____ Sometimes _____.

44. Has your stuttering had any bad effect on:
    a. Your job?   Yes _____ No _____
    b. Your school work?   Yes _____ No _____
    c. Getting along with people?   Yes _____ No _____
    d. Making friends?   Yes _____ No _____
    e. In other ways?   Yes _____ No _____
       Which? _____

45. Does your stuttering keep you from doing your school work or job well?
    Yes _____ No _____ Tell me about this. _____
    _____
    _____

46. How do your friends react to your stuttering? (Do they ignore it, show embarrassment, laugh, give advice, etc?) _____
    _____

47. Were you ever ridiculed, teased, or punished for your stuttering at school, at work, at home, or with friends? Yes _____ No _____. If yes, by whom and in what situation? _____

_____

48. What were your reactions at these times? How did you *really* feel inside? _____

_____

49. What do you do when someone tries to help you with a word or when somebody turns away when you speak to them? _____

_____

50. Do you do anything to "get your speech going" such as trying to control your breath, moving your head, tapping your foot, saying "uh," etc. Tell me what you do. _____

_____

51. Can you give me some idea about the way you feel about your stuttering? Have you learned to live with it? Do you fear it, hate it, or just suffer? How do you *really* feel about your stuttering? _____

_____

52. Can you think of anything else that is important or significant about your speech or yourself that I ought to know to better understand your speech problem? _____

_____

_____

53. Do you *really want* to receive speech therapy at the present time? Yes _____ No _____ Not sure. _____.

Checklist of Physical Behaviors Accompanying Stuttering

Name _____ Age _____ Birth date _____

Clinician _____ Today's date _____ Evaluation number _____

Area	Behaviors	Check	Comments
Head	Bending head backwards		
	Turning head sideways		
	Nodding: moving head downward		
	Bobbing head: short, jerking motion		
	Furrowing forehead		
Eyes	Blinking eyes		
	Poor eye contact		
	Closing eyes		
	Squinting eyes		
	Enlarging eyes		
	Raising eyebrows		
	Frowning		
Nose	Nasal movements		
	Dilating nostrils		
	Sniffing		
Mouth	Lip tremors		
	Pressing lips together		
	Pursing lips		

Mouth, cont'd	Opening mouth inappropriately		
	Facial grimaces		
	Protruding tongue		
	Hard articulatory contacts		
	Pressing tongue against palate		
	Pressing tongue against or between teeth		
	Preformation of syllables or words		
	Jaw tremors		
	Jaw tension		
	Neck tension		
Vocal or Laryngeal	Clearing throat		
	Vocal tremor		
	Laryngeal spasms		
	Inappropriate pitch pattern		
	Inappropriate intonation pattern		
	Inappropriate loudness level		
Chest and Breathing	Holding breath		
	Inhaling irregularly		
	Exhaling irregularly		
	Gasping		

Chest and Breathing, cont'd	Speaking on exhausted breath		
	Noisy breathing		
	Lifting shoulders		
	Coughing		
	Sighing		
Arms and Hands	Moving arms		
	Moving hands or fingers		
	Clenching fists		
	Cracking knuckles		
	Tapping fingers		
Legs and Feet	Moving legs or feet		
	Tapping foot		
	Stomping foot		
Body	Body tremors		
	Moving body		
	Fidgeting		
	Body tension		
	Inappropriate posture(s)		

Other	Inappropriate rate: too rapid, too slow		

4. A Component Model for Treating Stuttering in Children

Glyndon D. Riley
Jeanna Riley

Overview

This chapter describes a method for differentially diagnosing and treating a child who stutters, based on the components that contribute to the child's fluency breakdown. The neurologic components that predispose a child to stuttering are defined along with the attitudinal and environmental conditions that place pressure on the marginal system. Treatment focuses on the components first, and then attends to any remaining abnormal disfluencies directly. Of 37 children treated and monitored for 2 years or more following treatment, 30 successfully maintained their normal speech.

History of the Therapy

"Children say the darndest things," and when we listen to them we usually learn a thing or two. Our approach was developed during the last 15 years from things taught us by children who stutter. We have learned that treatment of stuttering is not fundamentally different from treatment of other speech and language disorders; we diagnose and treat every possible aspect of the child's problem. We have learned (from these children) that a multidimensional approach is needed to accommodate the variety of problems that seem to constitute the syndrome of stuttering.

Others have come to the conclusion that stuttering is not a homogeneous disorder. Gavin Andrews (1981) reviewed the "state of the art" in stuttering and concluded that his would be the last state of the art summary because the future title should be "state of the arts, plural." Martin Adams (1982) came to the same conclusion in his address to the Second Annual Multi-Disciplinary Conference on Stuttering. He said:

For years, we have given shelter to the notion that stutterers are a homogeneous population, especially relative to causation. We have harbored this view in spite of the fact that the results of over 40 years of laboratory investigations show us clearly that stutterers are characterized more by their differences than their similarities. If we are to be guided by what our own research findings tell us, then we should be moving in the direction of probing for and examining stutterers' heterogeneity and the sources of it.

Operating from this context experimentally and clinically is not easy. Simple research paradigms must give way to multifaceted approaches. Clinically, differential diagnostic methods and remedial programs tailored to fit disparate diagnostic patterns may be needed (p. 183).

Others have reviewed the literature and reached similar conclusions (Beech and Fransella, 1968; Canter, 1971; Williams, 1978; Van Riper, 1982; Blaesing, 1982).

This multivariant line of thinking led us to predict the existence of subgroups, and we searched for them earnestly. We interpreted our first factor study, based on 100 children, as "promising" in its ability to define subgroups (Riley and Riley, 1972). After further definition and revision, we did a second analysis but the hoped for subgroups did not materialize (Riley and Riley, 1980). Four strong factors did emerge, however, and these were remarkably similar to factors reported by Andrews and Harris (1964). Our strongest factor was related to language dysfunctions, the second was related to oral motor discoordination, and the other two were related to auditory processing deficits. Andrews and Harris identified factors that implicated motor and language differences in stutterers. They concluded, as we did, that factor analysis does not lead to subgroups. Several other attempts to establish subgroups have been inconclusive as well (Berlin, 1954; Graham and Bramlick, 1961; Preus, 1981).

As an alternative to subgroups, we proposed a component model for diagnosing and treating children who stutter (Riley and Riley, 1979). This model allowed us to take a multivariant approach without categorizing each child according to a single factor.

The components that were traditionally related to stuttering were organized according to intrapersonal (within the child) and interpersonal (in the child's environment). At the intrapersonal level, high self-expectations were noted in 89 percent of the 54 children surveyed and manipulative stuttering in 25 percent. At the interpersonal level, the communicative environment was disruptive in 53 percent of the families. There were unrealistic parental expectations in 51 percent and an abnormal need for the child to stutter in 5 percent of the cases.

The model also shows four components which we regarded as neurologic, that is, the children have some neurologic dysfunction or difference that predisposes them to develop stuttering. Reference to Figure 4-1 shows that 69 percent of the children had oral motor discoordination (33 percent also had significant dysarticulation for their ages), 36 percent had attending problems, 27 percent had auditory processing problems, and 31 percent had sentence formulation problems.

This constitutional predisposition theory is consistent with recent genetic models (Andrews and Harris, 1964; Kidd, Kidd, and Records, 1978; Kidd, Heimbuch, and Records, 1981), and with twin studies (Howie, 1980; Van Riper, 1982). These neurologic dysfunctions are usually not severe enough to be of interest to a physician. The typical manifestations are subtle and show up only during complex functions such as language reception and production. Because they are subtle, careful observation is required to evaluate them.

Recently we surveyed 54 children enrolled in treatment at our private

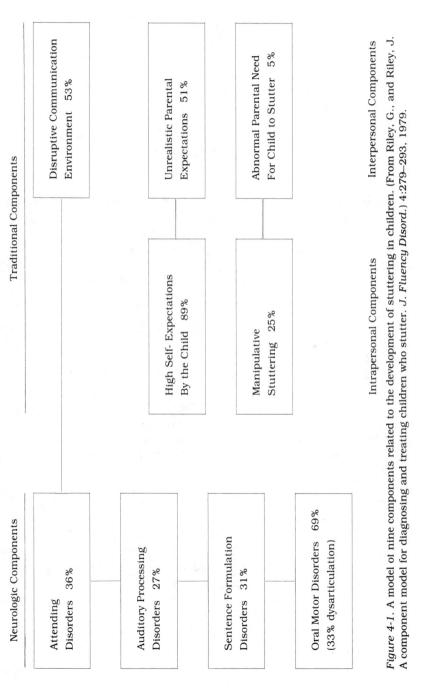

Neurologic Components

Traditional Components

Attending
Disorders 36%

Auditory Processing
Disorders 27%

Sentence Formulation
Disorders 31%

Oral Motor Disorders 69%
(33% dysarticulation)

Disruptive Communication
Environment 53%

High Self- Expectations
By the Child 89%

Unrealistic Parental
Expectations 51%

Manipulative
Stuttering 25%

Abnormal Parental Need
For Child to Stutter 5%

Intrapersonal Components   Interpersonal Components

Figure 4-1. A model of nine components related to the development of stuttering in children. (From Riley, G., and Riley, J. A component model for diagnosing and treating children who stutter. *J. Fluency Disord.*) 4:279–293, 1979.

practice. This group includes some children from the sample on which the component model was based. It is not a random sample because we have a higher than average number of clients whose stuttering is complex or severe or children who have failed to improve with traditional treatment. We were conservative in diagnosing the neurologic components; a rating scale of 0–4 was used (0 = not present; 1 = possibly present; 2 = definitely present to a mild degree; 3 = present to a moderate degree; 4 = present to a severe or profound degree). Only ratings of 3 or 4 were counted, and a child with these ratings was considered in need of treatment for the component identified. Given these criteria, 4 children (7.4%) had problems with all four neurologic components, 5 children (9.3%) had problems with three components, 23 children (42.6%) had problems with two components, 21 children (38.8%) had problems with one component (usually oral motor discoordination) and one child (1.9%) had no problem with any neurologic component.

With the component model in mind, we can look again at its relation to recent genetic models. The studies of Kenneth Kidd and his colleagues indicate that some children inherit a trait or traits that result in a reduced neurologic threshold which predisposes them to stutter. Boys with this genetic predisposition have a lower threshold than girls, which accounts for the fact that so many more boys stutter than girls. Kidd considers his findings compatible with a multi-dimensional model of stuttering development.

We have used the concept of a threshold of fluency breakdown to explain the operation of the components. A problem with this model is that many children have some combination of the components but do not stutter. It may be that more careful analysis of the psychological and environmental stressors will reveal some combination that reliably predicts stuttering in children with reduced neurologic thresholds. Jeanna Riley is currently exploring this possibility in her research. Her data show that stuttering children with neurologic components have higher self-expectations than children who do not stutter but have oral motor-based dysarticulations.

Assessment Procedures

"Component treatment" requires a comprehensive assessment of stuttering and its related disorders and of the components themselves. This assessment takes 2 or 3 hours to accomplish, but the time is well spent because it is a blueprint for therapy. Consider the analogy of trying to fill a case of empty soft drink bottles. One way is to pour a bucket of water over the bottles so that some water gets into each one, although much water is spilled. A better way is to insert a funnel into each bottle, fill it completely, and spill very little. Obviously, in this analogy the funnel represents the careful assessment, and the water represents hours of treatment.

DEFINITION OF TERMS

Some terms need to be defined at this point. Since all children are disfluent, but only a few stutter, we need to define normal disfluencies before defining abnormal ones. Normal disfluencies do not call attention to themselves; they stick out like *well* thumbs, unnoticed, and include the following:

1. Whole multisyllable word repetitions
2. Repetition of phrases of two or more words
3. Rephrasing or revision of sentences
4. Interjections that are otherwise fluent
5. Pauses for linguistic purposes or communication effect

Abnormal disfluencies are defined as follows:

1. *Part-word repetitions* of a sound or syllable are abnormal. Two variables are important in evaluating the severity of repetitions: first, the number of repeated attempts prior to success in saying the target word, and second, the degree to which the repeated syllables themselves are abnormal. They may contain the schwa vowel instead of the target vowel; they may be marked by separations instead of overlapping as with normal coarticulated syllables; or they may be accompanied by tension and struggle behaviors.
2. *Prolonged vowels* are abnormal when the duration is 1.5 seconds or longer. The longer a vowel is prolonged, the greater the number of abnormal elements, such as pitch rise, vocal fry, etc., it is likely to contain.
3. *Phonatory arrests* of 0.5 second or longer are abnormal. These arrests include complete blockage or severe constriction of the glottis, resulting in silent struggle or audible, nonvowel-like phonation.
4. *Articulatory posturing* of 0.5 second or longer is abnormal. These abnormally long postures include complete blocking or severe constriction, resulting in silent struggle or prolonged consonantlike sounds. The posture may be appropriate for the target sound except for duration.

Physical concomitants are accessory behaviors that are distracting to the listener. They include nonspeech sounds, movements of the head, arms, legs, or torso, and facial grimaces. Such behaviors as sniffing, clicking sounds, looking away, clenching fists, and making faces are examples of physical concomitants.

Other accessory features include behaviors and attitudes that are important although not necessarily associated with the moment of stuttering. They are part of the overall condition in which the stuttering occurs and include

1. The child's behaviors that indicate frustration with his ineffective ability to communicate
2. Avoidance of certain sounds or words
3. Avoidance of certain speaking situations

Listener behaviors in reaction to the child's stuttering can be negative and contribute to the overall pattern of abnormality. Examples of these behaviors include interrupting, rushing, criticizing, and teasing; or a listener (usually a parent) may simply over-react to the stuttering, showing delight with fluent speech, discouragement with every instance of stuttering.

ASSESSMENT INSTRUMENTS
We use two instruments to help assess stuttering: the Stuttering Severity Instrument (SSI) (Riley, 1980) and the Stuttering Prediction Instrument (SPI) (Riley, 1981). The instruments provide a way of quantifying observations; however, a great deal of each child's behavior and attitudes cannot be quantified. Both instruments require three phases of administration.

1. *The parent interview* provides for parent input concerning (1) the onset and development of disfluencies; (2) a description of the disfluencies when most severe; (3) a comparison of the examiner's sample with the child's "average" and "most severe" disfluencies; (4) an explanation of the feelings and reactions of the parents and other household members to the disfluencies; (5) a commentary on how other children react, especially any history of teasing or mimicry; and (6) observations of the child's reactions to his or her disfluencies, including any evidence of frustration such as word avoidance, situation avoidance, or distracting physical concomitants.
2. *An extensive conversational speech sample,* recorded on tape, provides 50 to 100 utterances that we later use to assess fluency, articulation, voice, and expressive language. In addition, while making the audiotape, an experienced speech pathologist takes notes which describe the child's stuttering behaviors that are primarily visual, such as silent phonatory arrests, silent articulatory postures, physical concomitants, and noticeable muscle tension.
3. *The examiner assigns numbers* on the SSI and SPI to each item based on the tape recording and related notes.

The SSI has three categories: (1) frequency, (2) duration of the three longest blocks, and (3) physical concomitants. Frequency of stuttering events per 100 words is counted from a section of the audiotape that is representative of the conversational speech. When the child has silent blocks, such as phonatory arrest or silent articulatory postures, the examiner's notes assume importance because they include words from the sample showing where the silent blocks occurred. For example, the notation [*(3 seconds)* æpl] indicates that the child opened his mouth and tensed his speech muscles, but no sound was emitted for 3 seconds. Without the notation there is no way to distinguish this silent period from a pause when the child stops to think.

To determine frequency, we simply count the number of stuttering events per 100 words and compute the total as a percentage. The test instructions and recording form provide a method for converting this percentage to a task score. To ascertain duration, we average the three longest blocks, estimating those under 10 seconds in length and timing those that are longer. The average duration then converts into a scale score according to SSI instructions. The examiner rates the physical concomitants during the actual examination because most of them are not evident from the audiotape. Of course, a videotape is more useful, but even then movement of the feet, legs, hands, etc., may be off-camera. The "physical concomitants" section of the SSI (see Appendix 4-A) provides a rating scale which the examiner uses to quantify the distracting behaviors. There are four areas to observe: distracting noises, facial grimaces, head movements, and body and extremities movements. Each of these areas receives a rating from 0 to 5 depending on the extent of distractibility.

0 = none
1 = not noticeable unless looking for it
2 = barely noticeable to casual observer
3 = distracting
4 = very distracting
5 = severe and painful looking

The overall reliability of the SSI is acceptable with frequency being the most reliable and physical concomitants the least. Details of reliability and validity are provided in the administration manual that accompanies the test package. Normative data for children and adults are also included.

The Stuttering Prediction Instrument (SPI) has more items than the SSI and relies on the parent interview, an audiotape recording, and the examiner's notes for rating each item. The parent(s) provide information concerning (1) onset and development of disfluencies, (2) the severity of the examiner's sample as compared with the most and least severe disfluencies exhibited by the child, and (3) any family history of stuttering. This information is not scored but is obviously very useful. Other information, which the parents provide, is rated in the following areas:

1. Parent's level of *concern* about the child's disfluencies
2. Child's level of *frustration* about any inability to communicate, as indicated by questions such as "Why can't I talk right?" or behaviors such as stamping the foot in anger, giving up, or running away because he can't get the words out
3. History of *teasing* about disfluencies by playmates, siblings, or others
4. *Word avoidance* as indicated by starting to say one word then changing it to another word in an apparent attempt to avoid stuttering
5. *Situation avoidance* such as fear of talking on the telephone or refusing to participate in "show and tell"
6. The presence of *physical concomitants* with the disfluencies as described

The clinician may use any of these six areas as part of the treatment plan. Such planning requires a detailed description of the treatment areas, not just the numerical ratings, to form base-line data and facilitate writing goals and objectives. Each disfluency type described in the definition of "stuttering" is rated by the examiner using the instructions in the SPI. Frequency is simply the number of stuttering events per 100 words.

Based on the results of the fluency assessment, the child either enters a treatment program or undergoes monitoring.

FLUENCY MONITORING PROGRAM

The Fluency Monitoring Program (FMP) is designed for children whose stuttering is nonchronic. We assume that these children will outgrow their stuttering without systematic intervention, but we believe that it is not safe to turn them away. We call their parents every 6 months to monitor their stuttering and related behaviors.

Based on a review of 95 children whom we considered to be chronic stutterers and 20 children who were considered nonchronic, we identified seven criteria which proved useful in placing a child in the FMP.

1. The child's disfluencies are free from phonatory arrests.
2. The child's disfluencies are free from articulatory postures.
3. The part-word repetitions are free from excessive tension, the schwa vowel, or abrupt separation of the repeated sounds or syllables.
4. The frequency of the stuttering is 3 percent or less per 100 words.
5. The stuttering is not accompanied by distracting physical concomitants.
6. The child does not substitute "safe" words for feared ones.
7. The child shows no evidence of frustration about failure to talk correctly, such as giving up speech attempts or asking "Why can't I talk right?".

Clinical experience and judgment must be used in applying these criteria. Though most children who need fluency monitoring rather than therapy will meet all seven, some are borderline and hard to diagnose. Severity of stuttering varies, so the clinician who is examining a child on a day when the stuttering is mild needs to rely on the parent's report to estimate the more severe periods of stuttering. We recommend a follow-up exam if there is any question about the chronicity.

The Fluency Monitoring Program maintains a file of test data, observations, and audiotape recordings for 2 years, during which time the parents contact the clinic if the stuttering increases or if they have questions. A speech pathologist telephones every 6 months and the criteria for FMP are reevaluated based on that telephone interview. Parent counseling is provided in three or four sessions. The goals of these sessions are

1. To reduce inappropriate reactions to the child's stuttering
2. To provide a healthy communication environment for the child
3. To modify the child's use of stuttering as a manipulative tool

ASSESSMENT OF COMPONENTS

A clinician using the component model approach assesses each of the nine components in addition to the stuttering behaviors already discussed. Standardized tests do not address some of the components and allow only a partial assessment of others; therefore we must rely on trained clinical judgments to develop a comprehensive description of a child and his disorders. The methods described here are applicable to most areas in our field. There need be no apology for using clinical judgments so long as the practitioner understands the criteria for them and has adequate experience in observing the behaviors in question. A problem arises only when we need to equate test scores with clinical judgments, but a set of rating charts simplifies this task.

Test results ordinarily are expressed as z scores, that is, we compute how far a test score is from the mean (average) and then express this difference in standard deviations (SD). For example, suppose a child scores 20 on a certain test for which the mean (in the test manual) is 30 and the SD is 5. Since the child's score is 10 points below the mean (-10) and the SD is 5, the z score is $\left(\frac{-10}{5}\right)$. Put another way, the child scored two SD below the mean.

The next step is to translate the SD into clinically meaningful terms. The following examples may help.

A z score of -1 SD equals the 17th percentile. That is, 17 children out of 100 do worse and 83 do better.

A z score of -2 SD equals the 2nd percentile (approximately). That is, 2 children out of 100 do worse and 98 do better.

Mean or above $= 0$
-0.5 SD $(z = -0.5) = 1$
-1.0 SD $(z = -1.0) = 2$
-1.5 SD $(z = -1.5) = 3$
-2.0 SD $(z = -2.0)$ or lower $= 4$

It is a simple matter to devise a similar scale for clinical judgments in which

No problem $= 0$
Borderline problem $= 1$
Mild (but definite) problem $= 2$
Moderate problem $= 3$
Severe problem $= 4$

Each of the components is assessed using a rating scale of 0 to 4 for each descriptor. A descriptor is a specific statement that defines some aspect of the component under consideration. The descriptors taken together define the component. The score for each descriptor is a product of clinical judgment or of a standard test. A rating chart is used for each component in which the rating of 0, 1, 2, 3, or 4 is used for each descriptor whether it is a test score (expressed in z scores) or a judgment of "mild," "moderate," etc. By using these rating charts we are able to obtain better reliability between clinicians. Familiarity with the specific descriptors improves reliability. We ask our students and clinicians in training to compare their judgments with ours as they learn to assess each component.

Attending disorders is the component assessed first. When a child cannot maintain attention, other assessment and treatment are very difficult. Thirty-six percent of the children on whom the component model was based had moderate to severe attending problems. To assess attending we use two subtests of the Burks Behavior Rating Scales (BBRS) (Burks, 1969) and three clinical judgments. The BBRS, which has 18 subtests with 5 to 8 specific behaviors in each, requires the parent or teacher to rate each of 105 behaviors on a scale of 1 to 5 where 1 means "not noticed at all" and 5 means "noticed to a very large degree." The results vary among mother, father, and teacher because each person sees the child under different conditions and is therefore likely to notice different behaviors. The two subtests related to attending disorders are poor attention and poor impulse control and these, along with clinical judgments of reduced attention span, distractibility, and impulsivity, assess the attending component. We are interested in length of time in which a child can perform a tedious task and also in the quality of the attention. Does he focus on the task easily? Can he ignore environmental sounds and sights? Does he try constantly to change activities? Hyperactivity may accompany distractibility and impulsivity, but it is not a defining characteristic. A method for rating BBRS scores along with clinical judgments appears in Figure 4-2, Attending Disorders Rating Chart.

Assume, for example, that a child's BBRS score is 13 in "Poor attention." The evaluator simply enters an *X* under column 3 which represents BBRS scores of 12 to 14 (moderate problem). "Poor impulse control" is charted in the same way and, with the addition of ratings for the three areas of clinical judgment, the chart yields a profile of five descriptors. The two highest descriptor ratings are then used to indicate the overall rating for attending disorders.

Auditory processing disorders were present in 28 percent of our sample. These children had difficulty receiving and manipulating auditory information. Auditory processing includes image retention, figure-ground distinctions, and selection of symbols from nonmeaningful auditory signals. The seven specific descriptors of this component appear in the Auditory Processing Disorders Rating Chart (Fig. 4-3). The first four (delayed responses, self-corrected responses, needed repetition of instructions, and needed cues to respond), observable during any structured, demanding testing procedure, require clinical judgments. Casual procedures do not usually elicit these behaviors. Three subtests of the Illinois Test of Psy-

Figure 4-2. Attending Disorders Rating Chart, based on Burks Behavior Rating Scales (BBRS) and clinical judgments (Cl. Jd.).

Attending Disorders Rating Chart

Descriptors	Ratings				
	0	1	2	3	4
*1. BBRS: Poor attention	5–6	7–9	10–11	12–14	15+
*2. BBRS: Poor impulse control	5–8	8–9	10	11–13	14+
3. Cl. Jd.: Reduced attention span	No	Border-line	Mild	Moderate	Severe
4. Cl. Jd.: Distractible	No	Border-line	Mild	Moderate	Severe
5. Cl. Jd.: Impulsive	No	Border-line	Mild	Moderate	Severe
Overall Rating Average of two highest ratings	0	1	2	3	4

*Use highest rating from mother, father, or teacher.

Auditory Processing Disorders Rating Chart

Descriptors	Ratings				
	0	1	2	3	4
1. Cl. Jd.: Delayed responses	No	Border-line	Mild	Moderate	Severe
2. Cl. Jd.: Self-corrected responses	No	Border-line	Mild	Moderate	Severe
3. Cl. Jd.: Needed repetitions of instructions	No	Border-line	Mild	Moderate	Severe
4. Cl. Jd.: Needed cues	No	Border-line	Mild	Moderate	Severe
5. ITPA: Auditory memory (scaled score)	36+	33–31	30–28	27–25	24–
6. ITPA: Sound blending (ss)	36+	33–31	30–28	27–25	24–
7. ITPA: Auditory closure (ss)	36+	33–31	30–28	27–25	24–
8. Other auditory processing test (z score)	Average+	−0.5 SD	−1.0	−1.5	−2.0
Overall Rating Average of two highest ratings	0	1	2	3	4

Figure 4-3. Auditory Processing Disorders Rating Chart, based on clinical judgment (Cl. Jd.) and the Illinois Test of Psycholinguistic Abilities (ITPA).

cholinguistic Abilities (ITPA) (Kirk, et al., 1968) serve as descriptors also. These are auditory memory, sound blending, and auditory closure. Note that on this chart the ratings represent scaled scores from the ITPA in which a scaled score of 36 is the mean (average) and the SD is 6 regardless of the child's age. So a rating of 0 is given for a score of 36 or above. Because the value of each subsequent rating varies by one-half of an SD, the rating scale becomes

33 (−0.5 SD) = 1
30 (−1.0 SD) = 2
27 (−1.5 SD) = 3
24 or lower (−2.0 SD) = 4

If other standardized tests of auditory processing are used, the rating levels compute in the same manner.

Sentence formulation disorders were present in 31 percent of our sample. The influence of syntax on stuttering was recently reviewed by Wall, Starkweather, and Cairns (1981). They found that young children stuttered more at clause boundaries than at other positions in the sentences. This syntax-bound locus of stuttering is consistent with several other studies (Bloodstein, 1974; Hall, 1977; Hayes and Hood, 1978; Kline and Starkweather, 1979; Wall, 1980). We analyze taped speech samples with at least 50 utterances to rate the first four descriptors on the rating chart (Fig. 4-4). These items reflect the number of fragmented or incomplete sentences, the number of word order errors, the instances of word finding problems, and the lack of appropriate complexity. Item 5 requires the clinician to provide key words and ask the child to make a sentence using the word(s). The clinician must use clinical experience to rate this task because normative data are not available. There are several useful, standardized tests that measure some aspect of sentence formulation. Examples

Figure 4-4. Sentence Formulation Disorders Rating Chart, based on a conversational sample of 50 utterances.

Sentence Formulation Disorders Rating Chart

Descriptors	Rating				
	0	*1*	*2*	*3*	*4*
1. Number of fragmented or incomplete sentences	0	Border-line	1	2–4	5+
2. Number of word order errors	0	Border-line	1	2–4	5+
3. Instances of word finding problems	0	Border-line	2–3	4–6	7+
4. Sentence complexity (verbs, pronouns, prepositions, questions, negative constructs)	Normal	Possible disorder	Mild disorder	Moderate disorder	Severe disorder
5. Ability to form a sentence given one key word	Normal	Possible disorder	Mild disorder	Moderate disorder	Severe disorder
6. Other test of sentence form (z score)	Average +	−.5	−1.0	−1.5	−2.0
Overall Rating Average of two highest ratings	0	1	2	3	4

are the Carrow Elicited Language Inventory (CELI) (Carrow, 1974), the Test of Oral Language (TOL) (Clark and Madison, 1981), and the Bankson Language Screening Test (BLST) (Bankson, 1977).

Oral motor discoordination was present in 69 percent of our sample. Many people who stutter have difficulty timing the laryngeal, articulatory, and respiratory events that support rapid, accurate syllable production. Reviews of the extensive literature appear in Van Riper (1982), and in Conture (1982).

Not all children who stutter have observable oral motor discoordinations. Among the populations we have studied since 1969, the percentage of children with this problem has ranged from 61 to 87. The lower percentage occurred in a population that includes public school cases, and the highest among private practice clients.

Every child who exhibits chronic stuttering needs careful assessment of his oral motor functioning. We use rapid syllable repetition tasks, a tongue laterality task, and judgments of intelligibility and saliva control to rate oral motor coordination. The child is asked to produce the syllable sets [pʌ], [pʌtʌ], [tʌkʌ] (and if the child is 5 years old or older pʌtʌkʌ). We model the tongue laterality task so the child can imitate it. Clinical experience permits the examiner to make allowance for the child's age. We also consider the child's intelligibility in conversational speech and watch for any saliva control problems.

After the child demonstrates the ability to perform each syllable set, we ask him to repeat the task 10 times at fast conversational rate. We rate the syllables using the following criteria for accuracy (Fig. 4-5):

1. Precision of consonant production
2. Smoothness of performance during 10 repetitions of each syllable set
3. Voicing errors (especially substitution of the voiced cognate for the voiceless, i.e., b/p, d/t, g/k)
4. Maintenance of syllable order without retraining

The examiner compares the taped syllable productions to normal conversational rate and assigns (mild, moderate, or severe reduction in speed) the appropriate rating. If more precision is needed, the child's maximum rate is compared to the normative data in Table 4-1. The examiner rates the speed of the tongue laterality performance using the same table. Fletcher (1972) developed some of the data; we extrapolated or estimated the remainder.

High self-expectations characterized a large percentage of our sample (89%). This component stems from the child's need to be perfect and a tendency to blame himself for any problems, perfectionistic attitudes which often lead to anxiety and poor self-image. Five of the 18 categories of BBRS relate to this component: Excessive suffering, excessive anxiety,

Oral Motor Disorders Rating Chart

The child should imitate the examiner's performance of each task. Train the child to perform each task 10 times "as fast as possible, but say it correctly."

Rate as follows

0 = No problem
1 = Borderline performance
2 = Mild problem
3 = Moderate problem
4 = Severe problem

Consider accuracy of production and ability to sustain accurate production during 10 repetitions of the task. Time with stopwatch and score according to rate table.

	$\overline{X}$	0	1	2	3	4
1. [pʌ]	Accuracy problems	No $\overline{X}$	Border-line	Mild	Mod-erate	Severe
	Rate _____		−0.5	−1.0	−1.5	−2.0
2. [pʌtə]	Accuracy problems	No $\overline{X}$	Border-line	Mild	Mod-erate	Severe
	Rate _____		−0.5	−1.0	−1.5	−2.0
3. [tʌkə]	Accuracy problems	No $\overline{X}$	Border-line	Mild	Mod-erate	Severe
	Rate _____		−0.5	−1.0	−1.5	−2.0
4. [pʌtəkə] (if 5 yr or older)	Accuracy problems	No $\overline{X}$	Border-line	Mild	Mod-erate	Severe
	Rate _____		−0.5	−1.0	−1.5	−2.0
5. Tongue laterality	Accuracy problems	No $\overline{X}$	Border-line	Mild	Mod-erate	Severe
	Rate _____		−0.5	−1.0	−1.5	−2.0
6. Reduced intelligibility		No	Border-line	Mild	Mod-erate	Severe
7. Saliva control problem		No	Border-line	Mild	Mod-erate	Severe
Overall Rating Average of two highest ratings		0	1	2	3	4

Figure 4-5. Oral Motor Disorders Rating Chart.

Table 4-1. Time in Seconds to Perform Each Oral Motor Task 10 Times for Ages 3 Through Eight

Oral Motor Task	Severity Scale				
	No Problem (0)	Borderline (1)	Mild (2)	Moderate (3)	Severe (4)
Task: pʌ					
Age 3 E/F	2.8	3.1	3.3	3.6	3.8
4 E/F	2.6	2.9	3.1	3.4	3.6
5 E/F	2.5	2.8	3.0	3.3	3.5
6 F	2.4	2.7	2.9	3.2	3.4
7 F	2.4	2.7	2.9	3.2	3.4
8 F	2.1	2.3	2.45	2.6	2.8
Task: pʌtə					
Age 3 E/F	5.4	5.9	6.4	6.9	7.4
4 E/F	5.2	5.7	6.2	6.7	7.2
5 F	5.1	5.6	6.1	6.6	7.1
6 E/F	4.9	5.4	5.9	6.4	6.9
7 F	5.1	5.6	6.1	6.6	7.1
8 F	4.2	4.6	5.0	5.4	5.8
Task: tʌkə					
Age 3 E/F	5.9	6.4	6.9	7.4	7.9
4 E/F	5.6	6.1	6.6	7.1	7.6
5 E/F	5.4	5.9	6.4	6.9	7.4
6 F	5.2	5.7	6.2	6.7	7.2
7 F	5.4	5.9	6.4	6.9	7.4
8 F	4.8	5.2	5.6	6.0	6.4

Task: pʌtəkə

Age						
3	—	—	—	—	—	—
4	—	—	—	—	—	—
5	—	—	—	—	—	—
6	F	10.3	11.7	13.1	14.5	15.9
7	F	10.0	11.4	12.8	14.2	15.6
8	F	8.3	9.3	10.3	11.3	12.3

Task: Tongue laterality

Age						
3	est.	9.5	10.0	10.5	11.0	11.5
4	est.	9.0	9.5	10.0	10.5	11.0
5	est.	8.5	9.0	9.5	10.0	10.5
6	est.	8.0	8.5	9.0	9.5	10.0
7	est.	7.5	8.0	8.5	9.0	9.5
8	est.	7.0	7.5	8.0	8.5	9.0

F = based on normative data developed by Samual Fletcher (1972); E/F = extrapolated from Fletcher normative data; est. = estimated from clinical experience.

excessive self-blame, excessive dependency, and poor ego strength. The scores for each of these categories are converted to a 0 to 4 rating as before (Fig. 4-6). In addition the parents comment on the child's self-expectations and frustration tolerance because sometimes this description picks up attitudes which the BBRS does not detect. The clinician also rates the child's need to be perfect and any lack of tolerance for routine frustration. The child who constantly asks, "Am I getting it right?" is demonstrating this attitude.

Manipulative stuttering was present in 25 percent of our sample and surfaced in comments made by parents in response to the statements listed in Figure 4-7.

Since these behaviors are difficult to rate, an experienced clinician will be able to ascertain whether or not a problem exists. The parent(s) must feel secure enough to talk freely, and assurances that "parents do not

Figure 4-6. High Self-Expectations Rating Chart, based on Burks Behavior Rating Scales (BBRS), parent's report (PR) and clinician's judgment (Cl. Jd.).

High Self-Expectations Rating Chart

Descriptors	Ratings				
	0	*1*	*2*	*3*	*4*
*1. BBRS: Excessive suffering	7–9	10–11	12	13–15	16+
*2. BBRS: Excessive anxiety	5–8	9–10	11	12–17	18+
*3. BBRS: Excessive self-blame	5–8	9–10	11–12	13–16	17+
*4. BBRS: Excessive dependency	6–10	11–12	12	14–18	19+
*5. BBRS: Poor ego strength	7–10	11–13	14–15	16–19	20+
*6. PR: Child is perfectionist	No	Border-line	Mild	Moderate	Severe
7. Cl. Jd.: Child needs to be perfect	No	Border-line	Mild	Moderate	Severe
8. Cl. Jd.: Low frustration tolerance	No	Border-line	Mild	Moderate	Severe
Overall Rating Average of two highest ratings	0	1	2	3	4

* Use highest rating of mother, father, or teacher.

Manipulative Stuttering Rating Chart				
Descriptors	*Ratings*			
	0 *1*	*2*	*3*	*4*
1. Child gets special privileges because he stutters.	No Borderline	Mild	Moderate	Severe
2. Child is allowed to dominate family conversations.	No Borderline	Mild	Moderate	Severe
3. Parents are extremely anxious about the child.	No Borderline	Mild	Moderate	Severe
4. Parents feel excessive pity for the child.	No Borderline	Mild	Moderate	Severe
5. Child is not told "no" appropriately because of fear of stress on the child.	No Borderline	Mild	Moderate	Severe
6. Family members all become silent when the child speaks, but not for others.	No Borderline	Mild	Moderate	Severe
Overall Rating Average of two highest ratings	0 1	2	3	4

Figure 4-7. Manipulative Stuttering Rating Chart, based on parent's report.

cause stuttering" are helpful. Frequently, the mother has read traditional explanations of the origins of stuttering and assumed her own guilt. We explain that stuttering does not "start in her ear" but that the child is vulnerable to develop stuttering. The parents do play some part in its development and maintenance. Manipulation depends on the reaction of the audience so modification involves changes in parental responses. The assessment interview sets the tone for later attempts to change these reactions.

Disruptive communication environment was present in 53 percent of the families in our sample. The attitudes and behaviors that disrupt the child's communication are probably well-known to most speech pathologists. The ones that seemed most important to us are listed in Figure

4-8. As mentioned above, the tone of the interview needs to be accepting and nonthreatening so that the parents feel free to share their perceptions of the communicative conditions in the home. We also like to observe the child and parents engaged in conversation and play. If possible the examiner videotapes the parent-child interaction for use in modification of any disruptive behaviors. From the parents' report and the clinician's observation, we rate the descriptors in Figure 4-8.

Some of the disruptive conditions that contribute to the child's stuttering may be subtle and indirect. For example, when the child is formulating an answer to one question, an unthinking listener may interject a second question. The child with delayed-processing or sentence formulation problems is trying to form a response to the first question while deciding what to do with the second one; yet during this time he has

Figure 4-8. Disruptive Communication Environment Rating Chart, based on parent's report (PR) and clinician's judgment (Cl. Jd.).

Disruptive Communication Environment Rating Chart

Descriptors		*Ratings*				
		0	*1*	*2*	*3*	*4*
1. Child has difficulty	PR	No	Borderline	Mild	Moderate	Severe
getting parents' at-	Cl. Jd.	No	Borderline	Mild	Moderate	Severe
tention.						
2. Family members	PR	No	Borderline	Mild	Moderate	Severe
rush the child's	Cl. Jd.	No	Borderline	Mild	Moderate	Severe
speech.						
3. Family members in-	PR	No	Borderline	Mild	Moderate	Severe
terrupt or "butt in"	Cl. Jd.	No	Borderline	Mild	Moderate	Severe
while the child is						
speaking.						
4. Child is teased about	PR	No	Borderline	Mild	Moderate	Severe
his speech problem.	Cl. Jd.	No	Borderline	Mild	Moderate	Severe
5. People make critical,	PR	No	Borderline	Mild	Moderate	Severe
negative or sarcastic	Cl. Jd.	No	Borderline	Mild	Moderate	Severe
comments about the						
child's speech.						

Overall Rating	0	1	2	3	4
Average of two					
highest ratings					

said nothing at all. From the child's point of view, impatient parents do not accommodate his speech disorders.

Indirect critical reaction is evident too when the child starts to answer the phone and another family member rushes to prevent it. The interception conveys the message that the child's speech will cause embarrassment to all concerned.

The clinician's understanding of the child's perspective will help him to explain the interrupting situations from the child's point of view, thus making the parents' report more reliable. The descriptors in Figure 4-8 are rated by evaluating the parents' report and behaviors observed in the clinic.

Unrealistic parental expectations (Fig. 4-9) were present in 51 percent of the families in our sample. In a nonthreatening interview the parents will provide reasonably accurate information. The clinician rates each descriptor based on parents' reports and observations of behaviors in the clinic. We develop the goals of parent conferences from these initial ratings, but they are revised when additional insights into the family ex-

Figure 4-9. Unrealistic Parent Expectations Rating Chart, based on parent's report (PR) and clinician's judgment (Cl. Jd.).

Unrealistic Parent Expectations Rating Chart

Descriptors		Ratings				
		0	1	2	3	4
1. Parent expects child	PR	No	Borderline	Mild	Moderate	Severe
to be a "little adult."	Cl. Jd.	No	Borderline	Mild	Moderate	Severe
2. Child's accomplish-	PR	No	Borderline	Mild	Moderate	Severe
ments are never good	Cl. Jd.	No	Borderline	Mild	Moderate	Severe
enough.						
3. Parent expects per-	PR	No	Borderline	Mild	Moderate	Severe
fection from himself	Cl. Jd.	No	Borderline	Mild	Moderate	Severe
or herself.						
4. Parent expects child	PR	No	Borderline	Mild	Moderate	Severe
to stop stuttering	Cl. Jd.	No	Borderline	Mild	Moderate	Severe
soon after treatment						
begins.						
Overall Rating		0	1	2	3	4
Based on two						
highest ratings						

pectations are forthcoming. Actually, the modification of these expectations begins with the first interview. When the parents understand that certain attitudes are unrealistic, they begin to change them. For example, some parents praise fluent speech without realizing that, from the child's point of view, such praise implies that disfluent speech is unworthy of praise. We encourage the family from the very beginning to turn the stuttering over to the clinician so they don't need to worry about it.

Abnormal parental need for the child to stutter was present in only 5 percent of the families in our sample. The component proved difficult to rate with accuracy at the time of the initial interview because the parents usually tried to say what was expected. Later, when contradictions surfaced, it was evident that one parent (usually the mother) was not able to tolerate improvement in the child's speech, and a pattern of sabotaging the therapy became obvious. This attitude is rare, which is fortunate, because it is a powerful force against successful treatment. Figure 4-10 shows the specific descriptors used in evaluating this component.

To supplement the assessment of these descriptors, we sometimes consult with a qualified psychologist or psychiatrist who may diagnose the parent as having a severe neurosis, a psychosis, or a borderline or psychopathic personality. If this happens, we assign an overall rating of 4 for this component regardless of the speech pathologist's ratings of the individual descriptors.

Reporting the results of these clinical assessments to parents is an important step in the treatment process. Both parents should attend this session, if possible. In this meeting, we review the nature of the child's stuttering and explain with lay terms any neurologic dysfunctions that may have predisposed the child to develop it. We also discuss the attitudes and behaviors of the child, the family, and others to develop parental awareness of any unrealistic demands or expectations for the child's speech performance. The concepts that the child has a reduced threshold for fluency breakdown and that attitudes and environmental pressures can push him over this threshold help to explain the parents' role. They do not "cause" stuttering, but they do play an important part in its development and in its treatment.

Description of the Therapy

THERAPY GOALS

The component approach to treatment of stuttering has two goals:

1. To modify the impact of the components that accompany abnormal disfluencies
   a. Environmental (interpersonal) influences
   b. Attitudinal (intrapersonal) influences
   c. Neurologic influences

Abnormal Parental Need for the Child To Stutter Rating Chart

Descriptors	Ratings				
	0	1	2	3	4
1. Parent thinks about child's stuttering "every waking minute."	No	Border-line	Mild	Moderate	Severe
2. Parent denies treatment gains and claims child is getting worse.	No	Border-line	Once mild	Once moderate +	2 times
3. Parent threatens to take child out of treatment when child is improv-ing.	No	Border-line	Once mild	Once moderate +	2 times
4. Parent is threatened by clinician-child relation-ship.	No	Border-line	Mild	Moderate	Severe
5. Parent understands an important aspect of treatment one day, then can't remember it next session.	No	Border-line	1 time	2 times	3 + times
6. Parent brings child to treatment late, misses sessions, and refuses home assignments.	No	Border-line	2 times	3–5 times	6 + times
7. Parent's behavior is bi-zarre.	No	Border-line	Mild	Moderate	Severe
Overall Rating Average of two highest scores	0	1	2	3	4

If the parent is diagnosed by an appropriate specialist as having a severe mental disor-der (e.g. psychosis; psychopathic or borderline personality; severe neurosis) assign a rating of 4 for this component.

Figure 4-10. Abnormal Parental Need for the Child to Stutter Rating Chart, based on parental behavior during child's treatment.

2. To further reduce abnormal disfluencies to zero so that the speech after therapy should have
   a. Normal rate (with no treatment artifact)
   b. Normal rhythm (with no timing artifact)
   c. Normal flow (with normal disfluencies)

THERAPY METHOD

Specific Techniques, Procedures, Activities

Sequencing of treatment is accomplished first. With a multidimensional approach such as ours, the number and nature of the variables determine the organization of therapy. Our model requires treatment in four major areas:

1. Modification of the environment
2. Modification of the child's attitude
3. Modification of any neurologic components
4. Direct modification of remaining abnormal disfluencies

We set up the sequence of therapy in such a way as to address (1) attending (before any other component) in the child; (2) environment (early in therapy); (3) the child's attitude (relatively early); (4) oral motor discoordination (relatively early since it requires short, intensive sessions over a long period of time); and (5) any direct modification of abnormal disfluencies last. Table 4-2 may help visualize the organization. There are five steps in the treatment sequence, and there are four major areas of intervention represented by the columns. During the first step, we begin parent conferences and modify any attending problems in the child. No other treatment is attempted until attending is improved to the point at which the child can focus on therapy activities for at least 5 minutes.

During the second step, we continue parent conferences, we begin work on any attitudes of the child that need changing, and we start using short segments of therapy time to modify oral motor discoordination.

During the third step, we continue parent conferences as needed, modify any auditory processing component the child may have, and continue attitude modification.

During the fourth step, we modify any sentence formulation difficulties the child has. We continue attitude modification as needed.

During the fifth and final step, we employ direct methods to modify any remaining abnormal disfluencies.

Obviously, because treatment is individualized, the sequence of components varies slightly from program to program. For example, if a child has oral motor discoordinations (OMD) and sentence formulation problems, we proceed with OMD modification during step 1; attitude modi-

Table 4-2. Treatment Sequence for Component Model Therapy

	Environment Modification	Attitude Modification	Component Modification	Direct Modification of Abnormal Disfluencies
Step 1	Parent conferences 1, 2, and 3		Modification of attending problems	
Step 2	Parent conferences 4, 5, and 6	Modification of high self-expectations	Modification of oral motor discoordination	
Step 3	Parent conferences as needed	Modification of high self-expectations as needed	Modification of auditory processing problems	
Step 4	Parent conferences as needed	Modification of high self-expectations as needed	Modification of sentence formulation problems	
Step 5	Parent conferences as needed			Direct modification of abnormal disfluencies

fication and the first three parent conferences are also conducted in the same time frame. If, however, the child has attending problems, we modify the attending as indicated in Table 4-2 during step 1 and wait until step 2 to begin OMD modification and attitude modification. Also, step 3 may not be necessary if auditory processing is normal. The number of hours for parent conferences and attitude modification are only approximate, so we sometimes need to adjust the sequence to accommodate these differences.

Many people, including parents, school districts, insurance companies, and the speech pathologist need to know the estimated number of treatment hours an individual child is likely to require. To obtain data from which to calculate the average length of treatment, we analyzed 19 cases using intake summaries, reports of service from each treatment session, and progress reports to determine the number of hours needed for each component of treatment (Table 4-3). These numbers are only averages based on a small sample, and therefore do not guarantee treatment length. The ranges for each treatment area are instructive merely as averages. The average total number of treatment hours was 48, the standard deviation 25.6, and the range from 10 to 111 hours, so variation was considerable. In addition, we discovered certain variables that predicted longer than average treatment, such as severity of attending disorder

Table 4-3. Number of Treatment Hours for 19 Children with Several Patterns of Components Related to Their Stuttering

Area Modified	1 No Neurologic Components	2 OMD Only	3 OMD SF	4 OMD AP	5 ATN OMD	6 ATN OMD SF	7 ATN OMD AP SF	Overall
Environment (ENV)	4		4	7	8	6	12	
Attitude (ATT)	9	12	11	9	20	19	4	
Attending (ATN)						12	4	
Oral motor discoordination (OMD)		16	14	18	17	17	16	
Auditory processing (AP)				12		17	6	
Sentence formulation (SF)			7				8	
Abnormal disfluencies	12	8	5	4	7	27	10	
Total mean	25	40	43	50	61	98	60	47.9 SD = 25.6
Total range	10–39	23–54	30–51	28–111	30–88	NA	NA	
Number of subjects	2	5	4	3	3	1	1	

(r = .40) and oral motor discoordinations (r = .42), which were the best predictors. Interestingly, the severity of stuttering was not related to treatment length.

Environment modification, always started early in treatment, consists of a series of four to 12 1-hour sessions with the parent(s). The counseling is conducted by the clinician who works with the child and is concurrent with other aspects of therapy (See Table 4-2). Although the exact nature of the counseling varies with the training and personality of the clinician, these sessions provide the opportunity, not only to explore feelings and behaviors that may relate to stuttering, but also to elicit additional information. Most of the time we deal with concerned, loving parents who are willing to accept guidance from a professional and who can provide useful observations from their vantage point as parents. Sometimes members of the extended family (siblings, a grandparent, etc.) participate in some sessions, as well.

The first goal of parent counseling is to reduce the sense of guilt about "causing the stuttering." Most parents are well aware of the admonition that stuttering is aggravated or even caused when they pay attention to it. They may have tried to ignore it, but it has developed anyway so they feel they have failed. We tell them simply, "Parents do not cause stuttering." Most children who stutter have some organic predisposition toward stuttering (91 percent of our sample had at least one neurologic component). When a child is vulnerable, some completely normal and otherwise harmless family behaviors may act as a catalyst for a speech problem. So while the parents do play some part in the development of the stuttering, their role does not deserve blame.

Another goal of parent counseling is to identify and reduce disruptive behaviors in the communication environment. Some examples of specific behaviors that rush or frustrate a child's attempts to communicate include (1) difficulty in getting the parents' or siblings' attention, (2) interruption by family members if the child stops to think, and (3) critical comments or teasing about the child's speech. The child's other components of stuttering are usually tied into the environmental disruptors, and these relationships can be explored during parent sessions. For example, a child may have difficulty forming sentences, and the fast-paced family conversation may frequently catch him midway in the process of deciding how to put his ideas into words. With such information, the parents usually find it easier to allow the child enough time for sentence formulation.

The clinician uses whatever techniques that seem appropriate to help the parents identify and change their disruptive behaviors. The parents can usually describe conversations in which the child felt rushed or frustrated, but they have trouble describing their own behaviors. They can tape-record some family conversations which are then used in the clinic to help illustrate the interactions between parent and child. Once a parent learns to identify a specific behavior, he can learn to self-monitor and eliminate or reduce it. The behaviors that rush and frustrate a child are not usually eliminated entirely, but they are modified to the point that the child can accommodate and accept them. It is also important that the communication rules that allow the child who stutters time to talk apply to other members of the family.

A third goal of parent counseling is to reduce any unrealistic parental expectations, especially those related to fluency (about one-half of our parents were unrealistic in this area). It is natural for them to accept a child's self-imposed, perfectionistic attitudes. Parents need information about the child's abilities to help them align their perspective with what is realistic. They need to know that stuttering comes and goes even when the child is in treatment, and that they should not be overly pleased with periods of fluency or displeased when the stuttering returns. Ideally, they develop an attitude that allows them to turn the stuttering over to the clinician so they can channel their energies toward enjoying their role as parents.

A fourth goal of parent counseling is added if the child uses stuttering to manipulate the family (25 percent of our sample did this). This behavior is almost impossible to modify directly with the child because he is getting what he thinks he wants. Modification comes when the parents and others stop responding to the manipulative behaviors, such as:

1. Giving the child special privileges because he stutters
2. Allowing the child to dominate family conversations
3. Feeling extreme anxiety about the child's problem
4. Feeling excessive pity for the child
5. Not telling the child "no" at appropriate times because of the fear of placing him under undue stress
6. Becoming silent when the child is speaking in a family conversation but not reacting the same way when other family members speak

Once the involved family members identify these behaviors and feelings and recognize the pattern of manipulation, they usually can alter the actions and, to some extent, the feelings that reinforce the stuttering.

Attitude modification usually begins early in the treatment process, but enters into other aspects of treatment as the child exhibits a readiness to discuss his feelings. Speech pathologists should not expect to do the job of psychotherapists, who in one way or another restructure the child's ego defenses, but they can expect to reduce the child's need for perfection, especially with regard to fluency.

Generally, it is advisable to focus on modification of some behavior that is not related to speech first. In this way, the child can experience the therapy process with a behavior that is not as threatening as speech, then apply the process more directly to stuttering. If, for example, the child exhibits frustration or fear that he is going to fail at a task, the clinician begins by talking about what the child does when things do not go right. Then, assuming the role of the child, the clinician role plays a situation which represents potential frustration for the child. Before demonstrating that frustration, however, the clinician stops to offer alternative reactions to it, including the behavior which the child ordinarily exhibits. Next, the child role plays the same situation with several alternative reactions. In the next phase of attitude modification, the clinician observes the child in some therapy task that is usually frustrating to the child. Just before the child actually reacts with frustration, the clinician intervenes and reviews the alternatives with the child. The child is then asked to select the old behavior or one of the alternatives. The new alternatives are, of course, less demanding for the child and permit the child to accept his mistakes as a normal part of learning new tasks.

The next goal is to reduce the need for perfect fluency. The child needs information at this point about normal and abnormal disfluencies (see Assessment Procedures). The clinician models the normal disfluencies of speech and asks the child to bring to therapy examples of these from television, radio, friends, and family members. The message is that "nobody's perfect." Next, the clinician models speech with both normal and mildly abnormal disfluencies, and encourages the child to accept, even welcome, normal ones and tolerate mildly abnormal ones simply because they are better than severe stuttering blocks. As the child realizes that many of the disfluencies which he considers "bad" are either normal or "not very bad," he is better able to tolerate them. He focuses less on perceived failures in his speech and gradually develops better self-acceptance and less need for perfect fluency.

Another goal of attitude modification is improving the child's self-concept. Our approach is to help the child appreciate that all children have "good" and "bad" points. To achieve this, we sometimes identify one child who our client considers a hero and one he considers a dud. We then focus on helping the child discover good and bad things in each to help him recognize that it is all right for him to have some problems. Then we help our client discover good things about himself to counterbalance the undeniable fact that he stutters. The result of this process is illustrated in a real incident which happened a few years ago. A third-grade boy, who had been in stuttering therapy the previous year, asked his teacher if he could say something to the class on the first day of school. She was surprised, but said yes. So the boy stood up and announced rather formally and with an air of confidence, "I stutter. Everybody has got sumpin' wrong with 'em, and I don't want to hear no more about it." And he didn't.

Attending problems are treated with a combination of behavior modification and, in some cases, medication. The use of medication depends on our findings and the assessment of the child's family doctor or pediatrician. Some parents do not want medication used as an adjunct to speech therapy for their child, which is their right, and we honor it. We do explain to them, if we have entrée, that gaining the child's full attention will shorten the course of treatment. A child who is neurologically distractible but able, with the aid of medication, to edit incoming stimuli will receive more benefit from each treatment session than the same child without medication.

The program to improve attending employs a systematic program using *immediate, positive,* and *primary* reinforcement. The aim of the program, outlined below, is to increase auditory attending and decrease visual distractibility. The child should be seated in a higher chair than the clinician so that their eye levels are approximately the same, but they should sit side by side rather than across a table from each other. The clinician uses a stopwatch and some age-appropriate items that are visually attractive.

1. The child will look at the clinician, put both hands on the table, and wait 1 second for the clinician's next auditory command. The auditory command may be anything appropriate to the child's age, such as repeating digits or words. Do not reward fluency or punish disfluency. Reward only for attending, i.e., waiting 1 second for the next auditory command. Repeat the task until the child has been successful three successive times.
2. Same as 1. Increase waiting time to 2 seconds.
3. Same as 2. Increase to 4 seconds.
4. Same as 3. Increase to 8 seconds.
5. The child will look at the clinician, put both hands on the table, and wait 1 second for an auditory command while a visual distraction is introduced into the child's line of sight.
6. Same as 5. Duration 2 seconds.
7. Same as 6. Duration 4 seconds.
8. Same as 7. Duration 8 seconds.
9. The child will perform an age-appropriate task (such as counting or naming pictures) for 2 seconds while a visual distractor is introduced into the line of sight.
10. Same as 9. Duration 8 seconds.
11. Same as 10. Duration 60 seconds.
12. Same as 11. Duration 120 seconds.
13. Same as 12. Duration 180 seconds.

Objectives 11 through 13 are lengthy so the child needs to perform tasks that can sustain interest for up to 3 minutes. The tasks themselves should be well within the child's ability level and only attending should be reinforced. Reinforcers include pats on the back, verbal praise, and, if necessary, bits of food. Reinforce each successful performance at first, then reduce reinforcements gradually to random reinforcement of one-third of the successful performances. Success criteria are three correct performances at a given level before moving on to the next. If the child cannot perform on the next highest level, the clinician uses smaller time increments or less demanding visual distractors.

This program improves impulse control, strengthens resistance to distraction, and increases frustration tolerance. Increase in the attention span beyond 3 minutes will occur as a result of other aspects of treatment. In other words, while you are engaged in oral motor training or auditory process training, you also are increasing the attention span. For a child who is distractible, the clinician will need to monitor the attending during all other phases of treatment.

Oral motor discoordination (OMD) is treated in the same way it was evaluated, that is, we employ a systematic syllable training to improve oral motor skills. We view oral motor timing as a feed-forward, motor planning process aimed at an acoustic target. About 150 muscles must be coordinated in order to initiate and terminate each syllable. In addition, the syllable timing overlaps because of varying transmission times for different muscle groups. Laryngeal timing is the most difficult because the nerves that serve the larynx are so much longer than the nerves that serve the tongue, lips, facial muscles, and velopharyngeal areas. When a child is speaking at a rate of 2.0 to 3.5 syllables per second, he is executing thousands of neurologic events per second; all of which must be precisely timed. Our task is to reprogram the child's "subcortical computer" so that this timing is accomplished with greater accuracy.

We theorize that improved oral motor planning tends to normalize voice onset and termination times and to improve transitional formants. If this is so, the child's *fluent speech* should improve, and the modification of remaining stuttering events should be simpler. In addition, we theorize that the changes in the child's basic oral motor system are likely to facilitate maintenance of treatment gains.

We began our treatment approach using the sensory-motor program described by McDonald (1964). Since then, we have modified it several times so that we now use a systematic syllable training program that manipulates five variables related to syllable complexity. These variables are (1) number of syllables in the set, (2) number of different vowels used, (3) number of different consonants used, (4) number of unvoiced consonants per set, and (5) number of consonants between vowels. Performance criteria are the same as those used in testing OMD:

1. Precision of consonant production
2. Continuity of performance for 10 repetitions of each syllable set
3. Accurate voiced/unvoiced distinctions in consonant production
4. Order of syllables maintained
5. Rate within normal limits for age

For each syllable repetition we attend to accuracy first and then ask the child to say the syllable set slowly two times, then three, and so on up to ten times. When the child can produce the set accurately and smoothly at a slow pace, the rate is increased until the criteria in Table 4-1, column 1, are reached.

We start with easy, all-voiced syllable sets of one or two syllables. For example, the first training syllable can be [ba]. It has *one* syllable in the "set," *one* vowel, and *one* consonant. All sounds are *voiced*, and there is *one* consonant between vowels when the set is repeated, thus [bababab a . . .]. Other single syllables such as [gu] and [vu] can be practiced in the same way, but avoid using sounds that the child cannot articulate easily at this point in syllable training.

Once the child has mastered sets of one syllable, expand the sets to two as with [babu babu babu . . .], for example. Other similar syllable sets can be generated easily and practiced until the child can perform at this level. Each syllable set is produced in chains of ten until it has been performed with 90 percent accuracy in three consecutive chains. We employ five sets of one type before increasing the difficulty by adding another syllable to the set or by adding an unvoiced consonant or adding another consonant between the vowels. The following outline details a sample sequence of training:

I. Easy syllable sets using the voiced consonants [b, d, g, m, n, v] and the vowels [i, æ, ʌ, a, oʊ, u]
   A. One-syllable sets: [ɖi, ɖæ, ɖʌ, ɖa] etc.
   B. Two-syllable sets: [baba, bʌda] etc.
   C. Three-syllable sets: [bʌbʌbʌ, dædæbʌ] etc.
II. Moderately difficult sets introducing one unvoiced consonant [p, t, k, f] per set
   A. One-syllable sets: [pʌ, tæ]
   B. Two-syllable sets: [pʌgi, duta]
   C. Three-syllable sets: [bʌbʌt, kaguni]
III. Difficult syllable sets using two or three unvoiced consonants per set
   A. Two-syllable sets: [tutu, pikæ]
   B. Three-syllable sets: [pæpæda, pʌkʌmu], (and of course the famous [pætækʌ])
IV. Very difficult sets that introduce two consonants between the vowels when said in serial fashion
   A. One-syllable sets: [bukbukbuk. . .]
                         [tʌnʌtʌn. . .]
   B. Two-syllable sets: [bʌkdækbʌkdæk. . .]

The child should overlearn at each level of difficulty and proceed to more difficult levels until he reaches a level that he cannot accomplish without undue frustration. Younger children usually do not reach level

IV. However, there is some overlaping between IIIB and IVA so, even if a child reaches his ceiling in level IIIB, he is given an opportunity to perform IVA syllable sets. Also, considerable variation in difficulty is possible within a given level, as with IIIB for example, which we can subdivide into three levels:

1. Less difficult: [pæpædɑ]
2. Moderate level: [pɑdipɑ]
3. More difficult: [fupɑki]

Children vary in what they find easy or difficult, so several trials at different levels are necessary to determine that the child has reached the limits of his ability. Oral motor training takes between 6 and 22 treatment hours with an average of 14.3 hours.

Auditory processing treatment methods are well known to most practicing speech pathologists and so no attempt will be made to describe them in detail. Therapy methods for aphasic adults and children with receptive language disorders include thorough descriptions of them. The goals for treatment of auditory processing depend on the exact nature of the child's problems. They may include

1. Reducing the need for repetition of instructions by requiring the child to perform after only one presentation of the instructions. Start with very easy instructions and progress to a level of complexity commensurate with the child's age and potential.
2. Reducing the need for extra cues.
3. Reducing the need for self-corrected responses. Only one response is permitted, and only correct responses are reinforced.
4. Increasing auditory memory for words and following directions.
5. Increasing the child's ability to make auditory closure by requiring him to perform a task with progressively less auditory information and fewer contextual cues.

An indirect result of these improvements is that there is less delay in the auditory processing system. We cannot directly program a decrease in response delay time because the child is responding as rapidly as he can. If the child's responses are still somewhat delayed after auditory processing treatment, we encourage him to accept the fact that he needs extra time. This type of self-understanding often helps him avoid undue frustration and anxiety during the delay.

Sentence formulation is another treatment area that is well described in language pathology literature. Several well-devised commercial programs equipped with appropriate stimulus materials and other aids are available; and we recommend programs that are based on generative grammar and not just length of utterance. A careful analysis of the child's syntax and morphology is necessary in order to devise a program that will train the child to produce sentences at his level of language ability. The goals are

1. To eliminate fragmented or incomplete sentences
2. To reduce the number of one word responses
3. To reduce echoic responses
4. To eliminate word order errors by training specific syntactic constructs
5. To increase the ability to form a correct sentence given one, two, or three words to include in the sentences
6. To increase sentence complexity by adding more complex verb constructs, using more pronouns and prepositions and adding negative constructs
7. To reduce word retrieval problems by providing cues, then gradually fading them out
8. To help the child take the time he needs to formulate his thoughts and provide strategies for coping if he is interrupted during this time, e.g., statements such as, "Wait a minute, I'm thinking."

Remaining abnormal disfluencies are modified after the nine components of the component model have been treated. To assess the need for direct modification, we readminister the Stuttering Severity Instrument (Riley, 1972). Among the cases subjected to detailed reevaluation, the average severity had diminished since the initial assessment from 22.8 to 9.9. This reduction occurred even though fluency itself had not been reinforced or treated directly. After direct modification, the average severity was reduced even further to 4.3.

Thirty-seven percent of the children needed no direct modification. This need correlated with the age of the child, however. Among children who entered treatment by age 3 or 4, only 20 percent needed direct modification of their remaining abnormal disfluencies; by age 5 the percentage was 67; and by age six the percentage was 83. All of the children 7 and older needed direct modification. Perhaps for younger children we assist some natural process which helps them to "outgrow" their stuttering without direct treatment. Environmental changes, neurologic development, and the individualized coping methods devised by each child are just some of the factors involved in this natural process, and component-based treatment may take advantage of these factors and strengthen them in these very young children who stutter.

Children whose stuttering is more firmly established need direct modification of the fluency itself after the components have been modified. Their remaining disfluencies are carefully described in terms of core behaviors, physical concomitants, and word avoidance. The type of modification deemed appropriate depends on the patterns of these remaining behaviors, but we employ four direct modification approaches on the basis of their compatibility with our stated goals. They should (1) result in normal (unmonitored) rate without any treatment artifact; (2) result in normal rhythm without artifact; (3) result in natural flow of speech; and (4) not require expensive equipment which may not be available in some clinical settings. The direct modification system employs four programs:

1. Physical concomitant modification
2. Avoidance modification
3. Simple program to modify core behaviors
4. Complex program to modify core behaviors

The number of treatment hours for direct modification ranged from 0 to 27 and averaged 8.1 with a standard deviation of 8.8 so there was wide variability. Children who needed avoidance treatment and complex modification of their core behaviors required more hours.

Physical concomitant modification is necessary if the child has distracting facial grimaces or abnormal movement of the head or extremities. Only one of our 19 children who participated in the detailed analysis of their treatment needed this program. He blinked his eyes tightly during stuttering blocks. Physical concomitants are learned behaviors that are readily extinguished using operant principles. We first train the child to identify the behavior, and then require him to signal in some nonverbal way when he is engaged in it. This signaling requires on-line monitoring, and together the monitoring and signaling serve as adversative negative reinforcement. Generally, the behavior is extinguished after two to four sessions in the clinic, but for the child previously mentioned, who monitored the tension around his eyes and then signalled his awareness by raising a finger, treatment time was less than 1 hour. This included 30 minutes to learn to identify the behavior and then 10 minutes in each of two subsequent sessions to signal his monitoring to the clinician. At this point, the monitoring transferred outside the clinic without further programmed reinforcement and was easily maintained.

Avoidance therapy was needed in three of the 19 cases. The dynamics of avoidance learning have been described extensively elsewhere (Sheehan, 1970; Van Riper, 1973; Starkweather, 1980). In each of these discussions, the author stresses the importance of modifying avoidance before modifying the core behaviors. As Starkweather (1980) says,

An avoidance response, once learned, tends to occur almost indefinitely, regardless of external conditions. The reason for this is that the reinforcement for the response is the nonoccurrence of the aversive event. . . .In stuttering, clients continue to struggle and avoid because each time they use these behaviors they believe that their speech would have been worse had they not done so. Avoidance behavior is automatically self-reinforcing, and this makes it tend to continue, regardless of current conditions (p. 329).

Novak (1975), who further supports the need to modify avoidance, states his finding that the 44 percent of adults who maintained fluency gains a year after treatment had a high incidence of "logophobia" (word fears). In other words they used their fluency management techniques to avoid rather than modify the stuttering.

Our methods of treating word avoidance, based on Sheehan (1970) and Van Riper (1973), demonstrate the high cost of avoiding and train the child to identify instances of word (and/or sound) avoidance in his speech. After learning to identify this avoidance in the clinic, the child's homework consists of observing his use of the behavior and logging it in a notebook (family members write for him if he is too young). During treatment sessions, the child's conversations are tape-recorded, and the clinician transcribes sentences from these to use as examples in which circumlocution obscures meaning. When the client is prepared to handle it, the clinician reads one of the meaningless sentences to the child and asks, "What was this person trying to say?" In one example, a child had said, "I went to, uh, the place and, uh, we had big water there." The clinician and the child finally agreed that "the person" wanted to say, "I went to the beach with Bobby," but was afraid of the [b] words, so the meaning was lost. After 10 or more similar sentences, the child realizes that avoidance ruins conversations, and is then ready to collect examples of words he wants to avoid but doesn't, first in the clinic, then at home or school. Soon after, he comes into a treatment session and announces, "I didn't change any words this week."

Avoidance is then monitored by a simple probe in each of the next six to ten sessions. Sometimes when avoidance modification is complete, we observe a dramatic reduction in core behaviors as well. Probably the reduction of tension during the period of indecision just prior to the stuttered word explains this sort of change.

Simple modification methods were used with five of the twelve children who needed direct modification of abnormal disfluencies. Children who received this type of therapy had relatively mild part-word repetitions, and some had vowel prolongations with little or no tension. All of these children were perceptually free of airflow breaks in their part-word repetitions, and they had no phonatory arrests or articulatory posturing. Their mean SSI score was 8; their range was 5 to 10. We used a binary "easy" versus "hard" description to rate their stuttering events, which is similar to the dichotomy that Williams (1971) describes in his more elaborate system.

We begin the modification by helping the child understand that some incidents of disfluency are harder to cope with than others. Using the child's word for such incidents, words such as "sticking," "stumbling," "blocking," "getting stuck," "bouncing," "bubbling," we ask the child to identify the easy blocks and the hard blocks. Many of the children have learned about normal disfluencies during component modification, so this is a natural extension of that process for them. At first the child just signals that a block is hard or easy, but later we ask him to substitute an easy block for a hard one. The clinician encourages the child to "do it the easy way when you can," and models the two ways for him. If a sentence contains a hard block the child can say it again, deliberately substituting one that is easier for him. This voluntary disfluency provides the child with a sense of control. When the child can use the easy blocks 90 percent of the time, he may need some method of reducing their severity further. He can use a very mild form of whole-syllable repetition to accomplish voluntary bouncing to a degree that is almost a normal disfluency. From these easy, mild repetitions, then, it is a small step to whole-word repetitions with normal coarticulation and rate.

Complex modification, used with seven children, is employed when the stuttering is more severe or resistant to binary treatment. The children needing this program had a mean SSI score of 16 with a range of 11 to 20 after component modification. Age was not a factor in distinguishing the simple and complex groups; the simple group averaged 7.1 years and the complex group averaged 6.3 years. The main criteria for placing a child in complex therapy were the presence of airflow breaks in the part-word repetitions, phonatory arrests, or articulatory postures. The purpose of this particular treatment was to improve airflow and facilitate easy onset and easy transition from one syllable to the next.

A system for accomplishing these goals was described recently by Conture (1982), who uses analogies to help the child visualize where his air-stream is blocked: It is like a "garden hose" that may have water cut off at the faucet (larynx), a kink in the hose (articulators), or at the nozzle (lips). He also employs an analogy of a frog hopping from lilypad to lilypad (syllables) to demonstrate that landing too hard (airflow breaks) or jumping up and down (syllable repetitions) can cause a frog to sink to the bottom. While these analogies seem like excellent cognitive learning tools, they were not available for use with the children under consideration in 1974 through 1980.

We use several means to help the child identify specific airflow disruptions associated with his stuttering. We first describe the blocks verbally; then we ask the child to describe them. When a child is not sure what he is doing with his lips or tongue, we offer a mirror which is usually accepted. Videotaping these sessions facilitates off-line monitoring, which is easier and allows repeated viewing of a certain behavior. Video equipment is not a mandatory part of treatment, however.

Laryngeal blocking is more difficult to visualize, so we have the child feel surface throat muscles with his hands first and learn to identify the feeling of tension inside when the surface muscles tighten. The child should not rush through this identification phase of therapy for he will find it difficult later to modify behaviors he does not understand. When the child is familiar with these details of his stuttering, we move on to modification of the behaviors. A few children seem so anxious to finish their sentences following the stuttering block that they appear to fit Van Riper's (1973) description of the need for fluency as a reward for the struggle. The child's anxiety and intensity are easy to recognize even though exact behavioral criteria are not used. When a child uses this reward of fluency, we remove it by using cancellation. That is, immediately after the stuttered word, we insist on 5 seconds of time-out before we allow him to continue speaking, which separates the struggle behavior from the immediate reward of fluency. For a comprehensive description of cancellation see Van Riper (1973).

In the next phase of treatment we use various methods to initiate and sustain airflow. To reduce tension while initiating a vowel the child starts from a sigh or a yawn, and then tries to keep that same open, relaxed feeling while initiating [ɑː]. He progresses to other isolated vowels, then to single words beginning with vowels, then to phrases with reinforcement from us for easy open onset. When he does block on a vowel, he slides off it by reducing pitch (and tension) as soon as he can gain control. To initiate consonants in an easy, relaxed way the child slights the articulatory contact and uses an open, breathy voice to get into the next vowel. For example, [tu] is produced with light contact between the tongue and the alveolar ridge followed by an aspirated release into the vowel. We use a number of one-syllable words, including words on which the child has stuttered in prior treatment sessions.

Once the child has mastered the skill with single words, he begins to work with phrases. To sustain airflow in phrases, the child can use Conture's (1982) analogy of a frog jumping from lilypad to lilypad in a smooth, even way without landing too hard or stopping to jump up and down. Sometimes, additional instruction to "keep the speech flowing easy" is helpful. The clinician, however, needs to be aware of the child's ability level and response to these various methods to improve airflow in order to select an approach that meets the child's needs. At this point in the treatment process, this kind of selection is easier since the stuttering patterns are usually rather weak and the ability of the clinician to communicate with the child is very strong.

PHYSICAL BEHAVIORS
Recognizing the importance of distracting physical behaviors which often accompany stuttering, we described an approach to their treatment in the *Physical concomitant* section, above.

ATTITUDINAL WORK
Attitude modification is a central goal of our treatment program, and we have described it in previous sections dealing with *Environment modification, Attitude modification,* and *Avoidance therapy.*

TRANSFER AND MAINTENANCE

We use parallel transfer to encourage the child to use each new skill at home and at school as soon as possible. When a skill is stabilized in the clinic setting, we send an age-appropriate assignment to the parents. The children do their assignments for about 5 minutes twice a day. The parents listen to their child perform the assignment and report the results to the clinician. They make judgments which are well within their abilities. Sometimes they receive special training so they can make more specific judgments, but they are never asked to train new skills. We call the system "parallel" because the child transfers each skill as it is learned.

No maintenance program is employed because none of the 54 children on whom this program was tested needed maintenance within 1 year of treatment termination. However, 2 of the 37 children whom we were able to follow for 2 to 4 years relapsed into significant stuttering and they were readmitted for additional direct modification of their abnormal disfluencies.

FOLLOW-UP PROCEDURES

We telephone parents and teachers every 6 months for 2 years after a child terminates treatment. We include all children who have received 24 hours of treatment in this follow-up even if the child was removed before all goals were accomplished. The rationale for this procedure will be explained in the Evaluation of Therapy section of this chapter.

EQUIPMENT AND MATERIALS NEEDED

The clinician using this program does not need any special equipment other than a good audiotape recorder and a stopwatch. Videotaping equipment is very useful but not required. We have recommended certain commercial tests used to assess the stuttering and its components; however, a clinician using other, similar tests will probably get the same results. The components are defined by specific descriptors which are not test bound.

CLINICIAN SKILLS AND TRAINING REQUIRED

In addition to training in the specifics of stuttering behaviors and their treatment, clinicians who plan to use a component model approach need a solid, broad-based education in speech pathology. They need training in the recognition and treatment of communication environment problems, attitude problems, and subtle neurologic dysfunctions.

CLIENT REQUIREMENTS

Children between the ages of 3 and 12 with normal intelligence are candidates for component model stuttering treatment. We have not evaluated the effectiveness of this model with children having severe language disorders, developmental delay, or cerebral palsy. We have used this approach with older children and adults, but they often accommodate and mask out their neurologic components. Upon careful examination, we usually can find residual symptoms of oral motor discoordination or sentence formulation problems. We treat these residual components if they are considered severe enough to interfere with maintenance of fluency. In this age group, basic attitudes of unrealistic expectations are usually complicated by word avoidance and situation avoidance. Additionally, these clients often use their stuttering as a scapegoat for other perceived social inadequecies. Attitude modification is therefore longer and more complex than with younger children. We need further research into the usefulness of a component approach to special subgroups and clients older than 12 years.

Evaluation of the Therapy

RESEARCH STUDIES

In order to assess the effectiveness of using a component based approach to treat stuttering in children, we evaluated 19 children from our private practice caseload in detail. We assessed these children for each component and for stuttering severity when they first began our treatment program, when the components had been modified to the extent that was practical, and when the treatment terminated. We also assessed these 19 children as part of a larger sample (N = 44) 12 months after termination, and again 24 to 48 months after termination.

RESULTS

The ratings of each component at intake and after the component modification phase of treatment are shown in Table 4-4. The "environment" component includes both "disruptive communicative environment" and "unrealistic parental expectations" (see Fig. 4-1). The "attitude" component includes both "high self-expectations by the child" and "manipulative stuttering." Since each of the nine components in Figure 4-1 was rated on a scale of 0 to 4, these areas, reflecting two components with one rating, have a potential range of 0 to 8. All other components in Table 4-4 have a potential range of 0 to 4. The component phase of treatment resulted in ratings from 0.6 to 1.9 which equates with borderline to mild, but note, however, that the standard deviations are large, indicating significant variation. In all areas but one the improvement was about 50 percent. The environmental influences and attitude improved 56 percent on the average with very large standard deviations, but this amount of improvement seems reasonable given the level of intervention that was used. We did not attempt to restructure the child's basic ego defense mechanism nor the family psychodynamics. A deeper level of intervention was necessary in only a few cases where psychological pathology existed

Table 4-4. Clinician Ratings of Components Related to Stuttering in 19 Children Ages 3 to 9 at Intake and After Completion of the Component Modification Phase of Treatment

	Intake		After Completion of Treatment		Improvement	Percent Change	No. Treatment Hours	
	X̄	SD	X̄	SD	X̄		X̄	SD
Environment	3.9	2.3	1.7	1.9	2.2	56.4	6.2	2.9
Attitude	4.3	1.9	1.9	1.6	2.4	55.8	12.4	7.6
Attending	2.8	.7	1.5	1.0	1.3	46.4	7.5	4.5
Oral motor	3.3	1.0	.8	.7	2.5	75.8	14.3	8.5
Auditory processing	2.8	1.1	1.3	1.0	1.5	53.6	10.0	8.2
Sentence formulation	3.0	.8	1.5	.6	1.5	50.0	8.0	4.5

X̄ = mean; SD = standard deviation.

163

in the child and/or in the parents. Only one of the 19 cases had an "abnormal parental need for the child to stutter," and in this case, with the parent refusing psychotherapy, the stuttering therapy failed.

We modified attending an average of 46 percent. The children who benefitted most generally had been placed on an appropriate medication as an adjunct to the behavior modification. Auditory processing and sentence formulation improved 54 and 50 percent respectively, with the resulting averaged ratings of 1.3 and 1.5 indicating borderline to mild problems.

Oral motor discoordination improved an average of 76 percent, progressing from an average rating that indicated a moderately severe problem at intake to a rating that was almost normal after treatment. The most likely explanation for this high level of improvement is that all clinicians had received extensive training in the use of systematic syllable training to improve oral motor functioning, and that there has been a special focus, therefore, on this component.

The severity of stuttering was reduced from 22.8 to 9.9 on the SSI during component treatment, and dropped to 4.3 on the SSI during direct modification of abnormal disfluencies. At the time of termination of treatment, stuttering was reduced by 81.1 percent and was subclinical in almost all cases.

FOLLOW-UP INVESTIGATIONS
Fifty-four children ages 3.8 to 12.8 were treated between 1974 and 1978 using a component based approach. We were able to follow 44 of the 54 children for at least 12 months after termination, and, of this group, we followed 37 for 24 to 48 months.

Previous studies have demonstrated that untrained judges can make fairly reliable decisions regarding the presence or absence of stuttering (McDonald and Martin, 1973; Schiavetti, 1975; Culatta, 1977; Hulit, 1978). Parents are just such intuitive judges unless they have learned to attend too intensely to their child's stuttering. In order to learn to attend less intensely to the stuttering, parents were retrained as part of the environmental modification program. In other words, their intuitive judgments had to be reestablished. In most cases this type of modification was successful. In 2 of the 54 cases the mothers were not able to make reliable judgments so their reports were not used in subsequent research. One of several fathers who themselves were stutterers was prone to rate his child as a "mild stutterer" on speech samples considered normal by the clinician, so his reports were discounted, also.

All follow-up was done by telephone calls which resulted, when necessary, in in-clinic evaluations. The parents and teachers were asked if the child exhibited any stuttering at all. If the response was "yes," the staff member read them the criteria described at the bottom of Table 4-5 and asked them to judge the stuttering "mild" (score 1) or "significant" (score 2 or 3). All children with inconsistent reports or with ratings of

Table 4.5. Treatment Results for Children (ages 3 to 12 and 9 months)
After Completion of a Component Model Based Stuttering Treatment Program

Rating	Number and % at Termination of Treatment (n = 44)		Number and % 12–23 Months Postterm (n = 44)		Number and % 24–48 Months Postterm (n = 37)	
0	8	(18%)	19	(43%)	16	(43%)
1	28	(64%)	18	(41%)	14	(38%)
2	5	(11%)	4	(9%)	3	(8%)
3	3	(7%)	3	(7%)	4	(11%)
4	0		0		0	

Rating criteria
0 = No stuttering reported at home or at school; speech sounds normal.
1 = Mild residual stuttering reported at home or school but it is not considered
a problem by the child or his listeners; speech is otherwise considered normal.
2 = Significant residual stuttering reported at home or at school; confirmed by
clinic examination.
3 = Stuttering was only slightly improved compared to severity at beginning of
treatment.
4 = Stuttering was as severe or more severe after treatment.

"significant" stuttering were evaluated and rated by a staff clinician, and
the authors subsequently reviewed and rated the audiotape.

In Table 4-5, note that 12 children improved from a rating of 1 (mild
residual stuttering) to a rating of 0 (no stuttering) during the 12 months
following treatment; one child improved from a rating of 2 (significant
residual stuttering) to a rating of 1; one child regressed from 0 to 1; and
seven of the children in categories 2 and 3 (only slightly improved from
pretreatment baseline) remained in those categories during the 12 months
after treatment. Between 12 and 24 months after treatment, two children
returned to the clinic for six to eight sessions of additional treatment.
One, who had regressed from a rating of 1 to a rating of 2, was able to
reattain his rating of 1; but the other regressed from a rating of 1 to 3
when he reached age 14, and additional treatment had no measurable
impact on his stuttering.

Overall, children with ratings of 0 or 1 were considered treatment suc-
cesses while those with ratings of 2, 3, or 4 were considered treatment
failures. By this standard, 82 percent of the children were considered
successfully treated at the termination of therapy, 84 percent 1 year later,
and 81 percent 2 to 4 years later.

Reasons for Therapeutic Effectiveness
To examine the reasons for the success or failure of the component approach, we computed correlations between treatment results 2 years after
termination and all other variables. Treatment effectiveness was not related to the child's age nor was it related to the severity of stuttering at

the beginning of therapy. It was related however to the five variables listed below with the Pearson correlations given in parentheses.

1. Severity of stuttering at termination of treatment (.84). That is, the more stuttering could be reduced during treatment, the more likely it was to be rated "0" or "1" two years after treatment was terminated.
2. Severity of attending problems at termination (.80). Children whose attending problems could not be modified were more likely to stutter significantly after treatment.
3. Severity of oral motor discoordination at termination (.58). When the oral motor system was improved so as to be close to normal, the treatment was more likely to be successful.
4. Severity of high self-expectations at termination (.56). Children who could not reduce their unrealistic expectations to be perfect were less likely to succeed in our program.
5. Severity of sentence formulation problems at termination (.54). Children who were able to construct age-appropriate sentences were more likely to maintain their fluency gains.

The level of confidence is beyond .01 in all of the above relationships. In general it seems that those who were unable to reduce their attending, oral motor, self-expectations, or sentence formulation problems adequately during treatment were not able to achieve or maintain normal fluency. Only two of the 37 children who were followed for 2 years or more had actually regressed. The other five "failures" never had achieved adequate fluency.

Considering the number of components treated, the time investment seems economical. The children made progress in areas that helped their receptive language, their expressive language, and their speech output including articulation. The average treatment time was 47.9 hours with a standard deviation of 25.6, and the total number of hours related to the number of hours devoted to oral motor training ($r = .74$; $p = .001$) and direct modification of abnormal disfluencies ($r = .49$; $p = .02$). The total number of hours also related to the severity of unrealistic self-expectation ($r = .68$; $p = .001$), attending problems ($r = .40$; $p = .05$), and oral motor discoordination ($r = 42$; $p = .05$).

The age of the clients was an important factor in evaluating the component approach. Remember that only 20 percent of the 3- and 4-year-olds needed direct modification, but at age 7 and above all the children needed it. Age was *not* related to treatment success either at termination or 2 years later among children 3 through 8, so within this group, age was not critical.

We view stuttering as the product of a system that is, for various reasons, especially vulnerable to a breakdown of fluency. A threshold concept explains the possible relationship of the components fairly well. Imagine that a child inherits a faulty oral motor and/or language system. These problems will, in the threshold concept, lower the resistance to fluency breakdown. Additionally, the child may impose impossible standards on himself for fluent speech and for his performance in general, and environmental disruptors may add other pressures. His neurologic system cannot live up to his standards. Given such a reduced threshold and expectations to be better than he can be, it is easy to see how a child can be pushed over his threshold and stutter at least some of the time. This model explains the conditions for most of our children who stutter. It does not explain, however, the children with neurologic differences that result in oral motor and language problems but not stuttering. Perhaps further analysis of how the stuttering child puts pressure on himself will help explain this dilemma. Jeanna Riley (1983) conducted a study comparing three groups: (1) children with neurologic problems who stutter, (2) children with similar neurologic problems who do not stutter, and (3) normal children. All three groups were tested for evidence of "high self-expectations." The stutterers exhibited significantly higher self-expectations than the other two groups. These results indicate that an emotional component such as unrealistically high self-expectations may trigger stuttering in a vulnerable child.

We think the treatment approach is as effective as it is because it changes the child who stutters and not just the abnormal disfluencies. The child with improved oral motor and language functioning, with less self-imposed pressure, and with a family environment conducive to fluency seems to be in a good position to become and remain normally fluent. The resulting fluency does not need constant monitoring, and it contains normal disfluencies.

Advantages of the Therapy

Component based treatment is multidimensional and therefore the child who completes this type of program is improved in several areas. The child's stuttering is likely to be treated successfully and the possibility of future articulation or language therapy is reduced.

Children can be enrolled in this type of program while they are very young. Early intervention cannot be overemphasized because so much information in the past has advocated a wait-and-see attitude.

Recently, a 6-year-old boy with moderately severe stuttering was brought to our clinic by parents who were told by their physician that "Your child will outgrow his stuttering if you ignore it." As the boy had been stuttering since age 3, they decided to bring him to us anyway. Physicians and some popular literature both advise parents that their child's disfluencies are normal and he will outgrow them. The parents come to the speech pathologist in spite of this advice because they know intuitively that something is wrong. Their intuition usually is correct. Research suggests that about 36 percent of these disfluent children are indeed nonchronic (Glasner and Rosenthal, 1957; Ingham, 1983).

This system of "nonreferral" has resulted in several related problems. First, the parents blame themselves as they try to follow the traditional instruction, "Ignore it, or you will make it worse." The stuttering gets worse anyway. For a recent review of the literature on this problem see Shine (1980). Second, treatment is delayed for 2 to 5 years after the stuttering can be diagnosed as chronic which leads to the next three problems. Third, treatment for school-aged children is more difficult, more lengthy, and usually less effective than for preschool children. Fourth, the child is more likely to suffer socially during school years, as verified by a comparison of our 20 preschoolers with 24 children in grades one through three. Only 5 percent of the preschoolers had experienced serious teasing while 33 percent of the school-aged children had been teased about their stuttering. Fifth, word avoidance (circumlocution) is rare at the preschool level, but common in first- to third-grade stutterers. In the same population referred to above, 15 percent of the preschoolers compared to 46 percent of the primary children had begun using word avoidance to a significant degree. Word avoidance alone can require many hours of treatment (Sheehan, 1970; Van Riper, 1973; Starkweather, 1980).

If every child who exhibits chronic abnormal disfluencies could begin treatment within a few months of stuttering onset, *almost all stuttering could be eliminated before the primary school years.* The possibility of added time and expense is suggested by those who argue for later intervention because some children will receive therapy who would outgrow the stuttering without therapy. These possibilities do not seem to us very persuasive given the benefits described.

As with any approach to treating people who stutter, the road to success is always under construction. We are dealing with a complex system involving various vulnerabilities and sources of breakdown. Since this system is not yet well understood, it seems likely that the component model will undergo many changes. The specifics of each component may be altered, some components may be subdivided, new components may be added and old ones deleted, but all these improvements need not change the fundamental objective. The complexities of each child's stuttering can be described and individualized treatment designed to fit his particular needs.

References

Adams, M. R. Fluency, nonfluency, and stuttering in children. *J. Fluency Disord.* 7: 171–185, 1982.

Andrews, G. Stuttering: A state of the art seminar. Paper presented at the annual convention of the American Speech-Language and Hearing Association, Los Angeles, 1981.

Andrews, G., and Harris, M. *The Syndrome of Stuttering*. London: Heinemann Medical Books, 1964.

Bankson, N. W. *Bankson Language Screening Test*. Baltimore: University Park Press, 1977.

Beech, H. R., and Fransella, F. *Research and Experiment in Stuttering*. Oxford, Eng.: Pergamon Press, 1968.

Berlin, A. J. An exploratory attempt to isolate types of stuttering. Northwestern University Ph. D. Thesis, 1954.

Blaesing, L. A multidisciplinary approach to individualized treatment of stuttering. *J. Fluency Disord.* 7: 203–218, 1982.

Bloodstein, O. The rules of early stuttering. *J. Speech Hear. Disord.* 39: 379–393, 1974.

Burks, H. *Burks Behavior Rating Scales*. Los Angeles: Western Psychological Services, 1969.

Canter, G. J. Observations of neurogenic stuttering: A contribution to differential diagnosis. *Br. J. Disord. Commun.* 6: 139–143, 1971.

Carrow, E. *Carrow Elicited Language Inventory*. Austin, Tex.: Learning Concepts, 1974.

Clark, J. B., and Madison, C. L. *Clark-Madison Test of Oral Language*. Tigard, Ore.: C. C. Publications, 1981.

Conture, E. G. *Stuttering*. Englewood Cliffs, N.J.: Prentice-Hall, 1982.

Culatta, R. A. The acquisition of the label "stuttering" by primary level school children. *J. Fluency Disord.* 2: 29–34, 1977.

Fletcher, S. G. Time-by-count measurement of diadochokinetic syllable rate. *J. Speech Hear. Res.* 15: 763–770, 1972.

Glasner, P., and Rosenthal, D. Parental diagnosis of stuttering in young children. *J. Speech Hear. Disord.*, 22:288–295, 1957.

Graham, J. K., and Brumlik, J. Neurologic and encephalographic abnormalities in stuttering and matched non-stuttering adults (abstract). *ASHA* 3: 342, 1961.

Hall, P. K. The occurrence of disfluencies in language disordered schoolage children. *J. Speech Hear. Disord.* 42: 364–376, 1977.

Hayes, W. O., and Hood, S. B. Disfluency changes in children as a function of systematic modification of linguistic complexity. *J. Commun. Disord.* 11: 79–93, 1978.

Howie, P. M. A twin investigation of the etiology of stuttering. Paper presented at the annual convention of the American Speech-Language and Hearing Association, Houston, 1976.

Hulit, L. M. Interjudge agreement of identifying stuttered words. *Percep. Mo. Skills* 47: 360–362, 1978.

Ingham, R. J. Spontaneous remission of stuttering: When will the emperor realize he has no clothes on? In D. Prins and R. J. Ingham (eds.), *Treatment of Stuttering in Early Childhood*. San Diego: College-Hill Press, 1983.

Kidd, K. K., Heimbuch, R. L., and Records, M. A. Vertical transmission of susceptibility to stuttering with sex-modified expression. *Proceedings of the National Academy of Science* 78: 606–610, 1981.

Kidd, K. K., Kidd, J. R., and Records, M. A. The possible causes of the sex ratio in stuttering and its implications. *J. Fluency Disord.* 3: 13–23, 1978.

Kirk, S. A., McCarthy, J. J., and Kirk, W. D. *The Illinois Test of Psycholinguistic Abilities* (rev. ed.). Urbana: University of Illinois Press, 1968.

McDonald, E. *Articulation Testing and Treatment: A Sensory-Motor Approach*. Pittsburgh: Stanwix House, 1964.

McDonald, J. D., and Martin, R. R. Stuttering and disfluency as two reliable and unambiguous response classes. *J. Speech Hear. Res.* 16: 691–699, 1973.

Novak, A. Results of the treatment of severe forms of stuttering in adults. *Folia Phoniat.* 27: 278–252, 1975.

Perkins, W. et al. Stuttering: Discoordination of phonation with articulation and respiration. *J.Speech Hear. Res.* 19: 509–522, 1976.

Preus, A. *Attempts at Identifying Subgroups of Stutterers.* Oslo, Norway: University of Oslo Press, 1981.

Riley, G. *Stuttering Severity Instrument.* Tigard, Ore.: C. C. Publications, 1980.

Riley, G. *Stuttering Prediction Instrument.* Tigard, Ore.: C. C. Publications, 1981.

Riley, G., and Riley, J. Clinical sub-types of stuttering among 100 children. Paper presented at the annual convention of the American Speech-Language and Hearing Association, San Francisco, 1972.

Riley, G., and Riley, J. A component model for diagnosing and treating children who stutter. *J. Fluency Disord.* 4: 279–293, 1979.

Riley, G., and Riley, J. Motoric and linguistic variables among children who stutter: A factor analysis. *J. Speech Hear. Disord.* 45: 504–514, 1980.

Riley, J. *A causal-comparative study of psychological behaviors in stutterers and nonstutterers who exhibit organic factors.* California Graduate Institute Ph. D. Thesis, 1983.

Schiavetti, N. Judgments of stuttering severity as a function of type and locus of disfluency. *Folia Phoniatr.* 27: 26–37, 1975.

Sheehan, J. G. *Stuttering Research and Therapy.* New York: Harper & Row, 1970.

Shine, R. E. Direct management of the beginning stutterer. *Semin. Speech Lang. Hear.* 1: 339–350, 1980.

Starkweather, C. W. A multiprocess behavioral approach to stuttering therapy. *Semin. Speech Lang. Hear.* 1: 327–337, 1980.

Van Riper, C. *Treatment of Stuttering.* Englewood Cliffs, N.J.: Prentice-Hall, 1973.

Van Riper, C. *Nature of Stuttering* (2nd ed.). Englewood Cliffs, N.J.: Prentice-Hall, 1982.

Wall, M. J. A comparison of syntax in young stutterers and nonstutterers. *J. Fluency Disord.* 5: 321–326, 1980.

Wall, M. J., Starkweather, C. W. and Cairns, H. S. Syntactic influences on stuttering in young children. *J. Fluency Disord.* 6: 283–298, 1981.

Williams, D. E. Stuttering therapy for children. In L. E. Travis (ed.), *Handbook of Speech Pathology.* Englewood Cliffs, N.J.: Prentice-Hall, 1971.

Williams, D. E. Differential diagnosis of disorders of fluency. In F. L. Darley and D. C. Spriestersbach, *Diagnostic Methods in Speech Pathology.* New York: Harper & Row, 1978.

Appendix 4-A. Physical Concomitants Form

Physical Concomitants

Evaluating scale
0 = none; 1 = not noticeable unless looking for it; 2 = barely noticeable to casual observer; 3 = distracting; 4 = very distracting; 5 = severe and painful-looking

Distracting sounds	Noisy breathing, whistling, sniffing, blowing, clicking sounds	0 1 2 3 4 5
Facial grimaces	Jaw jerking, tongue protruding, lip pressing, jaw muscles tense	0 1 2 3 4 5
Head movements	Back, forward, turning away, poor eye contact, constant looking around	0 1 2 3 4 5
Movements of the extremities	Arm and hand movement, hands about face, torso movement, leg movements, foot tapping or swinging	0 1 2 3 4 5

Total physical concomitant score

Source: G. Riley, *Stuttering Severity Instrument*. Tigard, Ore.: C. C. Publications, 1980.

5. Assessment and Fluency Training with the Young Stutterer

Richard E. Shine

Overview

This chapter describes a direct fluency training approach for managing young stuttering children (aged 3 to 12), emphasizing the rationale that the earlier the intervention the better the prognosis for success. Assessment procedures include an operational definition of stuttering in which stuttering disfluencies are differentiated from nonstuttering disfluencies, a comprehensive assessment protocol as well as a technique for self-training and the training of significant others to assess stuttering. Parent counseling techniques and fluency training procedures and activities give specific guidelines for developing an effective environmental program, defining the criteria for success and failure, and also organizing the steps and activities involved in establishing, transferring, and maintaining fluency. These assessment and fluency training procedures evolved from success with the beginning stutterers for more than 16 years. A 5-year follow-up study of this direct fluency training approach reveals that young children are able to establish and maintain normally fluent speaking patterns with rare instances of recurrent stuttering.

History of the Therapy

The rationale for this fluency training approach can be traced to the academic/philosophic training of my undergraduate and master's degree programs, specifically to the curriculum developed by Verne Ahlberg (1961). The curriculum emphasized the works of forerunners in our profession who could now be deemed ahead of their time, given our current knowledge of stuttering. Among these were both researchers and clinicians (Avery, Dorsey, and Sickels, 1928; Travis, 1931; West, Kennedy, and Carr, 1937; Berry, 1937, 1938; West, Nelson, and Berry, 1939; Berry and Eisenson, 1942; Backus, 1943; Backus and Beasley, 1951). Backus (1943), who presented a rationale for understanding stuttering that proved to be predictive of current research data, did not concern herself with theories that proposed stuttering as a learned behavior, a neurosis or psychosis, an emotional or psychological problem, or a neurologic problem, but rather stressed the importance of "known facts" quoted from her textbook as follows:

1. Stuttering is a disorder of childhood. 2. More boys than girls stutter. 3. Stuttering has certain hereditary aspects. 4. Stutterers as a class do not differ in respect to

mental ability. 5. The so-called speech organs are just as normal structurally in stutterers as in nonstutterers. The organs perform just as normally their basic functions of chewing, sucking, swallowing, sobbing, smiling, etc. 6. The stutterer's articulatory muscles show a slowness of diadochokinesis. In repetitive movement of the jaws, brows, etc., he cannot move these muscles as fast, as continuously, or as independently to one side or the other, as a nonstutterer can. 7. The proportion of certain chemical elements in the blood is found to be different in stutterers as a class from nonstutterers as a class. 8. During a stuttering block, a serious disorganization of the integrating centers of the central nervous system takes place. 9. A relationship between laterality and the occurrence of stuttering has been demonstrated to exist, if not in all stutterers, at least in many. 10. There is also the possibility of what has been called lack of vertical dominance associated with stuttering. The higher center for integration of the central nervous system is the cerebral cortex. The next lower center is the thalamus and striate bodies, which control emotional responses. Still lower centers exist. Ordinarily, the cerebral cortex is in control of voluntary motor activity. It may be, however, that for some reason the thalamic or even lower centers suddenly grasp control and, thus, interfere with the normal integration of cortical action. 11. Marked differences in the breathing pattern of stutterers have long been noted. Since these anomalies have been quite clearly demonstrated as reactions to the stuttering blocks rather than causes for them, attempts to change these patterns through breathing exercises have been mostly discarded. 12. Stutterers exhibit a lack of vocal inflection. This is due probably to their reduced ability to make rapid shifts in movement between sets of muscles, as required for the process that we call fluctuation in pitch. It may account, in part, also for the fact that most stutterers can sing without the occurrence of blocks or spasms. 13. Bilingualism has been shown to be an irritating factor in many clinical cases (Backus, 1943, pp. 202-206).

The above information is humbling if one considers that the profession has taken almost 40 years to provide evidence that supports what were viewed as "known facts" in the late 1930s and early 1940s.

Even though my undergraduate and master's degree training emphasized that theories of stuttering were not empirically substantiated and that "known facts" and empirically tested clinical procedures were most important to the effective clinician, my own initial beliefs, derived from the literature of the late 1950s and 1960s, were as follows: (1) Young children (aged 3 to 6 years or even 8 years of age) were normally nonfluent. (2) Stuttering did not become a problem until it was diagnosed, usually by a well-meaning mother or significant other. (3) The primary method of treatment was an indirect approach directed primarily at the child's disrupted environment. A colleague and I even wrote the following statement in a speech improvement text for classroom teachers: "It can truthfully be said that the way to treat a young stutterer in the primary stage is to let him alone, and treat his parents and teachers," (Shine and Freilinger, 1962). My beliefs changed, however, as a result of clinical experience in the schools and I quickly returned to known facts and empirically tested clinical procedures that were emphasized in my university training program.

INCEPTION OF THE CLINICAL MANAGEMENT PROCEDURE
The primary motivation to develop direct rather than indirect fluency training procedures for the beginning stutterer stemmed from two experiences I had in the fall of 1964. Just before the beginning of school, a mother of a 4-year-old boy requested a stuttering evaluation. My beliefs at that time dictated that, following the evaluation, I would counsel the mother to avoid calling attention to the nonfluencies, to be patient, to listen attentively, to keep the environment calm, and provide her with a list of do's and don'ts.

During the evaluation the child exhibited severe stuttering behavior characterized by whole-word and part-word repetitions, numerous prolongations, struggle behaviors (such as silent and phonated blocking, head jerking, increased pitch and intensity, and so on). During one such stuttering block (struggle behavior), the child turned to his mother and said fluently, "Why can't I talk right?" I was shocked, first by the child's severe stuttering that could not be mistaken for normal nonfluency, and second by his realization that he had trouble talking. Needless to say, my typical counseling approach was inappropriate as the child contradicted most of the basic beliefs that I held about the beginning stutterer; and following this experience, I began to challenge the ideas presented in the literature and to question my own interpretations of them.

Two months later I met a kindergarten child who not only became the impetus for the development of direct fluency training procedures, but actually helped evolve them during clinical treatment sessions. In 1964 I was working as a speech and hearing clinician in the Scott County, Iowa public schools. At the beginning of that year, we screened all kindergarten children in the county for any articulation, voice, stuttering, and language problems to facilitate development of a classroom speech improvement program that would best fulfill the specific needs of each child. One 5-year-old child, J.U., passed the screening which included counting; identification of 15 pictures, necessitating the use of all English consonants; telling name, address and phone number; and reciting a nursery rhyme, poem, or other memorized material. I evaluated J.U. as having no communicative disorder which resulted in the teacher's question, "What about his stuttering?" Imagine my embarrassment in realizing that I had failed to identify what must have been an obvious stuttering problem, for in a reevaluation the child was found to have a moderate but handicapping stuttering disorder. The fact that J.U. was fluent during rote speaking behaviors, single picture identification, and repetition of phrases suggested the basic aspects of the approach that eventually emerged. I worked with J.U. for 30 minutes 2 times per week and he was able to overcome his stuttering by the end of the school year (7 months). Follow-up evaluations for 2 years and periodic contact with the mother for an additional 3 years, revealed that he had maintained normally fluent speaking patterns. Underlying the clinical procedures of the program that emerged were the "fundamental principles of good speech," which were developed by Backus (1943) and Backus and Beasley (1951) and perfected later by Ahlberg (1961). The treatment rationale required the use of connected speech and emphasized (1) voice and diction (a clear, resonant vocal quality and obvious firm articulation); (2) breath groupings (use of appropriate speech breathing patterns and length of breath groups); (3) smooth flow of speech and voice (the blending of words, somewhat characteristic of continuous vocal phonation but with appropriate intonation and near normal rate patterns, and the prolongation of voiced consonant continuants (VCCs) at the ends of syllables and words); and (4) effective prosodic patterns (appropriate use of strong/weak forms which include articles, prepositions, conjunctions, pronouns, auxiliary verbs, and adverbs to enhance the meaning and effectiveness of communication by facilitating appropriate syllable stress, intonation, and rhythm of speaking). Student clinicians in courses taught by Ahlberg (1961) were required to achieve mastery of these speaking patterns and subsequently model them for clients.

The actual fluency training procedure, then, incorporated the "fundamental principles of good speech" into speech activities that controlled both the spontaneity and the length and complexity of utterances. The basic assumption was that young children could speak fluently if they (1) changed their speaking patterns significantly (primarily reducing rate and intensity and emphasizing widely variable intonation patterns while maintaining relatively normal stress patterns); (2) controlled the length and complexity of verbal responses; and (3) focused initially on imitative responses. We found that children with severe stuttering problems were, nevertheless, able to identify single pictures and imitate from one to four phrases without stuttering by speaking quietly and slowly. As a result we devised a syntax oriented procedure with activities built around pictures, story books, picture matching, and a "surprise box" (tin canister filled with toys and objects). The fluency training procedure proved successful with preschool and young school-age children in the 10 years before its initial emergence as a clinical training manual in 1974; and with its increasing acceptance from public schools and other clinical programs, it eventually was published (Shine, 1980b).

DEVELOPMENT OF THE THERAPY
The original therapy procedure grew out of the need for direct intervention (fluency training) with the beginning stutterer. It was my belief, as well as that of others (Glasner, 1970; Van Riper, 1971) that the earlier the intervention with any communicative disorder, the better the prognosis would be for success. Because I viewed stuttering as a coordinative disorder and had no fear of exacerbating the problem by helping the child

speak in a more acceptable way, I pursued a direct approach. I reasoned that having worked successfully with preschool children who have other communicative disorders, I could work with preschool stutterers as well; and almost 16 years of experience working with the preschool stutterer has revealed that the young stutterer is no different from any other young child with a communicative disorder. Direct intervention, which for lack of a better way to express it, appreciates the "whole child" (personal, social, physical . . .), has proved beneficial and in no way harmful to the preschool stutterer. What is more, clinical experience has demonstrated without a shred of doubt that direct fluency training (which historically has been referred to as "calling attention to the speech/stuttering/problem") is actually necessary for the beginning stutterer. Children who speak differently from their peers are aware of that difference extremely early in life, and even a 3-year-old child with an obvious stuttering problem (a problem which calls attention to itself) will realize that he talks differently from his peers and be ready to receive help. This does not suggest that either parents or clinicians should ever overtly label a child as a stutterer, but it does require that we convey to the child that we are going to help change the way he talks, explaining that there are acceptable and unacceptable ways of speaking, not only in the clinic but outside it as well. We can expect the child to change his manner of talking and thereby establish fluency initially in the clinic and gradually transfer fluent speaking patterns to other environments.

The formalized clinical approach (Shine, 1980b) resulted from 16 years of clinical experience with beginning stutterers, knowledge of stuttering literature and related areas, and repeated input from colleagues and graduate students in training. The approach evolved from the view that stuttering is neither a learned behavior nor a symptom of a deep inner neurosis or psychosis caused by emotional or psychological problems or by environmental interpersonal pressures, stresses or conflicts, but is, in fact, a coordinative disorder resulting from a predisposing neurophysiologic difference which may be genetic or the result of prenatal, natal, or neonatal complications (Shine, 1976, 1980a). In general, the predisposition may be neuromotor (a preprogramming-based motor deficit) or neurolinguistic (a language-based deficit) or more likely a combination of both.

Recent literature has acknowledged differences between stuttering and normally fluent individuals, such as "faulty monitoring" (Toscher and Rupp, 1978) and "faulty motor programming" (McFarlane and Prins, 1978); and hemispheric processing differences have emerged for both auditory and visual stimuli (Jasper, 1932; Moore, 1976; Plakosh, 1978). A contemporary hypothesis is that the stuttering individual may tend to rely on the right hemisphere (a nonsegmental processor) in order to process incoming auditory stimuli and to program (motorically) outgoing segmental linguistic units (Zimmerman and Knott, 1974; Sussman and MacNeilage, 1975; Yeudall, Moore and Boberg, 1982; Moore, Craven and Faber, 1982).

A logical deduction from current research is that fluency results from changes in manner of speaking; however, it would seem that if numerous speaking conditions do bring about fluency, that fluency probably is not simply the result of a modification in the acoustic, physiologic, aerodynamic, linguistic, or motoric speaking variables but, more likely, is the result of more central neurologic integration processes which govern fluent speaking behavior. One might conjecture that such central neurologic integration generates an interactive hemispheric balance which could involve primarily a harmonious interaction between the basic rhythm assignment (right hemisphere) and the complex aspects of neuromotor preplanning that are absolutely necessary for the maintenance of fluency. Thus, the system breakdown (stuttered speech) reflected in the acoustic aerodynamic parameters of speaking may be hierarchically related to the central processes of rhythm assignment and speech-motor preplanning and integration. This discussion has been directly influenced by the work of Logue (1983) who has formed conjectures about the central neurologic relationship between stuttering and developmental forms of dyspraxia of speech and nonfluent forms of anterior aphasia.

Assessment Procedures

Assessment may be defined as a process involving tabulation and notation of specified observations of behaviors in representatively selected environments, i.e., picture identification and selection, story telling, conversation, reading, and monologue. The statement by Backus (1943), ". . . observation is most fruitful when one knows clearly what to look for," appears simple but in reality is profound and critical in the assessment of communicative disorders. In assessing stuttering, the most critical aspect is to define stuttering operationally, that is, to know clearly what to look for.

OPERATIONAL DEFINITION OF STUTTERING

Ryan's (1974) operational definition of stuttering, based on the works of Johnson (1959), lists four identifiable types of stuttered words: (1) whole-word repetitions (WW) such as, "and-and," or "he-he"; (2) part-word repetitions (PW) such as, "lo-lo-lo-look", or "wo-wo-would"; (3) prolongations (PROL) such as, "ffffffun," or wwwwwwwwwent"; and (4) struggle behaviors (SB) that include any type of fluency disrupter that also involves muscle tension or associated physical concomitants, typically referred to as secondary behaviors (e.g., protrusion of the lips, stoppage of airflow, and inability to initiate phonation in attempting to produce the "w" in the word "went"). In addition Ryan's (1974) operational definition or classification system of stuttering reflects a *general hierarchy of severity* in which the primary type of stuttering exhibited by an individual were whole-word repetitions as the predominant stuttering behavior indicate a mild stuttering disorder, part-word repetitions and prolongations imply a moderate range of stuttering, and struggle behaviors suggest a severe disorder.

STUTTERING DISFLUENCIES VERSUS NONSTUTTERING DISFLUENCIES
As stated by Ryan (1974), the basic behavioral units to be identified are "the stuttered word and the fluent word," for in essence, one must be able to differentiate stuttering disfluencies from nonstuttering disfluencies. Numerous authors, including Van Riper (1973), Ryan (1974), and Wingate (1976), have stated that pauses, interjections, revisions, incomplete phrases and phrase repetitions are *nonstuttering disfluencies* and "are not counted as stuttering except in instances of 'starter devices' or in instances when the disfluencies are combined with oral muscular tensions that result in facial grimaces, increased pitch, intensity, and/or fixed oral postures (all identifiable as struggle behaviors—secondary behaviors)" (Shine, 1980a).

OBJECTIVES OF ASSESSMENT
Rather than attempting to determine whether the child is "normally non-fluent" (sic), the primary objectives, in the assessment of the beginning stutterer are (1) to differentiate the fluent words and nonstuttering disfluencies from the stuttering disfluencies (WW, PW, PROL, SB); (2) to determine the rate and severity of stuttering (stuttered words and syllables per minute, percentage of stuttered words out of total words spoken, and types of stuttered words); and (3) to determine the need for, and nature of, intervention by professionals, significant others (primary caretaker/s), or both, based on the overall comprehensive evaluation and the parent interview and interpretive summary. The need for and nature of intervention are not predetermined by a *theory* of stuttering but rather are determined from evaluation results, parent input, and the child's feelings and awareness (when discernible), combined with data-based criteria that specify ranges of normal fluency, borderline/at-risk stuttering, and handicapping stuttering.

EQUIPMENT AND MEASUREMENTS
Stopwatch and Tape Recorder
A stopwatch with a silent *on* and *off* switch or a digital display and a tape recorder are mandatory for assessment and treatment. We use the stopwatch to measure "talking time," to determine stuttered-word and speaking rates, and to calculate measurements; the tape recorder enables verbatim transcripts to be made that confirm rate and severity of stuttering and monitor the clinician's modeled speaking patterns during fluency training.

Talking Time (TT)
The actual time that the patient is talking includes all stuttering behavior such as prolongations and silent and phonated struggle behaviors ("blocking"). Talking time does not include prolonged pauses for thinking but generally will include quick pauses for inhalation. To make calculations (for the rate of stuttering, speaking rate, and so forth), record the exact TT in minutes and seconds and then convert the minutes and seconds into decimals. If, for example, the child talked for 2 minutes, 30 seconds, the TT would be 2.5 minutes (30 divided by 60); 2 minutes, 19 seconds would be 2.3 minutes (19 divided by 60), and so on.

Verbatim Transcript
During the course of the evaluation we identify the child's most representative connected speech sample including examples of his types of stuttered words, frequency, and severity of stuttering. We complete a 200-word verbatim transcript noting all stuttering (WW, PW, PROL, SB) and nonstuttering disfluencies (pauses, interjections, revisions, incomplete phrases, and phrase repetitions); breath groupings; and unintelligible utterances within the written copy. The duration of each instance of stuttering is recorded in seconds when that duration is significant for a particular client, and struggle behaviors are concisely described (see sample transcript in Appendix 5-A).

THE NEED FOR TRAINING
Previous experience in conducting staff development conferences has revealed that experienced, certified speech clinicians (as a group) obtain poor interjudge reliability scores in their identification of stuttered words for they tend to use a variety of standards for assessment that stem primarily from their previous academic training but which have evolved as well from self-training during clinical experience. While the issue concerning how to make reliable and valid judgements of stuttering has not yet been resolved in the literature, the following procedures, as outlined by Ryan and Van Kirk (1973), have proved overwhelmingly successful in training practicing clinicians, student clinicians, parents, and significant others.
Self-Training and Training Significant Others
In order to develop abilities for reliably and rapidly assessing stuttering, the following procedure for self-training is suggested:

1. Develop the ability to intellectually identify the four types of stuttered words and to differentiate stuttered words from nonstuttering disfluencies.
2. Videotape or audiotape 3 to 5 minutes of a young stuttering child's connected speech.

3. Play back the tape and select a section that includes approximately 200 words of the patient's most significant stuttering and demonstrates type, rate and severity. With some children two or three excerpts may be necessary in order to obtain a representative sample of 200 words.
4. Play back the selected sample. Identify and tally (⟡⟡ ⟡⟡ //) the number of stuttered words while using your stopwatch to record "talking time." Then, note the exact talking time in minutes and seconds and convert seconds to decimals.
5. Replay the selected sample a second time, write out a verbatim transcript (see sample transcript in Appendix 5-A).
6. From the verbatim transcript, identify and total the exact number of WW repetitions, PW repetitions, PROL, and SB; then compare this total with the total obtained in #4.

If the two totals of stuttered words are within plus or minus 1 of each other and you have made no fewer than 20 repeated judgments, your reliability can be considered excellent (at least for the one comparison). The validity is more difficult to determine, however, as it depends on whether you identified the same words as stuttered on both occasions and whether your identifications were truly stuttered words. While your totals may be the same or within plus or minus 1 of each other, your identification of the same stuttered words on each occasion may actually conflict as much as plus or minus 5, thus indicating poor validity. Such disagreement would result from not knowing which words are actually stuttered.

7. Replay the selected sample a third time and while listening to and reading the transcript, determine talking time.

A comparison of talking time with that determined in #4 will indicate any significant differences and a need for more practice. Stringent criteria have established repeated measures of talking time as reliable and valid if they are within plus or minus 10 seconds for a 200-word sample and plus or minus 5 seconds for a sample of 100 words.

Once the self-training is complete, the clinician is ready to undertake the training of significant others (parents, teachers, other clinicians, students) and may either develop materials or use the tape and manual included in the *Fluency Training Kit* (Shine, 1980b) to facilitate this instruction. The following procedure has proved effective with both individuals and groups:

1. Provide trainee(s) with an operational definition and examples of each type of stuttering behavior.

2. Read a transcript, imitating realistically each type of stuttered word; and ask trainee(s) to identify and tally each stuttered word.
3. After completion of scoring, write each trainee's total number of stuttered words on a chalkboard to demonstrate the possible range of disagreement among trainees and to compare with the actual number in the transcript.
4. Answer questions and review the types of stuttering.
5. Reread the transcript, and ask the trainee(s) to identify each stuttered word orally as WW, PW, PROL, or SB.
6. Repeat steps 1 through 5 with a second transcript and steps 1 through 4 with a third transcript for additional practice.
7. Reread the third transcript, this time asking the trainee(s) to score the stuttered words according to type by placing a tally mark under the appropriate heading (WW, PW, PROL, SB) across the top of the page. Then, provide additional training as necessary.

GENERAL ASPECTS OF ASSESSMENT
Talk to the parent or significant other prior to the evaluation to identify topics that are of interest to the child and likely to induce spontaneous talk when introduced (or mentioned) to him during the evaluation. Then during the evaluation, do not adhere vigorously to a structured assessment format, but rather maintain an informal atmosphere that will promote talking. If the child begins verbalizing when he should be naming a picture or repeating phrases, encourage the talk by remaining silent (which may actually prompt the child to continue talking) or by responding with stimulating facial expressions and comments.

Throughout the entire evaluation, the clinician's role is to observe and write down the following information: the types of stuttered words evidenced, the duration of each significant stuttering instance, the descriptions of struggle behaviors noting all physical concomitants, the body posture, the hand preference and gestures, extraneous sounds, breathing patterns, and phrasing. The clinician should also note any differences between the behaviors exhibited during fluency and those in evidence during stuttering, i.e., during fluent speech normal breath groupings are observed but during stuttering the patterns are aberrant. In order to time the durations of the longest instances of stuttering, with a reliable degree of accuracy, look at the stopwatch to note the position of the second hand as soon as the child begins stuttering (particularly during prolongations and struggle behaviors) and again as the stuttering terminates. Make note of the duration on the score form with a brief comment as to the type of stuttering and the physical concomitants involved (i.e., head jerk, closed eyes, lips pursed—which you may indicate as hd jk, clsd ey, lps prsd). Parents ought to observe a significant part of the evaluation in order to verify if the frequency and severity of stuttering exhibited during the evaluation were typical of the child's stuttering in his environment.

Many times the severity of stuttering is less severe during the evaluation because the child changes his physiologic speaking patterns and uses numerous short responses and phrases. If the parents are not available during the evaluation, they may evaluate the stuttering from your audiotape.

Generally we schedule a minimum of 1 hour to complete all assessment procedures (stuttering, language, phonology, and hearing screening), including the cursory tabulations of pertinent data, i.e., rate, percentage and severity of stuttering. The average time to administer all test procedures to the child is approximately 45 minutes, although the amount of time will vary according to how responsive and talkative the child is. An additional 15 to 30 minutes should be scheduled to conduct the post-evaluation conference with the parent or other individual.

ASSESSMENT INSTRUMENTS AND PROTOCOL

The following assessment instruments and protocol (which reflect inputs from many professionals) were developed over a period of 5 years during which clinical evaluations were completed on approximately 30 children between 2 years, 4 months, and 8 years, 5 months of age.

The overall design of the assessment protocol provides "checks and balances" to increase the likelihood of obtaining the true rate and severity of stuttering, and it is comprehensive because no one instrument alone is considered either infallible or ideal in revealing the true rate or severity of stuttering. The goal of assessment is to obtain spontaneous connected speech samples which reflect the rate and severity of the child's stuttering. If, for example, a child initiates conversation during imitative responses the clinician ought to encourage him to continue since these spontaneous utterances ordinarily amount to longer, more complex utterances with the most varied rate of speaking, which in turn result in the greatest degree of stuttering.

We are currently using the assessment protocol with children between 2 and 12 years of age and, with some revision of the stimulus materials, even with young teenage children. We administer the assessment protocol during pretest, posttest, maintenance, and follow-up testing (Shine, 1980b) and include the following: (1) The History of the Stuttering Problem, (2) The Rate of Stuttering Instrument, (3) The Stuttering Severity Instrument, (4) The Comprehensive Stuttering Analysis, (5) The Physiologic Speaking Processes Analysis, (6) The Parent/Child Communicative Interaction, (7) Other Assessment Procedures, and (8) The Parent Interview and Interpretive Summary.

History of the Stuttering Problem

The history is used to initiate the interview following assessment and is designed to elicit specific information regarding the onset and development of stuttering, familial history of stuttering or other communicative

disorders, and whatever action parents and others, including professionals, have taken to "help" the child overcome the stuttering. As the
clinician takes notes the parents are encouraged to comment further or
make additional inquiries; they are asked to provide as many examples
as possible of the child's problem.

Rate of Stuttering Instrument (RSI)

The RSI (Shine, 1980b), adapted from a similar procedure developed by
Ryan (1974) provides for the assessment of the stuttered word rate in a
variety of speaking behaviors including rote and imitative responses,
single picture identification, reading (when the material used is 3 grades
below the child's reading level), monologue, conversation, asking and answering questions, and communicative interactions with the parent or
other significant person. We then compute talking time and stuttered
words per minute (SW/M) for each of the following: reading (if applicable),
monologue, conversation, parent/child interaction, and overall SW rate.

Stuttering Severity Instrument (SSI)

The SSI (Riley, 1980), which is designed for both readers and nonreaders,
yields a single numerical task score of stuttering severity that is based
on standardization with 109 children and that falls within a range of 0
to 45, very mild to very severe. The determination of severity results from
(1) the frequency (percentage) of stuttered words (in which the range of
the task scores are 4 to 18), (2) the average length of the three longest
"blocks" or instances of stuttering (with a range of task scores that are
1 to 7), and (3) the observed physical concomitants (in which the range
of task scores are 0 to 20). Detailed instructions which are a part of the
evaluation instrument suggest that severity be determined on the basis
of 100 words obtained from a 150-word sample in which the first and
last 25 words are discarded; but in administering this instrument, we
have found it beneficial to obtain at least a 250-word sample of connected
speech that is fairly representative of the child's severity; we then analyze
the most representative continuous sample of 200 words.

In deriving the results we compute the percentage of stuttered words
from the 200-word sample, but establish the duration of the three longest
instances of stuttering and the physical concomitants from notes taken
throughout the entire evaluation. We suggest that this procedure seems
to provide a more realistic estimate of severity than one that determines
duration and physical concomitants from one sample of only 100 words.

The SSI, complete with manual, forms, and stimulus materials, is a
quick and easily administered procedure which in my more than 10 years
of clinical experience has provided valid and functional estimates of severity.

Comprehensive Stuttering Analysis (CSA)
The primary objectives of the CSA (Shine, 1980b) are (1) to attain additional descriptive data that are pertinent in diagnosis and remediation of stuttering, (2) to validate data collected with other test instruments, (3) to provide a basis for assessing physiologic speaking processes, prosody, and mean length and complexity of utterance, and (4) to quantify observations concerning the patient's overall effectiveness of communication (inclusive and exclusive of stuttering behaviors).

The CSA provides for the assessment of stuttered word and syllable rates, percentage of stuttered words, syllable and word rates of speaking, and frequency of each type of stuttered word. Computation of the mean length of utterance was added to the CSA following the statement by Adams (1980) that a child could be fluent during testing, by using a decreased length of utterance to maintain fluency. This is a logical conclusion as clinical experience has indicated that some children, who eventually were diagnosed as having severe stuttering problems, evidenced mild or moderate stuttering in the initial evaluation when they used primarily short utterances and never engaged in any prolonged, spontaneous, connected speech.

In completing the CSA, obtain a connected speech sample (from the tape of the entire evaluation) of at least 250 words, and from this select a sample of exactly 100 or 200 words that accurately reflects the patient's most involved stuttering behavior with regard to rate, severity, and type of stuttering. The selected sample will almost always be the patient's most spontaneous speaking behavior. Some children exhibit several such episodes during an evaluation, whereas others may do so only once or infrequently at best. Occasionally we have obtained samples from parent/child interaction, spontaneous interaction following the patient's imitation of a sentence during administration of the RSI, and so forth.

Once the spontaneous connected speech sample has been selected, transcribe the passage verbatim using the following guidelines: (1) Phonetically transcribe (narrow transcription, including diacritic markings) all stuttered words; (2) Include prolongations, specifically the phone that is prolonged, and note the duration in seconds; (3) Describe each struggle behavior in detail and note duration of each; (4) Indicate pauses and, if possible, note the pauses with and without inspiration. The use of a lavaliere microphone which can be attached to the child's clothing will sometimes reveal obvious speech breathing patterns as well as other inspirations and noisy exhalations. The notation of pauses will assist in determining length and functional appropriateness of phrasing and in some instances, breath groupings. (5) As part of the transcript, include detailed descriptive information of all physiologic speaking processes, tensions, and aberrations to assist in determining the type and severity of stuttering, the communicative effectiveness, the need for direct clinical intervention, and the nature of intervention. For example, one patient experienced particular difficulty in initiating phonation following a voiceless plosive and occasionally in initiating phonation on voiced plosives. Stoppage of air flow (silent blocking and tense silent pauses) was characteristic of the patient's stuttering/speaking patterns. Knowledge of the problems the patient was having in using correct phonatory, respiratory, and prosodic patterns enabled us to direct therapy toward exaggerated, prolonged durations of initial syllables—gentle onset (Webster, 1974)—of selected words initiated with plosives.

Physiologic Speaking Processes (PSP)and Analysis
The assessment of respiration, phonation, and articulation/resonance (RPA/R) implies the need to evaluate prosodic speaking variables such as stress, intonation, rate/rhythm (SIR). Assessment of the speaking variables begins with the child's first utterance (whether in the test room or some other environment) and is continued throughout the evaluation as observed behaviors are documented. The evaluation will address the use of RPA/A and SIR for both stuttered and fluent speaking behaviors, and a comparison of the fluent and stuttered utterances may actually serve to distinguish critical differences between the variables. Inadequacies noted during stuttering but not during fluent speech suggest that while the stuttering causes a functional breakdown, the physiologic speaking processes are generally intact. Such information may support the view that stuttering involves a generalized neurologic dysfunction.

1. *Phonatory Process.* *Phonation* refers to the production of voice, whereas *phonatory process* refers to the behaviors necessary for control of breathstream in the production of voiced and voiceless phones and during the production of sequential language. Phonatory process problems apparent in young stuttering children include: stoppage of airflow; hard glottal attacks and stops; tonic laryngeal patterns in which the vocal folds are "locked together" or in which the individual is unable to get the vocal folds together to initiate phonation; changes in pitch that are too high or too low; and glottal fry and monotone.

2. *Respiratory Process.* In addition to the respiratory aspects considered in the discussion of phonatory process, the inspiratory/expiratory speech breathing patterns of the individual demand separate assessment for normalcy and aberration during both fluent speech and stuttered utterances. Respiratory process problems include speaking on supplemental air, clavicular breathing, prolonged inspiration, audible inspiration, prolonged expiration prior to initiating speaking behavior, and the like. Assessment of respiratory function for speech purposes must be completed without the knowledge of the speaker,

for a comment such as "take a deep breath" almost always elicits unnatural respiratory effort from the patient. One way to assess speech breathing patterns, however, is to have the child count to 10 or higher (depending on his breath grouping abilities) five times in a row pausing between respirations long enough only to inhale. With this procedure, the clinician can then observe the patient's speech breathing behaviors, particularly between repetitions. What is more, by having the child place his hand on his abdomen (Webster, 1974) the clinician is able to observe the direction of movement during respiratory cycles involved in connected *speech* utterances.

If the stutterer's respiratory patterns prove to be adequate during fluent speaking and aberrant during stuttering, the change implies that there are no underlying speech breathing problems, but rather, suggests that the problems result from stuttering associated with physiologic incoordinations.

3. *Coarticulatory/Resonatory Processes.* As suggested by Webster (1974), the stutterer may use coarticulatory patterns, which are aberrant, too forceful, or too rapid. In assessing the coarticulatory/resonatory processes, the clinician must attend to each child's unique threshold of coarticulatory abilities, for within even the normal speaking population (if one exists) individuals exhibit different abilities. If we could obtain threshold measurements of each person's ability to speak as fast as possible while maintaining articulatory accuracy, we would derive subgroups of individuals for various rates. If the young stutterer attempts to speak as rapidly as other individuals in his environment, one could expect a breakdown in the system, particularly if the child has an underlying coordinative disorder. Coarticulatory/resonatory process problems include tense, forceful articulatory contacts, rapid movement patterns which exceed the child's unique threshold, inappropriate oral/nasal resonance, and so forth.

Parent/Child Communicative Interaction

Often young children in an unfamiliar environment will communicate more effectively when alone with parents than when alone with the clinician or with both the clinician and parent. Thus, the clinician might obtain a more typical and possibly more valid rate and severity of stuttering from an interaction between the parent and child only. From a tape of this interaction, the clinician would be able to determine the stuttered words per minute and the percentage of stuttered words. On occasion this type of sample results in the most involved stuttering behavior, not because there is a problem between the parent and child but rather because the two have an excellent relationship which results in the best, more complex, spontaneous language sample. The nature or content of the interaction between a parent and child must be evaluated with caution, however, for parents may not communicate in a typical fashion in a strange environment, particularly when they realize that what they do or say may be evaluated by a professional. As an example, one should realize that discipline and interaction between parent and child in the supermarket can certainly be different from the interaction that might occur under the same or similar circumstances in the home. Parents often are at a loss to engage their child in conversation when the clinician leaves the room; and if there are pictures lying around, they will resort to having the child name the pictures. On occasion the child will resist and insist on going home or going out for a hamburger or whatever it was that was promised, and all the parent can say is, "Not yet, we have to stay here and talk now." Such intervention ordinarily does not result in a good language sample.

To obtain the parent/child communicative sample, we suggest the following procedure: Arrange beforehand for the parents or significant others to engage the child in a private conversation without you. Then leaving the tape recorder on, excuse yourself from the room saying "The two of you can stay in here for a while and do whatever you want to. I'll be back in a little bit."

Allow sufficient time to obtain at least 2 minutes of talking time from the child (whom you can observe and listen to if you have a one-way window and monitoring speaker available). When you return to the room, have the parent or significant other leave, but mention at that time that the tape recorder was running while they were alone in the room.

Other Assessment Procedures
All children are routinely given a complete oral-facial exam, a hearing screening, a test of articulation/phonology, and a language test. Ordinarily we administer the Arizona Articulation Proficiency Scale (Fudala, 1974) and the Test of Auditory Comprehension of Language (Carrow, 1973) as well. If we have reason to suspect a motor speech disability, we administer the Motor Speech Protocol (Logue, 1976b,c); but we actually suggest that this instrument be given routinely, particularly for purposes of research with the young stutterer. All other tests are selected on the basis of need.

Parent Interview and Interpretive Summary
Prior to the interview, the parent will have completed a detailed case history form eliciting pertinent information with regard to birth history, developmental milestones, medical history, speech and language development, and general descriptions of all communicative and other problems.

We begin the interview by informing the parents (or other significant person) that before results of the evaluation are given, all questions pertinent to the child's case history must be answered before we summarize the results of the evaluation. We then review the detailed case history form with them and respond openly to their questions or need for clarification. After completing this form, we then work on the History of the Stuttering Problem (Shine, 1980b) with the clinician asking each question and writing down all pertinent parental responses. During writing there are periods of silence which parents generally feel obligated to fill by providing additional information or asking questions. We ask the parents to describe the problem further using examples to identify the onset and development, to specify any thoughts about the cause, to describe what has been done in the home and other environments to *help* the child overcome the stuttering, and finally to indicate whether the rate and severity of stuttering during the evaluation were typical of the child's ordinary stuttering behavior. If the parent did not observe a significant part of the evaluation, we play a tape recorded sample of the child's most significant stuttering (from the evaluation) so the parent can evaluate whether the stuttering behavior was typical or more or less severe. The evaluation results and the parent's evaluation of the severity will determine the direction of future intervention. Although in almost all instances there is agreement concerning the severity, the evaluation occasionally indicates a mild or moderate severity classification when the parent rates the stuttering as severe. Clinical experience (of almost 18 years) has revealed, however, that it is extremely rare that the parent's classification is wrong (see McDearmon, 1968, for discussion of parental evaluation). Parents are able to validly rate frequency and severity of stuttering, contrary to a significant portion of literature which suggests that they misdiagnose non-stuttering disfluencies as stuttering disfluencies. Generally it appears that the profession ought to heed the statement by West and Ansberry (1957): "Everyone knows what stuttering is except the expert." It is noted, however, that occasionally a parent and even trained clinicians will identify a child with a motor speech disorder (dyspraxia of speech) as having a stuttering disorder.

If the parent rates the stuttering as significantly more severe than is indicated by the evaluation results, we schedule another evaluation and/ or ask the parent to tape record the child's stuttering in the home environment and bring the tape in for us to evaluate. On occasion the evaluation will determine a mild rating for a child with a moderate to severe stuttering disorder if the child's speaking behavior consists primarily of very short utterances (rarely more than 4 words), or if he talks quietly and carefully in a manner that is compatible with fluency and incompatible with stuttering.

We generally can approximate the age of onset with greater accuracy if the parents associate onset with an important date or occasion such as Christmas, a birthday, or a vacation. In most instances, the description of the circumstances at the time of onset indicates that nothing unusual has happened though some case histories do place a significant event (i.e., parents' being involved in a divorce, a child experiencing a mild concussion from a fall, the father having a drinking problem, or a death of a favorite pet) near the time of the onset.

A major question to ask parents is, "What have you done to *help* your child overcome the stuttering?" Typically the parent will say, "We sometimes tell him to slow down, take it easy, or stop and start over." When asked what the child does when such things are suggested, the parent almost always responds, "He does what I ask him and it usually helps him." The child's reaction to such parental promptings should provoke neither surprise nor controversy if one considers the data presented by Mulder (1972) concerning parental intervention and remission of stuttering. While parents have intuitively been aware for centuries that having the child slow himself down has a beneficial effect, the profession has only recently concluded this, and many contemporary fluency training procedures for children and adults now begin by having the patient slow down their rate of speaking.

A few noteworthy publications concerning parental intervention and "spontaneous recovery" are recommended reading for all speech pathologists working with the beginning stutterer and counseling parents (Milisen and Johnson, 1936; Glasner and Rosenthal, 1957; Wingate, 1962, 1971, 1983; Shearer and Williams, 1965; Cooper, 1979; Andrews, et al., 1983; Ingham, 1983; Kent, 1983). The conclusion derived from this literature and from clinical experience is that the majority of children probably overcome stuttering because of parental intervention (i.e., "Slow down," or "Take it easy," or "Stop and think before you talk," etc.) or self-taught changes in speaking patterns rather than spontaneous recovery. (*The recent article by Zimmerman, Liljeblad, Frank, and Cleeland, 1983, is suggested as required reading for all clinicians who work with individuals who stutter.*) One might even conclude that having the parents refrain from giving directives to the child might actually be detrimental to the remission of stuttering. The beginning stutterer, like children with other communicative disorders, needs the direct intervention of a clinician, a parent (or significant other).

Once we have obtained the background information and completed the history form, we present the results of the evaluation. During the parent interview we summarize results and other information on a blank piece of paper and provide a copy for the parents to take home which enables them to present the results accurately to other individuals in the immediate environment and serves to educate lay persons.

The clinician begins by providing the parent(s) (or significant other) with an operational definition of stuttering (see p. 178) that is written down and includes examples of stuttering exhibited by their child during the evaluation. The writing allows the parent time to better understand and formulate questions about the information presented. We make it clear that we count stuttered words. Thus, if the child says, "I-I-I-I-I-I," that is only one stuttered word, the word "I"; and "we-we-we-we-we-we-

went" is one stuttered word, the word "went." We explain that we use a stopwatch during the evaluation in order to record "talking time" and thus determine the number of stuttered words during each minute of talking.

Determining the Need for and Nature of Intervention
We use three data-based ranges of fluency/stuttering as well as realistic considerations of the parents' concerns, the parent/child relationship (when determinable) and the general maturational and emotional makeup of the child. The child who perceives his stuttering as a problem or appears to be immature or emotionally sensitive warrants strong consideration for direct intervention despite contradictory data-based results. The data-based criteria incorporate the use of three ranges for stuttered words per minute (SW/M) and three for percentage of stuttered words(%SW) to interpret the rate and severity of stuttering and to assist in determining the need for and nature of intervention that is necessary. A prerequisite for understanding the following discussion is a thorough knowledge of the operational definition of stuttering (p. 178) and the general hierarchy of severity of stuttering (p. 179).

Based on SW/M the ranges are as follows: (1) *Normal fluency* ranges from 0 to 3 (Ryan, 1974), provided that the child exhibits no prolongations or struggle behaviors (Shine and Mason, 1981). (2) *Borderline/at-risk stuttering* ranges from 3 to 10 SW/M provided that the child exhibits no struggle behaviors, that the duration of prolongations is less than 2 seconds (Riley, 1981), and that the number of prolongations does not exceed the total number of whole-word and part-word repetitions (Shine and Mason, 1981). (3) *Handicapping stuttering* refers to speech with more than 10 SW/M, provided that types of stuttering are primarily part-word repetitions and prolongations and/or struggle behaviors. The child with only whole-word or part-word repetitions may be classified as exhibiting borderline/at-risk stuttering.

With regard to the percentage of stuttered words, the ranges and qualifiers (providing there are no prolongations or struggle behaviors, etc.) work similarly: *Normal fluency* ranges from 0 to 3 percent SW of words spoken (Webster, 1974); *borderline/at-risk stuttering* ranges from 3 to 10 percent SW of words spoken (Riley, 1981); and *handicapping stuttering* applies to speech with more than 10 percent SW. When the clinician's interpretation of the overall severity of the stuttering contradicts the data-based criteria, additional data must be inspected, including parent and child feelings, the overall effect of the stuttering on the family, and any other information deemed pertinent.

When counseling the parent of the child who is in the *handicapping stuttering range*, we do not provide the borderline/at-risk stuttering ranges because of a possible negative effect. The parent may resent their child's not being in the borderline range which suggests a better prognosis. Instead, we write down the ranges of normal fluency (0 to 3 SW/M and 0 to 3% SW) and their child's SW/M and percentage scores, and indicate that he has a significant problem. The contrast immediately makes it obvious to the parents that their child is significantly above the normal range and does indeed have a significant stuttering problem demanding professional remediation. While parents are understandably shocked by scores in the 20s to 30s, the clinician can handle this adequately by stating, "That's pretty high, but we get quite a number of children who score a lot higher." The parents then generally express some relief in knowing that their child is not the worst on the block.

In counseling the parent(s) of the child who falls within the *borderline/ at-risk range*, we do not assume prematurely that direct fluency training services by a professional are unnecessary. The prognosis for the child's overcoming the stuttering with only direct parental intervention may indeed be excellent based on the data collected overall, but for a number of reasons the parents may be unwilling to attempt to work with their child without having the clinician provide direct services as well. In spite of what the clinician might have concluded, the parents' concerns may be more significant than the stuttering data, for it is generally recognized that the speech clinician is an expert in changing the way children talk; and parents may feel much more confident if the expert helps their child. The parents may be concerned that if the child does not overcome the stuttering it could be because they have tried to help, when actually they should have turned that responsibility over to the clinician.

Cause of Stuttering

After the parents have gained an understanding of the need for and nature of the intervention prescribed, we discuss the cause of stuttering with them. Generally, the parents want to know, "Why does my child stutter?" My standard response to this question is "Years ago we used to think that children stuttered because someone, usually a mother, put too much pressure on the child to talk well or reacted negatively to the way the child spoke. It's amazing to me that we used to think that way and that some people still do because there is not one shred of evidence in any of our literature that has ever demonstrated that parents cause stuttering. This particular attitude gained acceptance during the 1950s when every bad behavior that a child exhibited was easily explained by blaming the parents."

"Since the late 1960s and early 1970s research has shown that the reason children stutter is because they're different, (*pause*) different like the child who has to wear glasses or the child who experiences problems with math or reading." (*Generally during the pause after the word dif- ferent, parents verbalize relief that they did not cause the problem. Our comments help not only to eliminate their sense of guilt, but also to instill in them the feeling that they can intervene directly and help their child rather than sit by helplessly amid suggestions to ignore the existence of a problem.)*

"If your child had a reading or math problem, what do you think you could have done to cause it? How about the 2- or 3-year-old who wears glasses; do you think the parents did something to cause the child to have to wear glasses? No, the child with glasses is different and the glasses help compensate for the difference. Your child is like the child who is clumsy and cannot control the muscles for running well or throwing a ball or riding a bike, except your child is clumsy in controlling the muscles for speech breathing patterns, the voice box to produce the voice, and the tongue, lips and teeth to say the sounds. All of these systems (*while speaking point to indicate breathing mechanism, larynx (voice box), and articulators*) have to be coordinated, and your child is having trouble doing that."

Finally, we explain that stuttering is a problem which can be dealt with very successfully, particularly if direct fluency training is initiated early (Glasner, 1970; Van Riper, 1973; Martin, Kuhl, and Haroldson, 1972; Reed and Godden, 1977; Thompson, 1977; Mason and Shine, 1981), and that we have had excellent success in teaching young children a new way of talking that enables them to compensate for the discoordination of their speaking system.

Description of the Therapy

THERAPY GOALS

The primary goal of this direct fluency training approach is to train the child to change his basic patterns of speaking in a manner that enables him to use physiologic and prosodic speaking patterns that are compatible with fluency and incompatible with stuttering (Webster, 1974), thus compensating for his generalized neurologic dysfunction, and to speak in a manner which both lay and professional persons regard as normally fluent. His new manner of speaking must be habituated as a "way-of-life" (Webster, 1974) rather than a means for controlling stuttering when it occurs or is anticipated; that is, the child's new pattern must involve accurate neurologic preprogramming of fluency rather than ongoing monitoring of stuttering.

The specific goals of fluency training are (1) to counsel and educate parents and other persons involved with the child concerning the onset, development and cause of stuttering; (2) to train parents and other significant persons to manage the child's stuttering openly and directly, to validly identify stuttered words and to establish an effective environmental program; (3) to select a variety of materials and related activities that can be used with children 3 to 9 years of age; (4) to select pictures that the child can readily identify and for which stuttering is unlikely; (5) to determine the child's fluent mode of speaking, whether it be a whispered speaking voice or a prolonged speaking voice; (6) to train the child to use a fluent easy speaking voice (ESV) that is compatible with fluency; (7) to train the child to use the ESV in a variety of structured speaking activities in which length and complexity of utterance is controlled within each session and from session to session, gradually approaching a terminal goal of spontaneous fluent conversation; (8) as part of and in addition to the therapy goal, facilitate transference of this general fluency to the child's immediate environment; (9) to facilitate the transfer of fluency to all speaking environments by providing an extratherapy generalization program involving the clinician, client, and other significant persons; (10) to initiate a maintenance program that will enable the clinician to follow up on the child and evaluate his fluency periodically for at least 1 year.

THERAPY METHOD

Specific Techniques, Procedures, and Activities

This fluency training approach, designed to train the child to develop a new manner of speaking, incorporates three major areas involving physiologic, prosodic, and linguistic variables and emphasizes the fundamentals or principles of good speech (Backus, 1943) all of which are applicable for individuals from 3 to 93 years of age. Although the variables are discussed separately, we realize that the modification of one variable may well demand an adjustment of another which can result in a complex learning task for the child. The task can be simplified for the child during the initial stages of training if evaluation of success is limited to only one variable with the addition of combined or more variables as the child makes progress.

1. *Physiologic speaking variables* include respiratory, phonatory, and articulatory/resonatory processes.

   Respiratory process involves breath stream management for appropriate airflow, breathing patterns, and breath groupings. We train the child by modeling phrases of varying lengths and by using repetition with certain rote speaking behaviors. For example, have the child count to 10 (or a number commensurate with the child's breath grouping ability) 5 times in succession, and evaluate the breathing behaviors between the repetitions. While we have found young stuttering children infrequently exhibit speech breathing difficulties during fluent speaking behaviors (see sections on assessment of breathing patterns, p. 186), we do provide verbal feedback on both correct and incorrect patterns and incorporate retraining procedures when necessary.

   Phonatory process involves management of the production of both voiced and voiceless phones and the smooth flow of speech and voice between syllables. A common characteristic of the young stutterer is his frequent use of hard glottal attacks and stops. We train the child to use an easy onset (Webster, 1974) which eliminates hard glottal attacks, and to use continuous airflow, smooth flow of voicing and blending between syllables which eliminates hard glottal stops. Once the child has established the easy onset we require its use every time he opens his mouth from that time on during clinical sessions. It appears that the neurologic mediation required to preprogram an easy onset before every utterance and after every pause during connected speech, greatly enhances control for fluency. We also monitor and modify intensity, pitch, and overall vocal quality thus promoting the best possible production of the patient's optimal speaking voice and avoiding any aberrant vocal patterns (i.e., a breathy voice, a monotone pitch, a high pitch) which, experience has revealed, interfere with generalization and transfer of fluency in the clinic and in the child's environment.

Coarticulatory/resonatory processes involve stressing "loose" or "light" coarticulatory contacts, which contrast with excessive contraction and/or "tight" contacts, as well as monitoring and modifying oral/nasal resonances. With many children we have them identify and point to their own "speech helpers" (lips, teeth, palate, larynx or voice box, tongue, airflow, nasal resonance, and ear), and practice contrasting "loose" and "tight" articulatory contacts.

2. *Prosodic variables* include stress, intonation and rate/rhythm patterns.

Stress patterns, which are concerned primarily with syllable stress, are a major contributor to prosody and particularly to normally fluent speaking patterns, and result in large part from the use of strong/weak forms of articles, prepositions, conjunctions, pronouns, auxiliary verbs, and adverbs. If for example, the clinician stresses the article "a" in the sentence as follows, "I see [eɪ] car," the meaning is, "I see 'one' car" and the intonation and stress patterns become stilted and generalization of fluency does not occur. In order to facilitate transfer, the clinician has to use an unstressed weak form of the article *a* in the sentence "I see [ə] car," placing the primary stress on *car*, *I*, or *see* depending on the communicative intent. The use of appropriate strong/weak forms and a vernacular type of conversational modeling enhances effective communication, and facilitates generalization of fluency to the real world. The child, then, should not practice the more formal statement ("I am going to go") but rather the vernacular ("I'm gonna go") if such generalization is to occur.

Intonation patterns refer to the ongoing changes in pitch/frequency during easy onset and connected speech production. We employ a variety of exaggerated and widely variable pitch ranges and intonation patterns which selectively stress different words in phrases, since clinical experience has clearly demonstrated that monotone interferes with generalization of fluency to conversational speech while variable intonation patterns facilitate generalization. In the phrase "I see a car," for example, we use duration and intonation to stress the word *I* initially and subsequently the words *see* and *car*. In addition we produce all potential strong/weak forms in an unstressed (weak) manner in order to carry the appropriate rhythm of the phrase.

Rate/rhythm patterns refer primarily to slowing the rate while maintaining the rhythm of speech production by increasing the duration of each syllable in direct proportion to its relative stress in a particular communication. Our primary goal is to effect a rate of speech that is analogous to a recording played at a slower speed: the more significant syllables would still demand greater stress/duration than the less significant ones.

While contemporary interpretations maintain that rate, intonation, and stress all interact significantly in changing the physiologic speaking patterns to effect fluency, my contention is that it is the neurologic mediation in which the child engages to modify these patterns that results in fluency. Logically then, it appears that it is the clinician's task to train the child to engage in neurologic mediation that would enable him to coordinate the cerebral hemispheres and compensate for the neurologic disfunction through functional preprogramming.

3. *Linguistic length/complexity and motor planning/preprogramming:* *Length/complexity of utterance* demands control in order to simplify linguistic and motoric preprogramming. Within each session, responses progress from the simple to ones that are increasingly more demanding, primarily on the basis of length; as the child makes progress from session to session both length and complexity are increased.

Motor planning/preprogramming is directed toward training the child to plan quickly and respond immediately to stimuli. We developed this area as a progression that moves from a "simple response paradigm" (SRP) to a "complex response paradigm" (CRP) as described by Underwood (1966). For the SRP, the child becomes aware through modeling and repetition that one stimulus and one response are required, and this enables him to preorganize a fixed response pattern (motor/linguistic preprogramming) to a fixed stimulus. A CRP, on the other hand, provides a choice of responses and thus the child is unable to preorganize a fixed response without engaging in additional processing time to make the choice. Inappropriate delayed latency periods between stimulus and response may signal linguistic word retrieval problems or motor preprogramming deficiencies, which generally cause a system breakdown and stuttering, but the repetitions of SRPs and CRPs and the establishment of rhythmic patterns and predictable rates of stimulation in which an immediate response is required, tend to minimize these problems.

Management of Antecedent and Consequent Stimuli
The most important component of the S-R-S paradigm is the *discriminative antecedent stimulus* (one which consistently evokes the desired response) because it must be identified before the consequent stimulus can be administered. A discriminative antecedent stimulus which consistently evokes fluency is easily identified with almost all children and thus fluency training involves gradually shifting stimulus control (McLean, 1970) to evoke fluency in conversational speech. The *consequent stimuli*, which are used to educate and motivate the child, are of two types, *verbal feedback* (which facilitates cognitive learning and neurologic preprogramming) and *token reinforcement* (which reinforces the child and motivates continued effort). The two types are managed separately with verbal feedback providing appropriate information concerning the correctness or incorrectness of a response as well as additional instructions, such as, "Great! That was a perfect, quiet, easy onset" or "No, that's not right. You started too loud and hard," and the "token reinforcement" (a chip, check mark, or a counter click) providing an immediate reward.

Token Economy System
A token economy system in which the value of tokens is clearly obvious to the client has three important aspects: a schedule of feedback, a system for administering the tokens, and minor and major back-up reinforcers.

The schedule for verbal feedback is 100 percent although this does not imply that explanations of correctness and incorrectness follow every response or even the majority of responses once the target response has been established. Instead, the clinician can respond simply with "great," "right," "super," "right on," "mm-hmm," or any other appropriate words of acknowledgment.

The schedule of token reinforcement begins at 100 percent but gradually decreases to 50 percent and even less as the child progresses. Tokens must not be easy to obtain and stringent criteria should be adhered to.

The system for awarding minor and major back-up reinforcers needs to be utterly clear to the child. He should realize that when he achieves certain levels on a selected graphing system, he will earn a back-up reinforcer, which must be immediately presented since waiting until the end of the session would obscure the correlation between the success and the reward. Edibles (generally not recommended) are not to be consumed during the session. We must follow stringent procedures in order to establish the value of the tokens (chips, check marks, whatever) with our clients. First, we administer the token only if the first attempt at a target response is correct; second attempts merit only the appropriate verbal feedback but not a token. Second, we strongly discourage awarding any back-up reinforcer unless it is truly earned because prizes following each session in which the child behaves well but fails to earn the specified level of proficiency actually weakens the strength of the token economy system.

Passing/Failing Criteria

Although the criteria for passing is fluency (0.5 or fewer SW/M, Ryan, 1974) at a particular response level for two consecutive sessions, this is a general criteria which can be inappropriate for individuals who progress more rapidly. Occasionally children become bored with one-word responses and will benefit by advancement to a higher level of imitated phrase responses. If they begin to experience failure at the higher level, the responses are simplified and appropriate behavior management is implemented.

Based on clinical experience, a child meets the criteria for failing if he does not attain fluency (0.5 or fewer SW/M) after three sessions. No more than three sessions are needed to realize that the clinician has not identified a true discriminative antecedent stimulus for fluency (i.e., the stimulus material or level is too difficult for the child or that his failure results from behavioral problems).

Children fail to meet fluency criteria for a number of reasons including (1) the need for additional training in speaking variables that are compatible with fluency; (2) the need for the clinician to change the pace of stimulation, such as slow stimulus rate that provides periods of silence in which the child initiates conversation and stutters, or fast stimulus rates which require quick responses that disrupt easy speaking; (3) the need to provide a rigorous structure that prevents the child from conversing spontaneously; and (4) the need to restructure or reprogram stimulus/response materials that are ineffective or inappropriate for the children in question.

SPECIFIC FLUENCY TRAINING PROCEDURES AND ACTIVITIES

We have outlined (Shine, 1980b) seven phases in fluency training with the young stutterer including the following: the environmental program; the picture identification prestep; the determination of a fluent speaking mode, either whispered or prolonged; the establishment of an "easy-speaking voice"; the establishment of fluency during four highly structured activities and spontaneous conversational speech; transfer and maintenance; and the follow-up research program.

The Environmental Program

We use the term *environmental program* rather than home or parent program, because clinical experience has revealed that although involvement of the parent is generally ideal, it is not mandatory and may not be possible particularly when job or family responsibilities or other significant problems are more important. The primary goal is to involve not simply the parent but rather any individual who spends or can spend a significant amount of time with the child and who also is important in the child's life (such as classroom teachers, peers, relatives, siblings, or others). Although the classroom teacher is in an ideal position to monitor the child's speaking behaviors and to expect the child to utilize a new manner of speaking, the best program might be one in which both the parents and a significant other are actively involved. The bottom line however, is that the speech clinician is an expert in changing speaking patterns of children and when necessary, she can manage the program entirely on her own.

Generally, the significant other(s) require two initial hour-long sessions without the child present and then whatever follow-up training appears necessary during the course of their observation of, participation in, or comments on the fluency training sessions. During the first hour we train them to identify and score stuttered words (see page 180) and during the second hour, we review counting stuttered words, using their child's audio recording and transcript, answer additional questions, and outline the steps involved in the environmental program (a copy of which is sent home) as follows:

1. We involve significant others in both the child's immediate environmental program(s) by having them count and record stuttered words during at least one and, if feasible, two or three 15-minute time periods each day.
2. We provide the significant other with a weekly record card and offer the following instructions for its use.
   a. Try to schedule your environmental sessions at about the same time each day. After participating in the recording sessions for 1 or 2 weeks, the child will begin to anticipate each session and begin practicing the "new manner of speaking," prior to and following the sessions.
   b. Have the record card clearly visible and indicate to the child that "It's time for us to do some talking so I can see how well you're using your new speaking voice" *(the terminology that you use with each child may vary because it is necessary that the child understand the concept being taught, i.e., easy speaking voice, quiet voice, turtle voice, little lady's voice, inside voice. The reason that the record card is clearly visible during environmental sessions is to insure that the child realizes that he is expected to utilize a new speaking voice and that talking with an inappropriate vocal pattern results in stuttering).*
3. We ask that the child deliver the record card to the clinician on a weekly basis in order to tabulate the following data to determine the progress or lack of it in the environmental program: the total stuttered words, the total number of sessions, and the average number of stuttered words per session (which is determined by dividing the total SW

by the total sessions). We also request that the significant other keeps a record of the total time that data are collected during each environmental session.

4. During at least every fourth session we discuss the data from both the environmental and the clinical programs with the significant other and attempt to solve problems in either program with functional solutions.

5. Initially, the significant other's environmental sessions will involve general conversational interaction; but as the significant other continues to observe clinical sessions and take over clinical activities under the supervision of the clinician, we encourage her to include similar activities in the environmental program.

The involvement of significant others in the clinical program is organized as follows:

1. We recommend that the significant other observe and/or participate in at least every fourth session. If facilities permit (one-way observation window) and the clinician deems it advisable, the significant other can observe and/or participate on a more frequent schedule.

2. As soon as the child attains fluency at one step or more in any one of the activities, we ask the significant other to participate in that activity during the next regularly scheduled training session. If, for example, during the third session the child attains fluency (0.5 or fewer SW/M) in the picture identification, the story book activities, but not in the picture matching or surprise box activities, we invite the significant other to participate in these first two activities at the next session.

   a. First, the clinician explains to the significant other that the child is "going to show you how well he can use an easy-speaking voice in some things we've been doing together and then he's going to teach you how to do it." Next, the clinician states, "I'm going to go through the entire activity one time and then I'm going to let you do it so I can make sure you're doing it right and help you if you need help." During these activities, the clinician observes to make certain that the child effects an appropriate vocal production (see the explanation of stimulus procedure for the specified step), that his responses are accurately evaluated relative to correctness/incorrectness, and that verbal feedback is provided.

   b. Then the clinician initiates the first activity in which the child is fluent and proceeds as though the significant other is not present. As happens on occasion, the child may present behavioral problems or may not use speaking variables that result in fluency. The situation should be handled strictly by telling the child, "If you can't use your easy-speaking voice (variables for fluency) or if you do that again (misbehavior) your (name of the significant other) is going to have to leave." While the child has only one chance, we nevertheless must be cognizant of the reason for failure in this particular situation. It is possible that the child does not want the significant other to be present and thus deliberately fails at the task. If we determine this to be the case, we reschedule the significant other for the next session, at which time we tell the child, "If you do everything like you're supposed to, we'll let your 'significant other' leave, but you have to do it right before she can leave." With some children who present problems we may decide to involve the significant other gradually or explore other procedures to involve her successfully in the clinical programs. By pairing the child and significant other after the child has established fluency in the clinical environment, we convey to the child that he can use an easy-speaking voice and be fluent in similar types of activities within his immediate environment and convey to the significant other that she can become an "expectant other," i.e., one who expects fluency from the child in similar environmental situations.

c. The significant other's participation in clinical sessions enables the clinician not only to observe verbal interaction but also to make recommendations concerning both the child's and significant other's use of variables for fluency. Finally, the significant other conducts an entire session on her own and begins to engage in similar fluency training activities within the child's immediate environment.

The Picture Identification Prestep

The objectives of this phase are to select approximately 50 pictures of monosyllabic nouns and in the process of selection eliminate pictures not readily known by the child, those which appear to present word retrieval problems to the child and those on which stuttering occurs. With one child, we initiated training with only 12 pictures due to the child's limited vocabulary, word retrieval problems and severe stuttering; but most children can spontaneously identify single pictures with little or no stuttering. Once the clinician selects the pictures she determines their order to be presented during fluency training according to the manner of production of the prevocalic phones, beginning either with voiced or voiceless continuants (depending on the child's stuttering patterns and fluent speaking mode) and progressing through voiced and then voiceless affricatives and clusters, and finally voiced followed by voiceless plosives. With most children we begin with voiced continuants to facilitate training in the use of an easy onset pattern.

The Determination of a Fluent Speaking Mode
(Either Whispered or Prolonged)
The objective in this phase is to determine whether the child can whisper fluently. While a majority of children can, some cannot; and we teach these children to use a prolonged speaking voice. To determine the speaking mode we ask the child to repeat 10 to 20 monosyllabic and polysyllabic words and then 10 to 20 four-syllable phrases, such as "I see a car," using a whispered speaking voice. If the child exhibits fluency, the clinician moves immediately to easy-speaking voice training. If the child exhibits stuttering during whispering, we introduce the prolonged speaking voice as follows: with monosyllabic words, such as "man," the clinician models a production characteristic of an easy onset (Webster, 1974), beginning with an almost inaudible intensity and gradually increasing intensity and pitch (a rising and falling intonation pattern) while producing a syllable approximately 3 seconds or longer in duration. To model phrases in the prolonged speaking voice, the clinician increases the duration of syllables proportionate to their relative duration in a conversationally spoken phrase, with the exception that the duration of the first syllable will be exaggerated by the proper execution of an easy onset which is required at the beginning of all utterances throughout therapy. For example in the phrase, "I see a car," the duration of the entire phrase would be approximately 6 seconds; and the breakdown would be as follows: "I" = 3 seconds, "see" = 1 second, the weak form "a" = ½ second, and "car" = about 2 seconds. If one were to measure the relative duration of each of these words in a conversationally spoken sentence, "car" would probably have the longest duration, except in this instance the easy onset, which is of primary importance in fluency training, must be exaggerated, particularly during beginning sessions.

The amount of time spent in determining the fluent speaking mode is the length of time it takes for a child to repeat 10 to 20 words and phrases in a whisper and, for those who cannot whisper fluently, the additional time it takes to repeat the words and phrases in a prolonged speaking voice. Rarely, if ever, will a child have trouble imitating the prolonged speaking voice; so once the fluent speaking mode is determined, the focus should shift immediately to establishing an easy-speaking voice (one that is compatible with fluency).

The Establishment of an Easy-Speaking Voice (ESV)
The objective in this phase is to establish a different speaking pattern encompassing physiologic and prosodic variables that are compatible with fluency and incompatible with stuttering. The ESV involves the modification of variables in the following ways: (1) a decrease in the rate of speaking, (2) a decrease in loudness, (3) a widely varying intonation pattern, and (4) an exaggerated easy onset (Webster, 1974) beginning with

an almost inaudible vocal intensity and gradually increasing in intensity with a rising-falling intonation pattern on the first syllable. ESV patterns will also influence breathing patterns, rate and volume of airflow, subglottal, glottal and supraglottal muscular contraction, coarticulatory movement patterns and any other system involved in speech production; and the degree to which each variable demands modification or exaggeration depends upon the child. Once the child has established a habitual function ability to produce the different speaking voice, the variables are modified only to the extent that is necessary in order for the child to maintain fluency. While children tend automatically to modify speaking patterns toward a normal production, one variable, the easy onset, needs to be continuously practiced even as fluency becomes more and more habituated. It appears that if the child engages in the neurologic mediation to effect an easy onset, it continues to enhance fluency.

The easy-speaking voice evidences the following: (1) a normal pause time between the stimulus and the child's response and a quick and inaudible inspiration; (2) an easy onset (Webster, 1974) that has barely audible initiation of phonation with rising-falling intonation and intensity patterns, and a normal duration of voiceless phones with the child moving quickly to prolong the vowel; (3) continuous airflow without pauses between syllables except for appropriate breath groupings; (4) a prosodic pattern that reflects the relative duration of each syllable when spoken at a normal rate; and (5) the unstressed form of strong/weak forms.

In training the child to use an easy-speaking voice, we have outlined eleven steps (Shine, 1980b) which progress from single words in a whispered or prolonged speaking voice to four-syllable phrases using an ESV. Although fluency during whispering does not transfer to a normal speaking voice, we prefer to use the whispered speaking voice to initiate ESV training since it conveniently conveys the concept of easy to the child and thus develops his understanding of a quiet ESV that subsequently applies to all fluency training activities in the clinic and environmental programs. In addition, the child tolerates the near normal rate of speaking used during whispering better than the slow rate used in a PSV, and the whispered voice can easily be used by the child during conversational interaction with the clinician.

The establishment of an easy-speaking voice (fluency) generally takes three or four 40-minute sessions, after which the four fluency activities are introduced. The easy-speaking pattern will vary from child to child depending on the severity of the stuttering as well as on the abilities of the child, but the objective is to teach the child an easy onset and to modify the rate and intensity of his productions to the degree that is necessary for continuous maintenance of fluency (0.5 or fewer SW/M).

THE THERAPY SESSION
General Aspects

The objective of each session is to have the child maintain 0 SW/M throughout the entire session. Our sessions run for 30 to 40 minutes two times per week (although three, four, or more times per week would be advantageous during the first 3 or 4 weeks of training). It appears that any session shorter than 30 minutes cannot be justified with children exhibiting significant communicative disorders. During fluency training at least 20 consecutive correct responses are required for each stimulus condition in order to assure that the child is stabilizing the target behaviors being practiced. This repetition along with the repetitious phraseology of sentences such as "I see a *(noun)*," including a different noun (naming the picture stimulus presented) each time, enables the child to habituate all aspects of preprogramming and production that are involved in fluent speaking patterns. It is recommended that sessions be scheduled for at least 30 minutes and preferably 40 to 50 minutes two times per week. Once the child has learned the easy-speaking voice, we expect him to use it at all times during the session. Some children need to converse during the sessions, however, and when doing so generally resort to their habitual speaking patterns that result in stuttering. Since using a habitual speaking pattern as well as stuttering are not allowed, we demand that the child who has an insatiable appetite to converse either whisper (if fluent) or use a prolonged speaking voice during extraneous speaking. Most children do not like to whisper and will generally begin therefore, to use an easy-speaking voice. Children who cannot whisper fluently must use a prolonged speaking voice during extraneous speaking. Meanwhile the clinician immediately becomes an "expectant other," who expects the child to use a fluent speaking pattern and kindly but firmly reminds him to do so. If the child begins talking without an easy onset, or too rapidly, or loudly, the clinician immediately says "Stop, what kind of voice are we supposed to use in here?" and the child should respond, "Quiet and easy" or something similar, and then continue to speak in an appropriate manner. Many times when the child is attempting to use the easy-speaking voice during conversation, he will not maintain fluency; and the clinician might have to suggest either whispering or no talking at all. For the child who can not tolerate the edict of "no talking," the clinician must provide a vigorously structured session in order to prevent speaking that results in stuttering. Of course, the general personality of the child will be most important in the management strategy that is used with a particular child. However, absolute control of the clinical sessions to effect constant fluency appears in fact to enhance the child's progress thus facilitating the development of behavior conducive to the establishment of fluency.

Establishment of Fluency During Structured Activities and
Spontaneous Conversational Speech
We have developed four fluency training activities (picture identification, story book, picture matching, and surprise box) as part of our systematic approach (Shine, 1980b) and *all four are included in every session.*

The objective of *picture identification* is to establish a fluent (0.5 or fewer SW/M) easy-speaking voice for single-word identification of pictures, for use in simple and compound sentences, and for story telling and conversation about given pictures, which is structured to be accomplished in 22 sequential steps. During the picture identification activities the length and complexity of utterances are gradually increased; however, we expect the child to speak fluently or with very infrequent whole-word or part-word repetitions. If prolongations or struggle behaviors are exhibited with any regularity during the structured activity, it suggests the need for additional training in establishing a fluent easy-speaking voice.

The objective in using *story books* is to establish fluency (0.5 or fewer SW/M) while engaging in the telling of an entire story. With preschoolers, stories about such familiar characters as the three bears and the three little kittens have proved quite successful because the requirement for the book selection is that the sentences are long. In this activity the clinician reads the story, omitting words at the end of phrases and sentences which the child must provide. Obviously, then, the clinician must read enough of a phrase or a sentence to provide adequate clues to the sentence ending. Initially, the child is required to fill in only the last word of a phrase or sentence but gradually the child provides more extended endings with two, three, and four to six words, whole sentences, and so on until he finally retells the entire story with only minimal cues from the clinician to prevent his omitting too much of the narration.

The criteria for progression is to retell the entire story fluently, and so the child will provide parts of the story during several different sessions before telling the story in its entirety. Since some children grow bored with the same story, we may abbreviate the procedure in order to complete the story ahead of schedule and introduce a new book which appeals more to the child's interests. Generally, our program employs a maximum of four books (which minimally involve about 20 to 25 sessions). If, as frequently happens, the child has achieved criteria for both the picture matching and story book activities, they are eliminated and we spend more time in spontaneous conversation about pictures and the surprise box.

The primary objective in *picture matching* is to establish a fluent easy-speaking voice for asking and responding to "wh" questions as well as for developing a normally fluent speaking manner during verbal interaction with the clinician and significant person (if one is involved). This activity includes picture boards with 8 pictures and matching single picture cards to provoke questions such as "Who has the *(noun)?*" and responses such as "I have the *(noun)*." The client and clinician (or other person) take turns selecting cards and asking or responding appropriately to the questions. Generally, the picture matching activity is the first to be eliminated which then allows more time for spontaneous conversation with picture identification and the surprise box.

The primary objective in using the *surprise box* is to establish a fluent (0.5 or fewer SW/M) easy-speaking voice which then is generalized to a new speaking voice through repetitions of standard phrases and topic-related conversation. The surprise box activity, introduced as the last segment of each session, is structured to facilitate generalization to everyday environmental speaking situations. The clinician and client alternate taking toys or objects from the box while uttering a prescribed phrase. The toy is then manipulated to elicit spontaneous utterances from the child. For example, when the client obtains a toy car from the box, the clinician will have him roll the car across the table and rolling it back to him will encourage him to do it once more. At this point the clinician may act very excited and try to roll the car past the child onto the floor making loud car motor noises in the process. We then ask the child, who we hope is excited, to retrieve the car, roll it one more time, and then to "park" the car (or other object such as a ball) and return to using an easy-speaking voice. The point of the activity is to excite the child and then demand that he control the speaking variables for fluency. With some children, use of the easy-speaking voice may break down immediately; and thus the clinician has to stage the activity in order for the child to progress systematically to stages of increasing excitement which he gradually learns to control. Our goal is not to control the stuttering but rather to control fluency by training the child to preprogram his manner of speech production.

The surprise box, as described by Ahlberg (1961), is limited only by the imagination of the clinician and has any number of imaginable uses (i.e., playing store, taking a trip, visiting the zoo, and so on). A particularly useful procedure for children who need to work on breath groupings, airflow, easy onset, and eliminating whole-word repetition of conjunctions is to play "I'm taking a trip; and I'm packing my suitcase with a horse and a car and a _____," continuing to name each item as he draws it from the box.

Another phrase which we use initially with every child who stutters is, "I close my eyes *(pause)*, reach in *(pause)*, and see what I get *(pause)*, a (noun)." At first the child imitates each of the four phrases after the clinician generally for 10 (and frequently 20) responses and then spontaneously produces the phrase while engaging in the motor activities described. We train the child to use an exaggerated easy onset (Webster, 1974) after each pause and as he repeats each of the four phrases to evidence a decreased (quiet) intensity, continuous airflow with appropriate, quick inspiration at each pause, smooth blending between syllables, appropriate stress (duration) contrasts among syllables, and a widely variable intonation pattern. In order to produce each phrase correctly, the child must make complex modifications but the most minimal difficulties with this are rare even for children as young as 3 years. It appears that the requirements necessary for preprogramming the modified speech patterns result in fluency rather than the slow rate, quiet intensity, or other identified patterns.

PHYSICAL BEHAVIORS

We do not work on the associated physical concomitants (secondary behaviors) of stuttering such as head jerks, lip pursing, tongue protrusion, facial grimaces, and the like during fluency training, for it has been our experience that when the child learns to use physiologic speaking patterns that are compatible with fluency and incompatible with stuttering, all physical concomitants are eliminated. The goal is to teach the child what to do to be fluent rather than trying to teach the child what not to do. For example, in working with an interdental lisp the clinician does not work on eliminating tongue protrusion but rather determines the normal pattern for a correct [s] production, then trains the child to produce that pattern. Rather than teach the child how not to jerk the head or grimace or improve eye contact, we teach the child how to initiate phonation, continue airflow, and use appropriate breathing patterns as well as other speaking patterns that result in fluency.

ATTITUDINAL WORK

Success is the most effective way to manage the child's attitude toward stuttering for, as someone once said, nothing succeeds like success itself. At the beginning we tell the child that we want to help him learn a new way of talking and that we start by talking in a rather funny way (slow and quiet speech) which we gradually change until we can talk and sound like anyone else. This kind of explanation is necessary only once and is not repeated. After we have trained the significant other to count stuttered words and to manage an environmental program, we meet with both the child and parent and say, "(child's name) I want (the name of the significant other) to sit down with you once a day for about 10 or 15 minutes; and while you're talking, she is going to remind you to use your easy-speaking voice and mark down if you have any trouble talking. I wanted you to know that (significant other) is going to do this for me, and I want you to bring this card back to me at the end of each week." If the child is aware of his stuttering and realizes that we are trying to help him overcome it, we add that the "significant other" is going to "make sure you are using our easy-speaking voice and mark down how many times you stutter." While we recommend at least one session per day, we obviously cannot be unyielding in this. Whereas some significant others conduct two or three sessions per day, we do have children with no significant other or with only a part-time helper.

The token economy system chart with designators marking occasions for receiving back-up reinforcers that reward success will influence the younger child's attitude, but with older children a chart that notes the overall stuttered words per minute for each entire session (with a line drawn across the chart at 0.5 = fluency SW/M) reflects success and will influence attitude.

On occasion, we deem it necessary to sit and talk with the child concerning how he feels about his problem and his progress. One 9-year-old child recently asked me, "Is there some kind of operation I can have to get rid of my stuttering?". Obviously the clinician has to be clinically skillful in recognizing and handling attitudinal needs of the child.

TRANSFER AND MAINTENANCE

Transfer involves intratherapy and extratherapy generalization of fluency to conversational interaction between the child and others (the significant other, the clinician, other clinicians and coworkers, peers, teachers, siblings, and anyone else designated as important in the child's life). The interaction between the clinician and the child facilitates the intratherapy generalization. The good clinician must be a "ham" or actress who makes the clinical sessions fun and exciting not only to motivate the young child but also to stimulate and excite him mentally and physically in order to insure that the child can maintain his easy-speaking voice while "excited." An easy-speaking voice (quiet and slow) can result in a deadly dull session, and the stereotypical animation of verbal feedback (Good boy! Great! I love that!) can become tiresome so the clinician has to use a contrasting voice for verbal feedback and to show excitement at the appropriate times. Variety is the spice not only of life but also of fluency training and the intratherapy generalization should be a daily business.

Throughout each fluency training session the clinician must continually evaluate all her speaking behaviors to determine whether the best possible procedures are being used to facilitate generalization into the real world. We always have a tape recorder running during the session which allows us to review our work to make certain we are doing the right things. There is nothing more revealing than to listen to what we thought was a great session at the time of the taping, for the sessions never seem as creative, dynamic, exciting, or valuable when played back on the tape recorder.

The fluency training procedures for the extratherapy generalization program are designed to transfer fluency to a wide variety of environmental settings that include the significant other and all other individuals who are important in the child's environment. Although approximately 40 children have completed the fluency training, only five children have required the structure of the extratherapy transfer procedures during the past 8 years since the majority of young children transfer fluency spontaneously.

We conduct the maintenance program for 1 year after releasing the child as fluent, i.e., the child is able to maintain fluency (0 to 0.5 SW/M with no prolongations or struggle behaviors) in the clinic as well as in his environment. Release from therapy generally results when the clinician and significant other agree that the child no longer stutters or that the stuttering (whole-word and part-word repetitions) is so infrequent and mild that it is no longer a problem. Even if the parents have not been actively involved in the environmental program, they will make it known when the child stops having trouble talking; and parents are valid judges of stuttering. A parent whose child had attained fluency in the clinic and surrounding environments eventually notified me that "This is our last semester. J.B. is talking all right now." We subsequently released the child, providing a maintenance program for the year, and the child maintained fluency.

During the maintenance program the significant other continues to monitor the child's environmental fluency, and the child is scheduled for six reevaluations within the clinic: twice during the first month and then once at the end of the second month, the fourth month, the sixth month, and after a full year. We do instruct the significant other to contact the clinic if the child begins to regress or if questions or problems arise.

FOLLOW-UP PROCEDURES
The initial follow-up study (see Evaluation of Therapy) was conducted from 2½ to 5 years following the maintenance program for 18 children. We plan to conduct another follow-up study within a year to relocate and evaluate every child who has received fluency training since 1974.

EQUIPMENT AND MATERIALS NEEDED
See page 179.

CLINICIAN SKILLS AND TRAINING REQUIRED
Clinicians need to understand the fundamentals of speech, including optimal vocal quality, breath groupings, smooth flow of speech and voice, continuous airflow, the use of voiced consonant continuants at the ends of syllables and words to increase duration and enhance blending from syllable to syllable and the use of appropriate strong/weak forms. Also needed is the ability to model an easy onset (Webster, 1974) and an easy speaking voice (decreased intensity, increased duration, widely variable intonation patterns) that maintains the relative stress and duration of conversationally produced phrases and sentences. Stilted speaking patterns are detrimental to success whereas vernacular speech is necessary to facilitate the transfer of fluency.

Although clinicians have reported success simply from following the programmed procedures (Shine, 1980b) a 2-day workshop and particularly a 3-day workshop in which demonstrations with young stuttering children is provided, helps to develop the understanding and skills that are necessary for success. No single publication can convey subtle findings from our years of experience, but the workshop training provides an excellent opportunity both for discussion and demonstration of our approach. The clinician must be able to validly identify stuttering words, complete a comprehensive evaluation, counsel parents and significant others that parents do not cause stuttering, and modify the speaking patterns of children to use speaking variables compatible with fluency and incompatible with stuttering. We proceed with the understanding that children must be taught to control for fluency rather than trying to control stuttering and, therefore, focus not on how to manage stuttering in difficult situations but rather on how to use speaking patterns that will result in fluency no matter what the situation.

CLIENT REQUIREMENTS

We have no specific requirements other than the child be mature enough to engage in a clinical program; the youngest child we have ever worked with was 2 years, 9 months of age when he first enrolled in therapy. Although the child demonstrated the ability to change his patterns of speaking and to speak fluently during most clinical sessions, we ultimately spent most of our time devising procedures to control the child's disruptive behaviors; and this left little time for fluency training. After two semesters of minimal progress by the child, the parents and clinician agreed to establish a home intervention program which is still in progress and, if necessary, the child will re-enroll in the clinical program in the future.

To date we have worked successfully with children who stuttered and also exhibited significant language disorders, phonological disorders, and both phonologic and language disorders. Generally the approach with children exhibiting handicapping language disorders has been to emphasize language while incorporating variables for fluency. With one child who had a severe language, phonologic, and stuttering disorder, we provided four 50-minute sessions per week for approximately 14 weeks of therapy (two sessions per week for language and two for fluency training). The following semester the child continued to receive fluency training in the clinic and language therapy in the school (kindergarten), and he was released at the end of the school year as fluent and with only minimal residual language deviations. To date we have not worked with any children who have been cognitively handicapped, but we have received verbal reports that the fluency training procedures are effective with such children if one modifies the language content and complexity.

Evaluation of the Therapy

RESEARCH STUDIES

Procedures

A study was designed (Mason and Shine, 1981) to determine if a direct fluency training procedure (Shine, 1980b) was effective in establishing and maintaining fluency in young school age and preschool children (ages 2 years, 9 months to 8 years). The study focused on 18 subjects (16 boys and 2 girls), all of whom had been released as fluent for periods ranging from 1 year, 2 months to 5 years. We evaluated the fluency of 14 of the 16 children located in interviews within the clinic or the school, or by means of tape recordings made by the mother. We even used one recording of a telephone conversation. Two parents located did not return taped samples. In addition, parents also provided subjective reports of each child's current fluency status.

We then completed descriptive data for all 18 subjects including pretreatment and posttreatment test results and mean, range, and standard deviation (based on age, length of treatment, and time since dismissal) for all 18 subjects. A Comprehensive Stuttering Analysis was completed for the 14 subjects included in the follow-up study.

Results

The results revealed that 13 of the 14 had maintained fluency, and that nine of the 14 subjects had attained fluency (3 or less SW/M with no prolongations or struggle behaviors) in 9 months or less. The average length of treatment was 10.4 months with a standard deviation of 7.9 months and a range of 1 month to 28 months. The mean number of 40- to 50-minute sessions was 56.7 with a standard deviation of 38.2 sessions and a range from 16 to 133 sessions. The length of time since "dismissal as fluent" was 14 months to 64 months with a mean time since dismissal of 38 months and a standard deviation of 15 months.

The one child who did not maintain fluency (E.W.) was a severe stutterer with a significant language disorder who also had an older brother who had stuttered but had attained and maintained fluency. E.W. was released with marginal fluency because the parents moved from the area, and although the stuttering had been severe, the child obtained a mild rating at the time of the follow-up study.

Reasons for Therapeutic Effectiveness

As stated by Van Riper (1973) and Glasner (1970), prognosis is excellent for the beginning stutterer. Glasner went so far as to say that prognosis was good only for the beginning stutterer for it appears, as with any disorder, that the sooner intervention is initiated, the better. Children at an early age are much easier to mold; and changing speech patterns before they become habitual or a part of the individual's personality is simply logical. The older the stutterer, the more he resists changing his speaking patterns because, as some individuals have stated, they feel phony when speaking in a different way. The young child up to about 6 years of age does not experience this feeling, but clinical experience suggests that by 9 years of age some children begin resisting the change although many do not.

The procedures are effective because they are direct. The speech clinician, who is an expert in changing speaking behaviors, is the person to be working with the child, not the lay person. We never question providing direct remediation for a 3-year-old child with a language or phonologic disability and we should not with the stutterer. Experience and research have demonstrated that direct remediation with the young, beginning stutterer is effective (Mason and Shine, 1981; Reed and Godden, 1977; Thompson, 1977; Ryan, 1974; Riley and Riley, 1979, 1980).

That fluency training, like language and phonologic training, can be effective without the involvement of the parents or without changes in the child's environment is recognized; however, in order to maximize the child's potential to overcome his communicative disorder, we always strive to develop an ideal intervention program through effective parental involvement and necessary reorganization of the child's environment: We also realize that seldom does life offer the ideal.

Advantages of the Therapy

Empirical testing has shown the procedures of assessment and fluency training to be effective (Mason and Shine, 1981); as systematically outlined these procedures can generally be followed with most children 3 to 9 years of age although the principles on which the approach is based apply equally with individuals 3 to 93 years of age. We find that the fluency training approach is easily learned because it requires competencies for which the clinician has already been trained, i.e., changing the child's physiologic and prosodic speaking patterns while controlling linguistic length and complexity. On the other hand the programmed format, which includes concisely written behavioral objectives and systematic procedures for accountability, enhances development of clinical competencies for students-in-training and facilitates development of individual education programs (IEP's) for children in the public schools. Since the approach stresses fluency or a positive rather than negative aspect of communication (Culatta, 1976) it is conceptually comparable to other intervention procedures within our profession and as such fosters the clinician's confidence in succeeding and eliminates her reluctance to implement direct fluency training for fear of causing the stuttering to become worse.

The background information on cause, development and environmental management of stuttering in children facilitates effective counseling with parents and significant others by immediately eliminating guilt, and this creates understanding that enables parents to become actively involved in direct management of their child's stuttering without fear of promoting or compounding the problem. In general the overall approach provides a means of implementing systematic procedures that most experienced clinicians have felt a need for or have previously experimented with in one form or another.

References

Adams, M. Personal Communication, 1980.

Ahlberg, V. Clinical Procedures in Assessment and Treatment of Communicative Disorders, Graduate Seminar, University Northern Colorado, 1961.

Andrews, G., Craig, A., Feyer, A., Hoddinott, S., Howle, P., and Neilson, M. Stuttering: A review of research findings and theories circa 1982. *J. Speech Hear. Res.* 48:226–246, 1983.

Avery, E., Dorsey, J., and Sickels, V. A. *The First Principles of Speech.* New York: Appleton-Century-Crofts , 1928.

Backus, O. *Speech in Education.* New York: Oxford University Press, 1943.

Backus, O., and Beasley, J. *Speech Therapy with Children.* Boston: Houghton Mifflin, 1951.

Beasley, J. Techniques of therapy for preschool children. *J. Speech Hear Disord.* 14:307–311, 1949.

Berry, M. A common denominator in twinning and stuttering. *J. Speech Disord.* 3 (1) 51–57, 1938.

Berry, M. Twinning in stuttering families. *Hum. Biol.* 9 (3) 329–346, 1937.

Berry, M., and Eisenson, J. *The Defective in Speech.* New York: F.S. Crofts Co., 1942.

Carrow, E. *Test for Auditory Comprehension of Language.* Boston: Teaching Resources, 1973.

Cooper, E., *Understanding Stuttering: Information for Parents.* Chicago: National Easter Seal Society, 1979.

Culatta, R. Fluency: The other side of the coin. ASHA 18:795–799, 1976.

Fudala, J. *Arizona Articulation Proficiency Scale* (rev.). Los Angeles: Western Psychological Services, 1974.

Glasner, P. Developmental View. In J. Sheehan (ed.), *Stuttering: Research and Therapy.* New York: Harper & Row, 1970. Pp. 240–259.

Glasner, P., and Rosenthal, D. Parental diagnosis of stuttering in young children. *J. Speech Hear. Disord.* 22:288–95, 1957.

Ingham, R. Spontaneous Remission of Stuttering: When Will the Emperor Realize He Has No Clothes On? In D. Prins and R. Ingham (eds.), *Treatment of Stuttering in Early Childhood: Methods and Issues.* San Diego: College-Hill Press, 1983.

Jasper, H. A laboratory study of diagnostic indices of bilateral neuromuscular organization in stutterers and normal speakers. *Psychol. Monogr.* 43: 72–174, 1932.

Johnson, W., et al. *The Onset of Stuttering: Research Findings and Implications.* Minneapolis: University of Minnesota Press, 1959.

Kent, R. Facts about stuttering: Neuropsychologic perspectives. *J. Speech Hear. Res.* 48:249–255, 1983.

Logue, R. Personal communication, 1983.

Logue, R. Disorders of motor-speech in children: Evaluation and treatment. *Commun. Disord:* New York: Grune & Stratton, 1978.

Logue, R. Motor-speech disorders in children. Paper presented at the annual convention of the American Speech-Language and Hearing Association, Houston, 1976a.

Logue, R. *Monitoring Articulatory Postures (MAP): A Speech Motor Training Program* (clinic manual). Greenville N. C.: East Carolina University, 1976b.

Logue, R. *Assess Speech Motor Behavior: An Examination Protocol.* (clinic manual) Greenville, N. C.: East Carolina University, 1976c.

McDearmon, J. Primary stuttering at the onset of stuttering: A re-examination of data. *J. Speech Hear. Res.* 11:631–637, 1968.

McFarlane, S., and Prins, D. Neural response time of stutterers and nonstutterers in selected oral motor tasks. *J. Speech Hear. Res.* 21:768–778, 1978.

McLean, J. Extending stimulus control of phoneme articulation by operant techniques. In F. L. Girardeau and J. E. Spradin (eds.), *A Functional Analysis Approach to Speech and Language Behavior.* ASHA Monogr. 14:24–27, 1970.

Martin, R., Kuhl, P., and Haroldson, S. An experimental treatment with two preschool stuttering children. *J. Speech Hear. Res.* 15:743–752, 1972.

Mason, D., and Shine, R. A Follow-Up Study of Fluency Training with the Young Stutterer (Ages 2-9 to 8-0 Years). Master's thesis, East Carolina University, Greenville, N. C. 1981.

Milisen, R., and W. Johnson. A comparative study of stutterers, former stutterers and normal speakers whose handedness has been changed. *Arch. Speech* 1:61–86, 1936.

Moore, W. Bilateral tachistoscopic word perception of stutterers and normal subjects. *Brain Lang.* 3:434–442, 1976.

Moore, W., Craven, D., and Faber, M. Hemispheric alpha asymmetries of words with positive, negative, and neutral arousal values preceding tasks of recall and recognition: Electrophysiological and behavioral results from stuttering males and nonstuttering males and females. *Brain Lang.* 17:210–224, 1982.

Mulder, R., The management of disfluency in its earliest developmental stages. In A. Weston (ed.), *Communicative Disorders.* Springfield, Ill.: Thomas, 1972. Pp. 199–219.

Plakosh, P. The functional asymmetry of the brain: Hemispheric specialization in stutterers for processing of visually presented linguistic and spatial stimuli. Ph. D. diss., Palo Alto School of Professional Psychology, 1978.

Reed, C., and Godden, A. An experimental treatment using verbal punishment with two preschool stutterers. *J. Fluency Disord.* 2:225–233, 1977.

Riley, G. *Stuttering Severity Instrument: For Children and Adults.* Tigard, Ore.: C. C. Publications, 1980.

Riley, G. *Stuttering Prediction Instrument for Young Children.* Tigard, Ore.: C. C. Publications, 1981.

Riley, G. and Riley, J. Motoric and Linguistic Variables Among Children Who Stutter: A Factor Analysis. *J. Speech Hear. Dis.* 4:504–514, 1980.

Riley, G., and Riley, J. A component model for diagnosing and treating children who stutter. *J. Fluency Disord.* 4:279–294, 1979.

Ryan, B. *Programmed Therapy for Stuttering in Children and Adults.* Springfield, Ill.: Thomas, 1974.

Ryan, B., and Van Kirk, B. Counting disfluencies, stuttered words, and total words: A tape recorded training program. Monterey, Calif.: Monterey Learning Systems, 1973.

Shearer, W., and J. Williams. Self-recovery from stuttering. *J. Speech Hear. Disord.* 30:288–90, 1965.

Shine, R. Direct Management of the Beginning Stutterer. In W. Perkins (ed.), *Strategies in Stuttering Therapy: Seminars in Speech, Language and Hearing*, New York: Thieme-Stratton, 1980a. Pp. 339–348.

Shine, R. *Systematic Fluency Training for Young Children: A Fluency Training Kit*. Tigard, Ore.: C. C. Publications, 1980b.

Shine, R. Systematic Fluency Training with the Young Stutterer, Paper presented at the annual convention of the American Speech-Language and Hearing Association, Houston, 1976.

Shine, R. and Mason, D. Direct intervention: A follow-up study of the beginning stutterer. Paper presented at the annual convention of the American Speech-Language and Hearing Association, Detroit, 1980.

Shine, R., Mason, D. Variables contributing to success/failure in fluency training with beginning stutterers. Paper presented at the annual convention of the American Speech-Language and Hearing Association, Los Angeles, 1981.

Sussman, H., and MacNeilage, P. Hemispheric specialization for speech production and perception in stutterers. *Neuropsychol.* 13:19–26, 1975.

Thompson, J. Suggestions for research: Young stutterers. *J. Fluency Disord.* 2:45–52, 1977.

Toscher, M., and Rupp, R. A study of the central auditory processing in stutterers using the synthetic sentence identification (SSI) test battery. *J. Speech Hear. Res.* 21:779–792, 1978.

Travis, L. E. *Speech Pathology*. New York: Appleton-Century-Crofts, 1931.

Underwood, B. *Experimental Psychology*. New York: Appleton-Century-Crofts, 1966.

Van Riper, C. *The Treatment of Stuttering*. Englewood Cliffs, N. J.: Prentice-Hall, 1973.

Van Riper, C. *The Nature of Stuttering*. Englewood Cliffs, N. J.: Prentice-Hall, 1982.

Webster, R. Behavioral analysis of stuttering: Treatment and Theory. In K. S. Calhoun, H. E. Adams, and K. E. Mitchell (eds.), *Innovative Treatment Methods in Psychopathology*, New York: Wiley, 1974.

West, R., and Ansberry, M. *The Rehabilitation of Speech*. New York: Harper, 1957.

West, R., Kennedy, L., and Carr, A. *The Rehabilitation of Speech*. Harper & Brothers, 1937.

West, R., Nelson, S., and Berry, M. The heredity of stuttering. *Q. J. Speech* 25 (1) 23–30, 1939.

Wingate, M. Evaluation and stuttering: I. Speech characteristics of young children. *J. Speech Hear. Disord.* 27:106–115, 1962.

Wingate, M. The fear of stuttering. *ASHA* 13:3–5, 1971.

Wingate, M. *Stuttering: Theory and Treatment*. New York: Irvington, 1976.

Wingate, M. Speaking unassisted: Comments on a paper by Andrews et al. *J. Speech Hear. Res.* 48:255–263, 1983.

Yeudall, L., Moore, W., and Boberg, E. Abnormalities in hemispheric functioning associated with stuttering, Paper presented at the annual convention of the American Speech-Language and Hearing Association, Toronto, 1982.

Zimmerman, G., and Knott, J. Slow potentials of the brain related to speech processing in normal speakers and stutterers. *EEG Clin. Neurophys.* 37:599–607, 1974.

Zimmerman, G., Liljeblad, S., Frank, A., and Cleeland, C. The Indians have many terms for it: Stuttering among the Bannock-Shoshoni. *J. Speech Hear. Res.* 26:315–318, 1983.

Appendix 5-A. Comprehensive Stuttering Analysis Verbatim Transcript

/wh—h:whats/ *(SB—2.1 sec, hard glottal stop, inappropriate pause—with prolonged whispered expiration, speaking on supplemental air)* this for? Oh yea, okay. It's got /wi'—h:wi'—h:wilson/ *(SB—8.5 sec, hard glottal stops, inappropriate pauses—with noisy aspiration, speaking on supplemental air)* and /ru–wrote/ (PW) on it /an–an/ (WW) I /hhhhhhhhit/ (PROL—1.5 sec) /t–two/ (PW) /nnnnnnnineteen (PROL—1.5 sec) home runs with it. /a—h: 'I/ *(SB—1 sec, inappropriate pause—with noisy expiration, hard glottal attack)* play base *(noisy inspiration, not stuttering)* ball. Last night it was so funny. I ain't kiddin'. /a'–h:—an/ *(SB—1.5 sec, hard glottal stop, noisy expiration, inappropriate silent pause—)* /'a—'I/ *(SB—1 sec, hard glottal attacks, inappropriate silent pause—)* got a man out /a–an/ (PW) /hi–hit/ (PW) my /bi–big/ (PW) toe and that guy *(implosion, stoppage of airflow)* can throw real /hu—'ard/ *(SB—1.5 sec, inappropriate pause with aspirated explosion)* and it's blue. /I–It's/ (PW) real sore. Toby Smith, Mark Jones, /Ju–Jim/ (PW) Bob Boone, /Ge'h:—Gary/ *(SB—2 sec, hard glottal stop, noisy, prolonged aspiration, inappropriate pause—)* Mason. /Tu–Toby (PW) and Gary *(um, uh—nonstuttering disfluency)* they go they go *(phrase repetition—nonstuttering disfluency)* to/hhhhhhhis/ (PROL—1 sec) school.

6. Vocal Control Therapy for Stutterers

Adeline E. Weiner

Overview

Vocal Control Therapy for stutterers has two main concerns: to provide a means of achieving reliable fluency and to create favorable psychophysiologic conditions to assure its successful use.

This chapter describes a phonatory approach to the fluency problems of stutterers and presents a brief review of behavioral desensitization techniques. Results of an ongoing evaluation are reported and some theoretical implications of a vocally oriented therapy considered.

History of the Therapy

In a recent study by Ragsdale and Ashby (1982), "Speech-Language Pathologists' Connotations of Stuttering," more than 200 public school speech-language pathologists were asked to respond to a semantic differential questionnaire concerning stuttering. The purpose of the inquiry was to elicit the thoughts of variously trained clinicians about seven concepts related to the disorder. The results clearly showed that attitudes toward stuttering disorders tended to be more positive than those toward stuttering *therapy*, regardless of the training or certification status of the clinician.

As others have noted (Wingate, 1971; Leith, 1971), these opinions reflect feelings of uneasiness, if not fear, about treating this complex disorder. Such marked inhibition toward treatment suggests an absence of security about method and with it a strong fear of failure. A test of efficacy for a particular therapy method might well include the attitude of the clinician towards its use: To what extent does it inspire clarity and confidence? It was just such uncertainties about the dominant programs of the day that led to the beginnings of Vocal Control Therapy (VCT).

In 1970, unhappy with the procedures and outcome of the conventional therapies of the time, I, along with successive groups of graduate students and several teaching clinicians associated with the clinical training program at Temple University, started a deliberate search for new and more satisfying approaches to stuttering therapy. As a first step, I called attention to Wingate's persuasive discussion (1969, 1970) of artificial fluency and vocalization change. Wingate's hypothesis stimulated us to

Appreciation is expressed to Lorraine Hansen Russell for her understanding and assistance as Director of Training, Division of Speech, Hearing and Language Sciences, Temple University, and for her perceptive editorial suggestions during the writing of this chapter. I am indebted to Dorothy Mewha and her staff for their generous technical assistance.

217

search for new treatment strategies. Operant conditioning methods for teaching speech behaviors were rapidly opening up new avenues of exploration, among them the use of fluency devices such as rhythm and delayed auditory feedback. The latter techniques had long been proscribed as artificial and misleading contrivances, but were now being utilized to induce fluent speech which was to be further maintained and expanded by contingent reinforcement procedures.

Furthermore, in a course on stuttering at Rutgers University, Ronald Goldman introduced me to the work of Joseph Wolpe on control of anxiety, which eventually led to an invaluable training experience in 1970 at the Behavior Therapy Institute, Temple University Medical School, under Dr. Wolpe himself.

This concurrence of events reaffirmed my conviction that remediation for stutterers rested with speech specialists, and not with psychologists, psychiatrists, or hypnotists. It was and is my belief that our profession is best suited to deal with both the physiologic and psychological nature of stuttering.

The original plan was to identify key speech motor controls which, when joined to systematic desensitization of speech anxiety, would bring about durable, natural fluency, the kind that could stand up to stress and the passage of time. We focused first on rhythmic speech, advocating a loosely rhythmic pattern, camouflaged by flexible phrasing and natural intonation, rather than the strict beat which Brady encouraged using the metronome (1971). Our approach proved to be somewhat vague, however, and few clients were able to master it. Those who nevertheless succeeded, complained that this technique held up only after phonation was initiated. Starting, they protested, was a constant hazard. As good speech-language pathologists, who knew how to manage that sort of problem, we offered a temporary strategy for voice onset: start to talk in a breathy or aspirate voice. That this worked well was soon clear. Moreover, it was found that use of a breathy voice replaced use of rhythm altogether: a voiced whisper was an equally powerful fluency condition to work from.

It was at this point, in 1972–1973, that M. F. Schwartz, a speech science professor in our department and an informal consultant to the experimental stuttering therapy program, arranged his first popular media interview, discussed his theory and therapy, and published a theoretical paper on stuttering (1974). His subsequent appearances on national television publicizing his "solution" to stuttering caused considerable confusion between his program and Vocal Control Therapy since both were associated with Temple University's Speech Department. Schwartz resigned in 1975 and published his book in 1976 in which he advocates a breathy release of expiration before initiating an utterance, as the "cure" for stuttering.

The artificial fluency we attained with aspirated voicing was clearly unacceptable for normal communication. No speaker could be expected to talk that way publicly, and since the breathy voice failed on its own to modify into normal volume, it qualified only as a temporary device. These findings led to a search of the literature on voice therapy which continues still. The goal was to experiment with ways recommended by voice specialists to manipulate phonational parameters so that normal intensity levels are obtained while essentially beneficial relationships within the vocal tract are maintained. The inclusion of desensitization using behavior therapy methods remained a constant part of the treatment program despite the changing speech controls.

The pursuit of suitable phonatory conditions led through thickets of trial and error along such variables as voice register, pitch change, and vowel lengthening. Sometime in 1973, we settled on a powerful and practical fluency generator—good vocal usage—a collective term for adequate breath support, appropriate vocal onset, and optimal voice quality. The therapy method to achieve good vocal usage for stutterers was dubbed "Vocal Control Therapy" (VCT), a program forthrightly devoted to and dependent on a vocalization hypothesis for remediation of stuttering.

At this point, I drew up formal plans for a trial therapy program which provided the substance of a report published several years after (Weiner, 1978). The basic tenets espoused then remain as originally formulated, except perhaps for a steadily deepening emphasis on phonation as the key to fluency.

In 1976, Temple University's Media Learning Center awarded me a grant to produce a series of 10 videotapes and one overview tape of VCT with excerpts from actual therapy sessions.* On completion of the tapes, I also prepared a VCT manual with exercises and source materials to accompany them. Since that time, I have included this series and a video record of pretherapy and posttherapy views of clients in training courses for graduate students in speech-language pathology at Temple University and in VCT workshops for speech-language professionals. In all, I have conducted an average of three such training courses and 1 or 2 workshops for area professionals annually since 1974.

PERTINENT RESEARCH

Although in one sense VCT developed independently through trial and error, the influence of the rapidly growing research on vocalization was immense during the 1970s. Among the major reports which lent support to a vocal approach were a series of indirect investigations of vocal tract behavior by Adams and his coworkers (Adams, 1974; Adams and Reis, 1971; Adams and Moore, 1972; Adams and Hutchinson, 1974; Adams and Hayden, 1976; Bruce and Adams, 1978). Even though the main focus of inquiry was related to phonational parameters of stuttering, Adams

---

*Produced and directed by Warren Schloss, formerly of the Office of Television Services, Temple University, with their support. Authors are A. Weiner and W. Schloss.

held that stuttering is in essence a failure to coordinate constituent parts of the speech system: respiration, phonation, and articulation (1974).

Direct evidence of aberrant laryngeal activity during stuttering emerged from use of electromyographic instrumentation, as reported by Freeman and Ushijima (1976, 1978) and was further supported by Shapiro (1980). Both studies described the phenomenon of co-contraction of the abductory and adductory intrinsic laryngeal muscles during stuttering, as well as the excessive glottal tonicity which in stutterers appears to accompany speech motor movement in general.

These findings were inestimably helpful in suggesting a hypothetical model that served to clarify and explain the precise behaviors we were observing. Envisioning the stuttering block as a stoppage due to the failure of reciprocal abduction/adduction processes at the larynx gave substance to our therapeutic strategy of voice and breath management.

Conture and associates (1977), using fiberoptic technology, revealed relatively consistent vocal fold patterns in respect to types of stuttering such as repetition and prolongation, which again appeared to corroborate the view of the glottis as the locus of disordered speech and the vibration of the vocal folds as the area of breakdown.

Although these studies (and many more) have enhanced our understanding of stuttering, we are still uncertain about the contribution of phonation other than that laryngeal misfunction is somehow implicated. Those of us who nevertheless undertake to treat stutterers must rely on insufficiently tested rationales as in the case of vocally oriented stuttering therapy. The distance that persists between theory and practice, on the other hand, has the effect of stimulating us to evaluate our therapy techniques with more rigor and curiosity.

The acquisition of an electrolaryngograph by the Temple University speech science lab prompted a study of still a third means for direct observation of stuttering behavior. This nonintrusive instrument permits the measurement of impedance between electrodes situated on either side of the thyroid cartilage. Rapid vocal fold movements are recorded as variations in impedance which in turn provide detailed information of phonation during stuttering.

The electrolaryngographic study (Weiner, in press) provided glottographs of 12 adult stutterers (8 men and 4 women) of which I examined samples of eight types of stuttering. From these I inferred that stuttering, regardless of the type of "block," consists of attempts to achieve steady state vibratory action of the vocal folds in an effort to phonate the vowel elements of speech. The few strategems that stutterers employ to overcome failure to initiate and maintain phonation appear stereotypical and automatic which suggests that these maneuvers are learned at an early age and maintained by peripherally controlled motor systems of loosely coupled oscillators (Polit and Bizzi, 1978; Fowler et al., 1980; Kelso, 1981). It appears that the child stutterer as he becomes aware of his unnatural speech, tries to repress it in trial and error fashion. These attempts, often counterproductive, remain largely intact and are gradually incorporated into a control motor speech program. According to Polit and Bizzi (1978), management of skilled motor activity that no longer requires central nervous system regulation is taken over by mechanisms peripheral to the center. For stutterers, the independence from top-down command of organ muscle systems may explain why both the stuttering behaviors and efforts to correct them appear joined in an "involuntary struggle" pattern, resistant to change segment by discrete segment. A further inference is that a therapy program would do well to retrain the originally faulty speech motor system as a whole rather than attempt to adjust its peripherally governed parts.

Assessment Procedures

The diagnostic format for VCT candidates followed at Temple University Speech and Hearing Center (TUSHC) is one used for all stutterers applying for therapy. The procedures are contained in the *Diagnostic Evaluation Form for Stutterers*, a checklist of items which is employed in conjunction with regular assessment practices.

Typically, a clinical team takes a case history and administers oral-peripheral and audiologic examinations along with tests for measurement and analysis of the disorder.

Clients make audiotape-recorded samples of elicited and spontaneous speech which are kept on file. (A videotape of the client speaking in five conditions, made just prior to entering therapy, provides the baseline of stuttering for VCT cases.)

CASE HISTORY INTERVIEW

In the case history interview the clinician obtains information concerning:

Time of onset (age, circumstances)
Periods of remission
Early stuttering characteristics
Early reactions of parents, teachers, and peers
Previous therapy (kind and length)
General health
Family history of speech, voice, language, or learning problems
Immediate concerns regarding education, job, social and personal goals

The clinician ascertains the client's view of his behavior and elicits a description of situations and variations: when he is most and least disfluent, how severe the stuttering is, and the type and loci of stuttering; the clinician also describes the client's voice and breathing patterns.

ASSESSMENT OF STUTTERING SEVERITY

To assess the extent of the stuttering problem, we administer the Stuttering Severity Instrument (Riley, 1972) which tests for frequency, duration, and the role of concomitant features. The scores from these tests are then given a percentile rating and categorized as mild, moderate, or severe stuttering.

The diagnostic team analyzes the type of stuttering displayed; tallies the frequency of repetitions, prolongations, and silent blocks occurring within 5- or 10-minute time segments, and takes counts of associated behaviors.

TESTS OF AFFECT

The client takes two pencil-and-paper tests, usually during the diagnostic team conference. Stutterers' Self-Ratings of Reactions to Speech Situations (Johnson et al., 1963) requires the person to rate on a scale of 1 to 5, the degree of avoidance, reaction, stuttering and frequency in a series of everyday speech encounters. The scores are compared with the norms for a group of young adult male stutterers, but these scores are probably less important than the information concerning specific speech conditions and their relative emotional effects. This information is useful for hierarchy construction for systematic desensitization.

The IPAT Anxiety Scale,* a 40-item questionnaire, taps the overall anxiety level of the prospective client. The instrument yields a stem score and norms for several population groups which serve as a measure of a generalized or habitual anxiety state.

The examiner then rates the client on an overall impression of tension on a scale of 1 to 10, using prepared tests if applicable. When possible, significant others provide estimates, also. We sometimes readminister these measures for posttherapy estimates of improvement, as well.

VOICE AND SPEECH INVENTORY
Respiration

Examiners determine if breathing pattern is clavicular, thoracic, or abdominal-diaphragmatic; they also distinguish the presence of audible inhalation, gasping, speaking on residual air, synchrony of breathing with speech, and other irregularities.

Phonation

Examiners estimate loudness (unsteady, too loud, too soft, appropriate), pitch (high, low, monopitch, normal), hyponasality or hypernasality, resonance (oral, pharyngeal, abnormal, normal), and quality (breathy, hoarse, harsh, glottal fry, dysphonia, constricted orality). We use a rating scale of 1 to 10, as well as verbal descriptions.

*Institute for Personality and Ability Testing, 1602 Coronado Drive, Champaign, IL 61820.

Vocal Onset
The Towne-Heuer Reading Passage for Vocal Analysis provides measurement of type of onset: the first part permits 100 opportunities for harsh or abrupt vowel initiation. This measure yields a percentage score for comparison to norms given for geographic area.

Speech Rate
The examiners determine rate by a count of words per minute during fluent productions (judged against a normal rate of 220 to 410 words per minute).

Articulation/Resonance
We observe the client's general precision, proficiency, and/or errors in intelligibility of consonant production, which we then test and measure if necessary.

Characteristics of vocal tract shaping of vowel elements are of considerable interest. We take note of oral functions such as tongue carriage, action of the mandible, oral-pharyngeal closure and openness, and efficiency of velopharyngeal action.

TRIAL THERAPY
The following procedures, which are wholly optional, are employed to induce artificial fluency: shadow talking, choral speaking, delayed auditory feedback with and without cues to prolong vocalization, metronome speech, and stretched syllables (prolonging the vowel).

A VCT clinician utilizes these maneuvers as a way to demonstrate to the client our facility in stimulating temporary fluent utterance. We then explain that this type of easy success is distinct from that which results from a serious program of retraining. Only the latter enables the speech system to produce and maintain genuine, stable fluency. Some clinicians regard the stutterer's sensitivity to these pseudofluency devices as prognostic signs of progress in therapy and, therefore, of possible significance in the evaluating process.

Trial therapy for assessing and introducing vocal subsystem function focuses on vocal quality and breathing.

Target Voice
Shape from a humming sound; cue for clear, full voice. Use delayed auditory feedback (DAF) to stimulate desired voice quality if necessary. The client is urged to count, say name, address and/or telephone number at target voice level, if successful. If not, the clinician should be able to offer a model and describe its characteristics.

Abdominal-Diaphragmatic Breathing
If the client can produce a correct respiratory pattern of exhalation, label and discuss this activity as necessary to support "good" voicing. If not,

the clinician again should model the correct movements of the upper abdominal wall for inhalation/exhalation.

During the diagnostic session, we usually do not ask the client to attempt the techniques of easy onset or vowel focus, but the choice remains open. If, however, the client can process large amounts of information, the clinician may explain all the vocal objectives by giving examples of each.

REPORT TO THE CLIENT

We report the results of the testing and observation, along with a characterization of the extent of severity and an estimate of the role of affective factors, to the client.

We also provide an overall description of and rationale for the VCT program, including the vocal and desensitization goals. In addition, within the limits of our knowledge, we answer any questions about the origin and nature of stuttering that our clients may pose.

COMMITMENT TO THERAPY

Both client and clinician express their degree of interest in and their expectations concerning the treatment program. The clinician discusses the conditions of admittance: the level of participation required by both parties; the number of sessions per week; the time and fee schedules.

We state our commitment to accept the client into therapy or make a referral to other VCT clinicians in other agencies or parts of the city, or to other types of therapy, if desired.

A written evaluation report is assured within 3 weeks, containing in full the information discussed and agreed upon in the assessment session.

Description of the Therapy

THERAPY GOALS

The chief object of therapy is to establish habitual speech patterns that will operate reliably in all types of speech situations. Starkweather (1980) suggests that the three major descriptors of normal fluency are continuity, a rate natural to the speaker, and ease of production. These characteristics are incorporated as objectives within the two main subgoals of the VCT program: (1) retraining of the vocal apparatus and its subsystems of respiration, phonation and resonation; (2) relieving speech anxiety through desensitization techniques employed in behavior therapy, such as systematic desensitization and behavior rehearsal.

THERAPY METHOD

The VCT method has two general features which are important to note in advance of a detailed description.

First, the approach is system oriented in the sense that the object is to reprogram a faulty schema of motor coordination by replacing it with a more efficient alternative. Initially, the program may focus on isolated aspects of the training just as instruction for any complex skill, such as driving a car or playing a piano sonata. It is only common sense to introduce new information slowly and a bit at a time. The aim, of course, is to attain integration of subsidiary skills in well-coordinated sequences of movements executed at one's normal rate of speed. The focus of therapy is on fluency, not on analysis or correction of separate stuttering events. This means that errors are not defined by incidents of stuttering, but are attributed to instances of improper phonation. Fluency failure is equivalent to a fault in the voice production process which, in turn, may sometimes be reflective of emotional stress.

The other general feature to note is that VCT is a *program* of therapy, but is not *programmed therapy:* there is no prescribed step sequencing or rigid procedural schedule, and the therapist has ample opportunity for creative invention. Clinicians, students in training, and clients themselves have all contributed ideas, exercises, and experiences to the shape of the program. We encourage choice by clinicians and clients in the sequence of skills, the stimulus materials, the amount of time spent on each target, and the types of transfer activities and home assignments. All parts of the program are adjustable both to the clinician's way of working and to the learning patterns, temperament, and preferences of the client. The requisite "bottom line" is fluent speech through optimal voicing and reduced communication fear.

SPECIFIC TECHNIQUES, PROCEDURES, AND ACTIVITIES
Acquisition of Vocal Skills
There are four main components to the process of acquiring vocal control for fluency: breath control through *abdominal-diaphragmatic breathing,* smooth initiation of phonation through *easy onset of voicing,* improved voice quality through *optimum oral resonance,* and a technique for maintaining steady state phonation during speech flow called *vowel focus.*

In view of the fact that voice therapy is a major source for the methodology of VCT, it is interesting to examine the list of facilitating techniques that Boone describes in a chapter on hyperfunctional voice problems (1977). Of the 24 strategies he lists for cases of vocal abuse and functional dysphonia, only 4 would be regularly unsuited to stuttering therapy. (An example is digital manipulation for pitch change.) Although we have developed original strategies for "stutterers only," so to speak, his methods have proved highly useful to practitioners of VCT. There exists a generous overlap with strategies derived from the voice therapy literature, which serves to underline the predominantly vocal content of this method (see References).

Target Voice

While fluent speech is the main purpose of rehabilitating the vocalization system of stutterers, the process itself results in a voice of good quality almost as a by-product. A good-sounding voice, then, notifies the speaker that optimal conditions for fluency prevail within the vocal apparatus.

For this reason, we emphasize a well-produced voice as the major target of therapy and at the beginning ask the client to attempt a brief sample of his best vocalizing effort. This sample is then identified (perhaps tape-recorded) as, at least, approximating the end goal of training. Most stutterers are able to manage this short task easily (as are most voice cases) either with the aid of appropriate cues or by imitation of a live or tape-recorded model provided by the clinician. We sometimes use delayed auditory feedback to effect those changes in volume and tempo that act to shape a better voice. (See Wingate, 1970, for a discussion of the Lombard effect on stuttering of auditory masking.) Whatever the techniques, the salient message to the client is that optimal voicing is the long-term goal of the speech control. The component factors that lead to habitual use of good quality phonation are then undertaken separately.

Breath Control

RATIONALE. Most stutterers exhibit, to some degree, deviant breathing patterns for speech, and some of these may be quite extreme (Bloodstein, 1981). When the question comes up in therapy, stutterers often express emphatic agreement, "Yes, I do have a lot of trouble with breathing when I stutter." Even if breathing aberrations are minor or absent, we find it mandatory to teach every client abdominal-diaphragmatic (A-D) breathing as the most effective source of energy for optimum voicing. The problem is almost always a matter of managing the exiting breath stream rather than inspiring sufficient pulmonary air for speech, and this requires firm A-D action.

Control begins at the moment of exhalation and requires active fixation or stiffening of the epigastric musculature (upper abdominal wall) in order to keep the airflow steady (Vennard, 1967). The main effect is to prevent a rapid loss of expiratory air at the beginning of the utterance which then is often followed by hasty grasping for control midway through the breath unit. Stutterers who resort to talking on residual air (when subglottal air pressure is low and vocal fold tension is reduced) especially need practice in taking charge of airflow at the start of exhalation and maintaining steady support throughout.

TECHNIQUES. We begin by describing in simple terms the basic principles of the breathing process and practicing passive easy intake of air through a slightly open mouth with little or no movement of the chest or shoulders.* Before the client begins exhalation, we emphasize controlled expiratory airflow with moderately active contraction of the upper abdominal musculature. After these trials with sustained silent outgoing breath, we introduce the phonemes [s], [m], and [a] (in that order), aiming for gradual increments of sustained sound up to and beyond 15 seconds. The client practices each of these phonemes in three positions: supine, standing, and then sitting. For the supine position, we use a pad or rug on the floor or perhaps, for a child, on a table surface. We then place a moderately heavy weight (a 2-pound book) on the stomach between the lower ribs as a visual-kinesthetic cue for slow smooth exhalation, but a hand is an equally effective cueing device for standing and sitting positions. Further increases in sustained phoneme duration, or better still, sit-up exercises for the upper torso help strengthen muscle tone in the upper abdominal wall. Jogging, running, swimming, and aerobic dancing are excellent activities for stutterers who are deficient in breath support and control; and for children, playing a wind instrument helps develop strong abdominal action. These activities, however, must be deliberately linked to breathing for speech, for clients seldom transfer this learning automatically.

Relaxed, upright posture in the sitting position is essential. When stimulus materials are used, they should be propped up so that they are easily visible. A client doubled over material that is lying flat on a tabletop is an example of poor logistics in breath control training.

> Seth, one of our college student clients, had breathing so erratic during speech that he was unable to keep a book on his stomach when it expanded for inhalation. His initial expiratory duration time, even on [s], was a shaky, uneven 4 to 6 seconds. His mother agreed to make him a 5-pound bean bag to practice with at home. He began jogging several times a week and in 2 months was able to achieve steady durations of 20 to 30 seconds on isolated sounds.†

As breath control develops, the clinician will typically introduce another subsystem of vocalization, that of smooth vocal initiation.

Easy Onset

RATIONALE. In the experience of the VCT program, glottal hypertonicity is a problem shared by most, if not all, stutterers, and the onset of phonation has a special place in the stutterer's list of vexations. If phonational in-

---

*A compilation of exercises utilized in the VCT program is contained in a supplementary manual, a mimeographed booklet produced in 1978 at Temple University.
†The therapy cases cited for illustration throughout the chapter are based on actual therapy logs although the names have been changed in the interests of anonymity.

tegrity is our main target, then the ability to induce a steady vocal tone promptly and smoothly is an important prerequisite.

One vocal initiation problem we examined early in the program was the relative frequency of harsh glottal attack (hga) in stutterers. It might be expected that due to laryngeal tension, stutterers would exhibit a significantly higher rate of hga than fluent speakers; yet this is not necessarily the case.

In a recent study, Heuer (1976) developed an instrument for measuring hga, and established norms for a population of native Philadelphians. As stutterers entered our program, then, we evaluated them on this point, using Heuer's reading passage, and they appeared by and large to share the speech patterns of their community with regard to evidence of hga. Nevertheless, the absence of harsh and abrupt initiation of voice did not belie the ever present, if less extreme, display of tense glottal onset in most disfluent speakers. Moreover, we realized early on that, due to the stutterer's frequent failure to initiate phonation, even the slightest hypertonicity in vocal onset would have to be regarded as a hindrance to fluency. Therefore, training in soft vocal fold adduction became a routine part of the retraining program.

Support for this approach is found in at least one other stuttering therapy program, "A Precision Fluency-Shaping Program" (Webster, 1975). From all indications, this therapy devotes the largest portion of the training to shaping "slow rise" onset of speech using the voice monitor, an instrument developed for that purpose by the Communications Research Unit, Hollins College, Hollins, Virginia. Boone (1977) describes this electronic device as a means of signaling to the patient the various levels of intensity with which abrupt voice onset is occurring.

In VCT we regard easy onset in Aronson's terms (1980) as "an even or static attack" on phonation with the vocal folds nearly at closure at the beginning of expiration. Initiation of vibration action can then be "smooth and instantaneous." Zemlin also suggests that complete approximation of the vocal folds is unnecessary for vibratory action to begin. Adequate closure may allow as much as a 3-mm space at the glottal chink and still afford sufficient subglottal air pressure to activate vocal fold vibration (1968).

In our program, to promote soft, simultaneous vocal fold closure, we rely on a number of methods, some of which follow.

TECHNIQUES. Head rolls: To stretch and relax the large muscles of the neck and throat, we instruct the client to allow his head to hang forward on the chest loosely. With the weight of the head pulling at the neck muscles, he then rolls the head slowly to one shoulder, to the back, then to the other shoulder, each for counts of 5. Repeat 5 times.

Yawn-sigh: To relax the muscles of the pharyngeal area, the client takes deep inhalations through a wide-open mouth, stretching arms to stimulate genuine yawning. He then exhales air slowly with a voiced sigh, using abdominal muscles to control the air stream.

Raising the velum (soft palate): To effect an immediate release of tension at the folds of the velum, the client begins by stretching the back of the mouth open while keeping the lips closed. This simulates a "hidden" yawn, as if one were bored but polite. After several practice trials, the client then draws in air through the mouth, stretching the velum upward and promptly producing the sound "ah." The client practices this series of gestures on isolated vowels at first but is encouraged to employ this maneuver whenever necessary.

The rationale for this strategy rests on the fact that it is the beginning of the yawn, at the point of optimal openness before the stretch becomes tense, that is really the "business" end of the gesture (Vennard, 1967). At the same time that the velum is in an upward stretch, the back of the tongue is lowered, forcing the larynx down. These simultaneous movements serve to enlarge the vocal tract (Sundberg, 1970) relaxing the conus elasticus membrane which rises from the cricoid cartilage to form the vocal ligaments (Borden and Harris, 1980). It is this reduction of tension which may be acting to free the folds for immediate easy oscillation.

Practice of vowel onsets with isolated vowels: To call attention to simultaneous activity at the laryngeal level, we instruct the client to take a comfortable breath and begin vibrations for "ah" in the throat. Beginning very quietly and easily, as if the edges of the vocal folds "were made of velvet," the speaker quickly builds up volume in a crescendo effect. Glottal control requires starting the voice at an "inaudible" level and rising slowly to a clear full sound. The client practices these approaches on vowels in isolation and then in nonsense syllables.

Auditory discrimination: To help the client judge the accuracy of his productions, we reject as incorrect productions that start with even barely perceptible signs of complete closure of the folds. These are heard as "clicks" and, however softly made, are remarkably discernible by the unaided ear. Aronson (1980) emphasizes the importance of auditory feedback from the act of voicing, since there is so little other sensory information issuing from the laryngeal area during vocalization. To heighten the client's awareness, the clinician may urge him deliberately to perform a series of hard laryngeal closures. This negative practice of incorrect muscle action, done with caution, provides an effective contrast between abrupt glottal stoppage and smooth initiation. In VCT experience, speakers soon hear the difference between the right and wrong ways to start to voice. Once that is learned they then rapidly develop the "knack" for bringing the edges of the folds together without clicks, or, in other words, with remarkable accuracy.

Using a voiced continuant: To promote control of adductory action at the glottis in a client slow to develop this skill, we sometimes introduce an intermediate step for producing easy onset of phonation. Our experience has been that using a breathy onset with [h] preceding the vowel is a comparatively inefficient procedure: one has always to return to the problem of setting up vocal tone from "scratch."

The strategy of sounding a voiced continuant before each vowel production, such as "is easy," "was easy," "has each," "have only," is a preferred approach (see Moncur and Brackett, 1974). From there, emphasis is on gradually reducing the [z] to silence, but sensing the start of glottal vibration just in advance of sounding the vowel, thus leading to gradual soft vowel onset.

Training proceeds with practice of vowel onsets of VC (vowel, consonant), VCVC words and phrases, and on into more complex speech environments.

> Doris was beset with a deeply-rooted habit of tense voicing of vowel initial words, easily the most troublesome part of her stuttering pattern. She especially feared any word that started with [eɪ]. When she brought clothes to the cleaners, she never gave her correct address because the number began with an *8*. She worked in an office in a responsible administrative position in spite of her difficulties with telephoning, but she complained of fatigue and severe tension which caused head and neck pain. After 6 months of VCT training in which she worked on eliminating the "clicks" before vowels, she became adept at detecting her errors and used "easy onset" speech at home, with strangers in therapy, and, on occasion, in her job. Her tension and anxiety were greatly reduced due to better breathing patterns, improved fluency and desensitization. After 60 sessions, Doris is now nearing completion of the program and is reporting over 90 percent fluency in transfer activities.

Almost 40 percent of our stutterers display tense glottal onset as a major problem. Still, we have found that merely correcting persistent prephonation closure is insufficient assurance against disfluency. Optimal phonatory function requires adequate breath control and easy initiation of voice, but most of all, promotion of full-fold laryngeal oscillation at the sound source.

Optimum Oral Resonance
This is probably the most distinctive component of the VCT program. A desirable quality of vocal tone, as perceived by the listener, serves as a measure of the functional integrity of the phonatory apparatus as a whole. In other words, the qualitative "goodness" of the voice reflects whether or not optimal conditions of breath control, vocal fold vibration, and vocal tract transfer obtain. This principle is the linchpin of vocal control therapy.

The meaning of the term *resonance* in this context is limited to perceived voice quality characteristics of oral cavity resonance. As Perkins (1977) states, the definition of voice quality is "mired in a terminological swamp" because it does not lend itself to quantification, as do the parameters of intensity and frequency. The absence of quantified data, Perkins makes clear, in no way denies the influence of physiologic factors on voice quality.

RATIONALE. We hypothesize that stuttering is chiefly a matter of failure to maintain steady state phonation, due very likely to involuntary disruption of vocal fold reciprocal action. If vocal fold activity can be initiated smoothly and sustained in a relaxed state of equilibrium, we believe that stuttering will be prevented.

Early in the development of this therapy program, good oral resonance was found to be a reliable fluency condition. When we observed its effects in light of the burgeoning laboratory research on stuttering and laryngeal function, we arrived at an hypothesis linking vocal fold behaviors to enhanced oral resonance. Though other important factors are known to be involved in producing optimum oral resonance (such as the size, shape and wall texture of the oral-pharyngeal cavity), what is considered paramount here is the effect of good oral resonance on the laryngeal mechanism. Full-fold laryngeal oscillation and valving constitute the best source for optimal sound wave amplification in the oral-pharyngeal cavity (Moncur and Brackett, 1974). Since we have little ability directly to manipulate vocal fold action (Aronson, 1980), we look to the *product* of well-coordinated vocal tract function, using our perception of a voice of "good" quality as our guide. Vennard (1967), an authority on the singing voice, also supports the larynx as the seat of vocal quality although the resonators often appear to be the source. By promoting improved oral resonance, we are teaching stutterers how best to influence the source of the voice in order to create stable laryngeal motor movement.

The next problem is to determine the best techniques for achieving the goal of optimum oral resonance. Here we look to the field of voice training in which actors, newscasters, and other public speakers have long received effective instruction. As with the issue of voice quality, we are again at a disadvantage due to the lack of precision and testing of the training strategies utilized. Still, these strategies have proved to be sufficiently effective and convincing to have remained with the VCT program since its inception.

TECHNIQUES. To identify the sensation of strong oral resonance, we have adopted Perkins' term *high vocal focus* to convey the feeling that the voice is located away from "low" points in the throat, and instead feels as if it is placed high behind the face, well away from the voice box (Perkins, 1977). To promote high vocal focus, some voice specialists teach the use of a falsetto (or loft) register voice and then scale the pitch down to normal levels to produce the desired effect. VCT, however, employs a humming sound [m] within the normal pitch range, from which the speaker is urged to create a mounting sensation of a progressively stronger "buzzing" sound or hum. These sympathetic or forced vibrations in the region of the lips, cheeks, bridge of the nose, and forehead are more strongly felt on nasal phonemes due to the coupling of the nasal and oral cavities, but a sufficiently clear vibratory sensation can be produced by any voiced continuant such as [z] or [v]. The real object of the exercise is to transfer the vibrant quality of the voice to all the vowel elements of an utterance. Vowel sounds will reflect the enhanced sound wave amplification in the oral cavity although the sensation of vibration in the head and face will have diminished somewhat with the open-mouth shaping of the vowels.

We instruct the client to hum until he feels strong vibrations at the lips, nose, cheek bones, and forehead. Next, we introduce nonsense syllables consisting of [m] plus vowel (NV) (nasal vowel) such as *may, mee, my, moh, mum;* and then we proceed to words with two nasal phonemes (NVN) such as *mine, man, mean.* The client initially says one word for each breath taken, but later works on three for each breath, sustaining the hum throughout. From there, we progress to NVC (nasal, vowel, consonant) words such as *mile, mass, made,* and then to NVNV, and NVNVC words such as *many, mini* and *manner, minute.* We introduce phrases such as *nine nouns, neon numbers,* or longer ones such as *mountainous morn, mineral mining,* and then sentences: *Mike was fond of mountain climbing.* Poems with lyrical, sonorous quality may be read to encourage temporarily exaggerated oral resonance, and at each level we provide intensive drills with ample lists of stimuli.

To avoid any tendency toward excessive nasality as a result of nasal phoneme emphasis, we alert the client to speak with an "open mouth." Open mouth positioning and activating the lower jaw will reduce the oral constriction which usually produces hypernasality. Stutterers who exhibit rigid mandible postures also need special attention to greater oral openness.

Our experience with the oral resonance segment of VCT has led us to an important observation: All clients, in spite of a lack of objective criteria for improved oral resonance, quickly distinguish "poor" from "good" quality voicing. Even children discriminate readily though the cue may be "Use your 'clear' or 'best' voice." We have found that every stutterer, even those with pleasant, adequate voice quality, needs to engage in oral resonance work to stabilize vocal fold action and inhibit phonatory failure. Clients, of course, vary in the ease with which they make a "good" voice an everyday practice, but the difference between acceptable and excellent voice quality has sometimes made the difference between continued stuttering and fluency.

At an early stage in the development of VCT, Alf, a severe stutterer, was engaged in training for breath control and easy onset. He was an active member of a choral singing society, but for him as with most stutterers, his singing had little relation to his stuttered speech. Alf had been making good progress, if a little slowly, and his stuttering had lessened; but he soon arrived at a plateau at which his disfluency persisted for weeks with little sign of change. Because his speaking voice was pleasant and his singing skills were apparently first-rate, we had chosen not to pursue the matter of good resonant voicing for speech. However, as soon as we made the decision to begin work on oral resonance, and he mastered the techniques of good quality voice for speech, his stuttering receded and a consistently fluent, natural conversational pattern emerged. He and we were equally surprised, and it was an important lesson in the development of VCT. We have since respected our own strategy which views *optimum* oral resonance as that level of vocal performance with which stuttering is incompatible.

As the client advances in mastery of the techniques of better voice production, he is oriented to regard voice quality as the centerpiece of the fluency program, subsuming previous techniques under one unified vocal control. There is still one further strategy available, however, as special insurance against breakdown: the vowel focus approach.

Vowel Focus
The fourth skill taught in the VCT program is one already familiar to the client. It combines the techniques of easy onset and optimum oral resonance for vowels, not just in vowel-initial words but in any position in the syllable.

The client practices presetting the vocal tract for the vowel that follows a "troublesome" consonant or blend. For example, the client who feels that he is likely to stutter on the word "box" will practice "ox, ox, ox" with smooth initiation and good resonance on each [ɑ] and then say "box" with care not to preset the articulators for the [b] sound. This exercise is practiced until the speaker acquires an habitual readiness for proper vowelization.

RATIONALE. The impulse for this maneuver came from our experience with stutterers who were convinced that, in spite of demonstrable gains in fluency, they were doomed sooner or later to stutter on certain consonants. And that is what appeared to happen. Because we originally attributed these behaviors to associated fear responses that interfered with an otherwise successful vocal approach, we undertook several special desensitization measures (covert positive reinforcement and biofeedback), but to little avail. On closer observation we found that the "difficult" consonants ("Jonah" sounds) were often not the ones anticipated and further, that the real difficulty appeared, not in *their* production—they were likely to be repeated or prolonged many times over—but in the voicing of the vowel that followed the feared consonants. Wingate (1976) states, "In the vast majority of instances of stuttering, the 'following' sound is invariably a vowel. The analysis here thus reveals that the focal disturbance in stuttering involves *vowels* and not consonants" (p. 257).

TECHNIQUE. The clinician is often able to demonstrate to the client that he in fact is saying the "problem" sound without hindrance and that where he is "getting stuck" is on the approach to the vowel that follows the consonant. The client may begin with a list of those consonant initial words he most fears and with proper technique practice the vowel nuclei *minus* the consonant. Later, practice includes the initial consonant which is added at the last moment before saying the whole word. We instruct him to maintain the oral set for the vowel sound and to resist presetting the articulators for the preceding consonant or blend. The client drills on list after list in this way until the principle of vowel focus is well established. This method has the advantage of ridding the stutterer not only of a primary source of disfluency, but also of some of his oldest and most baseless fears.

> Dave, a college student, found the news that he was not stuttering on [d] astonishing. He had spent most of his life in mortal fear of that sound, which appeared to set off a teeth-rattling tremor. Dave acquired good breathing and phonation patterns in therapy and had been one of the subjects in an aborted study on desensitization devices for "articulatory" breakdown. Among the first to try the new vowel focus technique, he listened to himself on audiotape in the act of stuttering on words like "desk" and "dessert" and was impressed that he was repeating the [d] sound without difficulty but was failing to say the rest of the word. Clearly [d] was not the culprit (nor were any other consonants he sometimes repeated helplessly). Dave made the suggested shift in attention to properly phonating the vowel nucleus. He was given lists of stop-initial words to practice, producing each word several times without the initial consonant but with easy onset and good resonance. He then worked on the entire word, adding the initial consonant with his mouth still "set" for the vowel. He practiced on carrier phrases and sentences and after many hours of home practice, reading, and talking with others, succeeded in overcoming his "bete noir." He reported that whenever he "blocked" he could feel it "down in his throat"—that's where he felt "stuck." This insight and his conscientious work on vowel

focus led Dave to believe, in his words, that he "now could lead a normal life." His current job is as an accountant in a large firm for whom he travels as a consultant.

For VCT clients learning efficient vowel phonation, we have found that lax (short) vowels ([ɪ], [ɛ], [ʌ], [ʊ]) appear to present less opportunity for full-fold oscillation of the vocal folds than tense vowels. Special attention is given, therefore, to producing a consistently strong level of resonant voicing that will fulfill whatever demand shorter vowels make on the stutterer's system. This does not require the speaker to keep track of which vowels are which as he speaks. All he needs to do is sustain a sufficient degree of "good" voicing to stabilize vocal fold equilibrium for all vowels, including the shorter ones.

> L.T., an early client in VCT, appeared to have achieved a usable level of fluency after relatively long-term therapy, but still various hangups persisted. On analyzing specific instances of stuttered words it became apparent that the stuttered syllables all shared the same feature: they were words with lax (short) vowel nuclei such as *Dex*ter, (his boss's name); *dif*ferent; *con*solidate. After intensive practice of easy initiation and full resonation of lax vowel nuclei in long lists of multisyllabic words, L.T. was able to make his posttherapy tape and terminate regular sessions.

Having observed the influence of lax vowel nuclei on vocalization in stutterers, we saw clearly why vowels in unstressed syllables (usually lax) often show the same effect. They also appear to offer frequent loci for breakdown. Again, the vowel focus technique proves effective by prompting better vocal initiation and production.

The issue of stuttering on weaker syllables has bearing on the claim that stuttering occurs overwhelmingly on syllables that carry linguistic stress (Wingate, 1976). Wingate regards the disorder of stuttering as occurring in association with the physical demands made on the speech and language system by the prosodic elements of speech: stress, intonation, and juncture. In a study by Weiner (unpublished), 18 subjects read in random order two lists, each with 16 bisyllabic words, that could be read with stress on either syllable (for example, *add*ress and ad*dress*). An analysis of the results revealed a 51 percent occurrence of stuttering on unstressed versus stressed syllables. Within the context of vocally oriented treatment of stuttering, this finding suggests that stutterers find the coordinations needed to produce unstressed syllables at least as taxing as stressed ones. In view of this, therefore, the point of entry for therapeutic intervention should be the management of the laryngeal/respiratory factors involved in phonation rather than concern with the processes involved in suprasegmental speech events.

Recent experiences with two very severe stutterers suggest that some speakers are so sensitive in the area of phonatory function that even semivowels appear to be a source of aborted voicing.

Jay is an undergraduate whose stuttering is so severe that he has spent nearly 4 years at school in almost total silence. At the beginning of therapy, his stuttering pattern was to block on almost every vowel in an utterance, regardless of its position in the word. In attempting the word *forty-four*, for example, he would repeat the [f] sound two or three times, fail to voice the [ɔ], and stand gaping with lower jaw in tremor and glottis locked shut, unable to sound the vowel. After training in breath control and voice production, Jay was observed to stutter a good deal on words such as *continue* or *butter*, evidencing a problem mainly with lax vowels. When the level of voicing improved further and he advanced to more communicative exchanges, he still stumbled on words such as *you*, *ready*, and *where*, unable to sound the first phoneme, a semivowel, through to the vowel. The glide [j] was particularly hazardous every time it appeared, as in *university*, or *year*, and vowel focus did not solve this difficulty until we realized that the brief presence of [i] in [j] before the glide into the vowel was the source of the glottal block. This bit of vowelization required the same easy onset and high focus resonance as the major vowel nucleus [u], and when vowel focus shifted to the [i] sound, the blocking ceased. Jay is now working to maintain onset and resonation at levels that will encompass all instances of voicing.

SUMMARY OF SUBSYSTEM SKILLS

The four skills discussed so far, breath control, easy onset, resonant voicing, and vowel focus, are the means employed to effectuate the goal of "fluent" voicing. The fluency condition is accomplished, not as a series of tasks that demand constant tracking, but as a unified vocal effort. The subsystem skills that promote fluency are themselves linked together both physically and functionally in a closely bound series of behaviors that fuse into joint, simultaneous activity of the vocal system as a whole.

Inasmuch as vocal competency demands a level of habituation strong enough to replace an old habit system with a more efficient and less laborious manner of speaking, a systematic method for practicing the unified parts as a single whole is a necessity. We call this integration.

Practice of an Integrated Control

RATIONALE. There is practice which, though mechanical, is nevertheless useful as a means to automaticity; but practice informed with thoughtful concentration is a superior way to acquire new learning. Bernstein's (1967) description of the process is illuminating.

Practice, when properly undertaken, does not consist in repeating the means of solution of a motor problem time after time, but in the process of solving this problem again and again, by techniques which we change and perfect from repetition to repetition.

TECHNIQUE. This period of drill establishes the use of unified vocal control through an intensive schedule of practice which we call "systematic massed practice (SMP)." At this stage drill begins with highly structured exercises that lead ultimately to unstructured, self-generated material.

Structured practice: The client is provided with many opportunities to automatize the desired vocal set: he will eventually practice on literally thousands of items such as serial speech and readings, with length ranging from short simple sentences to a role from a play script. Another set of drills promotes normally cadenced speech in informal phrases such as "Hi, how are you?", "Do you believe it?", "It blew my mind!" Still others address problems of volume for clients who in the course of training have fallen into habits of overloud speech or persisted in low volume utterance. In these exercises the client, working from a list of phrases, practices speaking at three or four levels of loudness so as to assure himself of control over all types of speaking situations: shouting for help, talking in noisy environments, speaking at the dinner table or in ordinary conversation, and whispering in the presence of a sleeper or someone who is ill. All of these (even low intensity levels) require the usual strong breath support, easy onset, and high focus resonance.

Formal structure gives way to less formal, but still structured, modes of practice. Many clients have more than just ordinary difficulty moving from structured to unstructured material, that is, from stimuli provided by the clinician to self-generated utterances, either of increasing propositionality or in casual "throwaway" speech.

Intermediate structured practice: To assist clients who require small increments of difficulty in moving toward self-generated speech, we employ a large body of transitional verbal tasks such as

Answering "Yes" or "No" to simple sorting tasks.
Providing one-word answers to word games or sentence completion tasks.
Completing carrier phrases such as "Here is a _____."
Providing whole carrier phrases in card games ("Here is a three of clubs.")
Generating brief statements about a series of pictures: "That's a woman," "She's pretty."
Calculating problems aloud from arithmetic flashcards.
Playing games such as table games (Lotto), word games (Twenty Questions).

Progressively increasing the number of statements made about a series of pictures (from one statement to ten statements per picture).

We have found a wealth of material in a series of aphasia workbooks (see References). Although these exercises are arranged for patients engaged in adult language therapy, stutterers can utilize them, provided they are selected sequentially according to length and complexity of utterance. These hundreds of drills have saved hours of clinician preparation time. Some examples: Name four things you need to boil an egg. Use *picnic* and *tomato* in a sentence.

Unstructured practice: To arrive at a new level of facility with vocal control, monologues and dialogues are introduced. These may be practiced along two dimensions, time and content. While initially the client may start with a 15-second speech on a neutral topic such as the weather, he might progress to a several-minute discussion of a topic such as "What are my good and poor qualities?" These activities will mesh into more complex exchanges, which bring the client to the threshold of transferring his newly learned skills to everyday speaking tasks.

DESENSITIZATION PROCEDURES

As previously stated, the engine that really powers successful transfer of fluency in this program is systematic desensitization (S.D.) but where for some reason that is undesirable, we utilize less formal methods of counteracting tension and anxiety. These auxiliary methods are behavior rehearsal, assertive responses, and desensitization in vivo.

The case for desensitization rests on the principle that stress and its train of physiologic fear responses are incompatible with the favorable respiratory and phonatory conditions requisite to fluency control. Because desensitization is usually indispensable to success, this part of therapy has parity with acquisition of vocal skills, both in emphasis and time allotted. In fact, there are cases in which neutralization of emotional tension is the main segment of treatment (Weiner, 1981).

Without a reliable method for eliminating the emotional penalties of stuttering, clinicians are reduced, by and large, to futile pep-talks or "reflecting" clients' feelings in time-consuming discussion. S.D. and auxiliary desensitization techniques, however, permit deeply learned anxieties to be systematically unraveled and cancelled out.

There is voluminous literature on the subject of behavioral desensitization, but the outstanding source for the theory and practice of systematic desensitization are the works of Joseph Wolpe, the creator of the behavior therapy school of psychotherapy (1958, 1976, and with D. Wolpe, 1981).

A condensed discussion of S.D. is offered here in the hope that this material will be useful to those who are able to procure the requisite training now readily available throughout the country.* This training is valuable to the speech-language pathologist for stress relief in any type of communication disorder, but it is described here only in its specific application to stuttering cases.

S.D. is a psychotherapeutic procedure designed to reduce and/or eliminate learned anxiety responses associated with external or internal stimuli that are intrinsically without noxious properties. The procedure is based on the principle of reciprocal inhibition between alternating states of autonomic excitation and calmness. In this way, a state of anxiety, which is incompatible with a deeply relaxed bodily condition will be neutralized and dissipated, provided that the negative emotion is consistently evoked at low levels of intensity. The major technique is to present to the deeply relaxed client a series of imagined scenes that in a sequence of gradual increase in anxiety will nevertheless produce a minimum of disturbance.

The S.D. procedure mandates a working knowledge of four techniques: deep muscle relaxation, hierarchy construction, use of a subjective anxiety scale, and scene presentation.

Deep Muscle Relaxation
The client learns the methods of progressive relaxation of muscle groups in various parts of the body until a zero tension level is obtained (Jacobson, 1938). The relaxation of the throat and chest areas receives special attention. In addition, we assign deep muscle relaxation for 15 minutes of home practice daily.

Hierarchy Construction
The client reports speech fears which he and the clinician arrange in hierarchical order from high to low levels, often grouping them under thematic headings such as "talking to strangers" or "talking on the telephone." We call them "hierarchies" and arrive at these lists of anxiety-evoking scenes after a thorough history-taking and a searching discussion between client and clinician. A good source for these hierarchy items is the Stutterers' Self-Rating Scale of Reactions to Speaking Situations (Johnson et al., 1963). We have found it useful to include clients' qualifying conditions for various steps: stipulations such as "good" or "bad" days, the mood of the listener, or whether one can be overheard by others.

Subjective Anxiety or Sud Scale
Sud stands for subjective units of disturbance. Used as items in a scale of numerical values, they are assigned to describe differences between

---

*For information write or call the Association for the Advancement of Behavior Therapy, 420 Lexington Avenue, New York, NY 10170, 212-682-0065.

internal states of emotional arousal. The range is usually given as 0 to 100, with zero as the point of greatest calm and 100 that of greatest anxiety. These substitutes for adjectival descriptions are then employed to rank hierarchy items from high to low.

Scene Presentation

Starting with the lowest item in the hierarchy, we present scenes from the ordered sequence to the deeply relaxed client, naming the scene and asking the client to signal when the situation is vividly experienced, by raising the index finger. The clinician asks the client to signal the sud level and then offers relaxation cues to bring the client back to a zero level of tension. In the presence of overwhelming physiological passivity, the bonds of negative emotional response are soon dissociated from the stimulus scene. After repeated presentations, when the client reports a stable calm, the clinician proceeds to the next scene of the hierarchy.

Use of S.D.

We recommend that S.D. be utilized at any time in the course of therapy when tension or anxiety is noted. If, for example, the client exhibits apprehension toward the therapy setting itself, S.D. or simply deep muscle relaxation may be used to facilitate initial stages of therapy. Typically, S.D. immediately precedes transfer tasks to prepare for carryover to extraclinical settings. To avoid needless recurrence of sensitivity to situations already desensitized (resensitization), the clinician will postpone scenes that contain speaking activity until vocal control is well established. Scenes for which the client harbors anticipatory fears, however, are appropriate at any time during the desensitization process.

Summary and Discussion

Contrary to wide belief, the ultimate purpose of S.D. is *not* to teach the client to relax in the presence of stress. The major achievement of Wolpe and his coworkers has been to discover a procedure that can bring about lasting psychophysiologic relief from anxiety. Feelings of stress experienced in the presence of an incompatible autonomic system response (deep muscle relaxation) will dissipate and dissolve. Whatever the neurophysiologic mechanism, the process results in the breaking of the bonds between the anxiety-evoking stimulus and the fear response, through the work that takes place in therapy sessions and reinforcing home practice. Given a brief lag-time (a week or so) the feelings of fear and tension will no longer recur in the given life situation. What is more, this effect tends to spread spontaneously to related stimulus situations.

One question that is often posed is "Why don't you just desensitize the client to stuttering directly and have done with the vocal control program altogether?" The short answer is that stuttering and anxiety are not considered to be in a cause-and-effect relationship in this program; so that if anxiety is reduced there is no assurance, as various studies have indicated, that stuttering will not continue, even if at reduced levels (Gray and England, 1972). It is our conviction that if one were to follow such a policy, a process of resensitization to a new series of noxious responses would ensue, and the old sad cycle would eventually return. Thus, caution must be taken to ensure that vocal control is in place so that speech flow does not fail even though stress has subsided.

> Jack, a truck driver, had worked for weeks on a subhierarchy of situations leading up to asking his boss for a raise. He was slated for this increase but was nervous and agitated about broaching the subject because he felt he was sure to stutter and ruin his chances. With fluency under good control, his clinician and he completed all the "wage-raise" items in his hierarchy and after a 2-week wait, the clinician asked Jack if he felt he could now approach his boss. To her astonishment, he casually remarked that just that week he had gone into the office and made his pitch and the boss, after a short argument, had agreed to the raise. Although disappointed at her client's offhand treatment of the matter, the clinician realized what many of us who deal with allaying anxiety soon learn—that fear cancelled is fear forgotten and that virtue must be its own reward. Jack had been so thoroughly desensitized with regard to negative feelings about approaching his employer that he felt free to act on an uninhibited impulse to confront the issue and demand his due.

Auxiliary Desensitization

Having a large repertoire of strategies for the relief of physical and emotional tension is the better part of wisdom in the treatment of stutterers. Methods other than formal S.D. are useful either as a substitute or as a reinforcing measure to this technique.

Three auxiliary methods frequently employed in VCT are behavior rehearsal, assertive responding, and desensitization in vivo.

Behavior rehearsal requires the repetition of scenes containing sensitive material concerning interaction with others. Client and clinician actually act out the parts, alternating roles in order to obtain information and insight into the client's perceptions and the interpersonal dynamics at work. The desensitization results from the repeated rehearsal of stress-filled material under conditions antagonistic to anxiety, thus gradually inducing calmer responses. The rehearsal format also provides occasions for practice of vocal control and in fact should not be undertaken until the speaker demonstrates consistent competence in its use.

> Ted, a 12-year-old boy, was preparing for his Bar Mitzvah and his rabbi was upset because he was quite disfluent during prac-

tice. Knowing this, the boy grew more and more tense, and the whole family was in a state of apprehension about what would happen when the actual ceremony took place. The clinician, who was totally unversed in both the language and the ritual, nevertheless prevailed on Ted and his mother to bring the prayers and text to the therapy session. There, with suggested imagery for feelings of calm and with diligent practice of good breathing and improved voicing, Ted was able to develop a correct vocal set and a relaxed state of mind. The rabbi was relieved and praised the boy warmly. After several "dress" rehearsals, his Bar Mitzvah went off without a hitch.

Assertive responding, a variation of behavior rehearsal, provides relief through systematic practice in making fear-contingent assertive statements.

Improvisation to explore possible reactions of others helps the client arrive at appropriate attitudes that reflect both his feelings and best interests. It is important to avoid formulations that are either too submissive or overly aggressive which may then result in negative repercussions for the client.

Role playing and rehearsal of suitably assertive material will help the client feel calm and comfortable about expressing formerly sensitive material in the anticipated event. Again, these are occasions for practice and use of vocal fluency control.

Fred, a mild stutterer, described a situation he often encountered: he became tense (and thus disfluent) in the midst of his weekly telephone conversations with his mother. Since there was little anticipation anxiety involved, behavior rehearsal with assertive responding was deemed more appropriate than S.D. Fred assumed his mother's place in the typical weekly exchange, as Linda, his clinician, took Fred's role. He produced an authentic version of his mother's approach in which there was a strong undercurrent of complaint and dissatisfaction. When, as the mother, the clinician reproduced the emotional coloring of the conversation, Fred clearly reacted as if this were reality: i.e., with discomfort and a loss of fluency. The two discussed several ways that he might respond which would express his feelings without upsetting his parent. They then set about practicing these until Fred was able to stay calm and flexible as well as able to retain his fluency. After a while, Linda, in the role of the mother, put additional pressure on her client, insisting on a longer visit than had been planned. As it happened, this is exactly what took place in a future phone call which, according to Fred, went smoothly and without the kind of guilty irritation that he habitually experienced at the expense of his speech.

Desensitization in vivo is a systematic process of desensitization to be used in reality situations, either as follow-up to S.D. or in its stead. The objective is to reduce anxiety with calm derived from pleasant, tranquil scenes recalled from the client's experience. It is prudent to check sud levels at frequent intervals as the target anxiety situation is being approached so that a sudden increase in tension level can be lowered before proceeding to the next step. Since control of unwanted environmental events is difficult, desensitization in vivo is best done as reinforcement to S.D. for more or less the same sequence of steps. Inasmuch as fluency is the main purpose of the activity, success in target speech tasks includes monitoring for vocal control as well.

With children, the presence of the clinician is often the major deconditioning agent. Fantasy figures, such as Superman or Luke Skywalker, evoke effective imagery, too; and comfort items (a favorite doll, blanket, or stuffed animal), material reinforcement (tokens, food), and praise are all useful adjuncts.

Since telephoning is a common fear among stutterers, a sample of steps for desensitization in vivo may be useful. In formal systematic desensitization, there is greater freedom to arrange imagined scenes according to the degree of tension evoked; therefore the sequence of steps for an actual phone call may vary somewhat from the original hierarchy of anxiety scenes. An example of sample desensitization in vivo uses telephoning for information:

Step 1. Ready oneself for vocal set and overall calmness.

Step 2. Run through process in the "mind's eye" before taking action.

Step 3. Check your sud level; it should not be over 5 suds at any step.

Step 4. Raise phone to the ear.

Step 5. Dial the number.

Step 6. Listen to the ringing.

Step 7. Operator answers.

Step 8. Ask for telephone number, using vocal control.

When sud level rises above five, hang up and resume calm before proceeding. Start again from the beginning of the sequence. After successful completion of the call, repeat the exercise several times and again on subsequent days.

MANAGEMENT STRATEGIES
Flexibility and the Individual Client

The comprehensive nature of VCT, which provides treatment for both speech motor skills and the emotional "fallout" of stuttering, demands flexible programming in order to shape the therapy to the specific needs of the individual. Although these may surface in part during the diagnostic process, inquiry regarding the abilities, feelings, and current concerns of the client must be ongoing. The structure of each therapy plan must reflect a careful analysis of the client's overall learning patterns and motivational system, remaining open to evaluation and change. For optimal results, the objectives and methods selected should be shaped with the client's full participation.

Use of Behavior Modification

Stuttering therapy is an exercise in teaching people to learn new behaviors. When I first published (Weiner, 1969), few people in speech pathology were aware of the advances in learning theory concerning behavior change. Today, knowledge of behavior modification is so widespread that most people assume its application to clinical teaching as a matter of course. Nevertheless, as any clinical supervisor will agree, student clinicians (and even professionals) require much guidance in the major tenets of this methodology.

In training graduate students, for example, we give considerable attention to the power of salient positive reinforcement, cost response, and maintenance of high levels of success. The students must encounter the paradoxical reality that a client has to know already most of what he is to learn at any given point, i.e., must at the start experience a 70 to 80 percent rate of success if rapid acquisition of new learning is to occur.

Counting Errors

In VCT attention focuses primarily on acquiring an overall means to fluency and not on modifying single instances of breakdown. Stuttering can thus be said to be circumvented, replaced, or discontinued as a system of communication. As the speaker learns new ways of "fluent" voicing, he will, of course, err as any new learner does while striving for top-notch performance. In VCT this may mean failing to initiate voice with easy onset or exhibiting glottal fry or losing control of the breath stream. These are the sorts of events that we tally as errors, not just the instances of stuttering. When stuttering does occur, it is regarded simply as confirmation that an error in one of the subsystem tasks has taken place and may possibly be identifiable. As a rule, the work continues on the current target, and the stuttering is counted as a routine mistake, easily fixed, and rendered harmless. The mild concern with instances of stuttering appears to relieve overall tension about fluency failure, and thus reduces some of its penalizing power, at least under therapy conditions.

This approach stands in contrast to those techniques which either "welcome" stuttering as proof that avoidance is being overcome or require the speaker to track every disfluency in order to modify it the moment after, during, or before it occurs.

The Therapy Session

In spite of our intention that the VCT program serve only as a set of guidelines within which individual therapists are free to develop their own expedients and personal style, there are definite common features to observe in the typical VCT session. The temptation for graduate students in clinical training to regard VCT as a step-sequenced, stage-dependent type of "programmed" therapy is prevalent, since individualized therapy requires a considerable amount of clinical expertise. Nevertheless, many of the best students have made imaginative contributions to VCT's development.

A VCT session tends to adopt a standard format, having two or three distinct segments usually of unequal length. The first segment is a period of "warm-ups" (and is a review of previously learned skills). Then in the next segment the focus is new learning which occurs with drills, desensitization, transfer tasks, or several of these activities; and frequently a parent or other significant person will participate in the session as well. In addition, a block of time is allocated to the practice of speaking outside the therapy room, in a gradual progression to areas beyond the clinic. At the same time, the clinician attends to certain ongoing concerns: tallying data and providing feedback, awarding contingent reinforcement, shaping more natural-sounding speech whenever possible, observing the effect of the stimulus materials, and preparing to shift when necessary. Most of these matters do not of course pertain exclusively to VCT, but in their specific application to our therapy are worthy of brief mention.

WARM-UPS. Begin with a variety of familiar exercises to promote a good vocal set for each session. For this purpose, a few minutes of warm-ups of the client's choice to check on the quality of home practice are needed. These warm-ups often make the difference between a stuttered or a fluent initial utterance from the client. They also teach the client how to achieve a good vocalization set on his own.

NEW LEARNING. The targets set for a particular session are based on the percentage of correct responses achieved in the previous one. The clinician sets a new goal of "expected percentage of correct responses" (EPCR) which she determines from questions such as "How did my client do last time? Can I expect him to do better this time? If not, why not? If yes, by how much?" Then, on the basis of the client's performance in that particular session, the clinician extends her questions to ask, "Why didn't he do as well as expected (or why did he do much better)? Does he need more practice in therapy? At home? Or, are we on the right track?" The purpose of such planning is not only to utilize time efficiently, but also to accept clinical accountability, which is an important standard of professional probity.

The corollary to this, of course, is the necessity of keeping accurate records as well as detailed anecdotal data, both of which are indispensable to scientific method.

NORMAL PROSODY. The discussion in VCT sessions often includes reminders of the client's ultimate goal: a relaxed voice of normal volume, rate, and intonation. As mentioned earlier, the clinician usually encourages the client to slow the rate and practice in artificial cadences at the beginning; but from time to time we urge even the unready client to attempt a normal rendition of easy onset or resonant vocal tone. Perhaps the clinician will choose to demonstrate how it will eventually sound. The aim is merely to keep the end goal of natural fluency always in sight. We have found, otherwise, that the client unwittingly develops the false impression that slow draggy speech or exaggerated volume will remain part of the final product.

HOME PRACTICE. When the clinician determines that the client has grasped the items covered in therapy sufficiently well to practice them independently, she assigns homework. Caution is taken, however, to avoid premature self-monitored exercising, for incorrect practice may be less helpful than none at all.

There is usually a considerable list of assignments: vocal exercises, relaxation, and desensitization scenes, commissions to talk to certain individuals with fluency control, and above all keeping records for reporting back. The clinician determines these tasks in advance, and then works them out with the client during the session, making certain to review and evaluate them at appropriate intervals.

REINFORCEMENT. VCT provides a clear system of positive reinforcement (Rf+), whether the client is an adult or child. When children are involved, we consult with the parents to set up a long-term contract, be it for earning a privilege (an outing with Dad to eat at MacDonald's) or a favored object (a new bicycle bell). These contracts can be very simple or highly complex, depending on the circumstances; their purpose, however, is always to assure the child's continued interest and cooperation. If the contract requires 2 weeks of negotiation to get all the details right, then we allocate time for that: The resulting pay-off is well worth the effort.

With adults, the problem may be both simpler and more subtle. The criterion here is the kind of reinforcement that actually reinforces. Without positive feedback, the person does not clearly perceive where he stands at the moment, may become confused or discouraged, and thus will fail to progress at an optimal pace. Clinicians tend to underestimate the beneficial effect of skillful and accurate verbal reward. There is a tendency to regard adults as not needing planned positive reinforcement, perhaps just an occasional "You're doing very well." The truth is that many of our adult clients watch the tally sheet and percentage scores with an eager vigilance and keep track of data as if it were money in the bank. They appreciate graphs and tables depicting their progress when these are offered in a serious spirit.

Cost response, an invaluable teaching tool easily applied to children receiving tokens or chips, is useful with adults as well. An effective device for inducing errorless onset of utterance, for example, is to require a penalty of timed periods of silence adjusted, of course, to the extent of the error. Contracts that stipulate fines as the penalty for failure to practice or carry out assignments are also effective. One client agreed that he would donate a certain amount of money to his least "favorite" charity, the Ku Klux Klan, if he missed over 5 days of daily practice a month.

STIMULUS MATERIALS. Finding sufficient variety of stimulating materials, especially for children, is a constant challenge to the imagination and ingenuity of the clinician. This is true more for stuttering therapy, perhaps, than for other types because of the amount of talking time that must be generated. A new source of drill material for adults and older children has been the workbooks for aphasic patients mentioned earlier. We often are hard put, especially with the shy, uncommunicative child, to create conditions for lively exchange between client and clinician especially as connected speech becomes the major focus of therapy. Here is an example of how an ardent interest in food was embellished to break the logjam with one nontalker.

> Matthew, a boy of 9 with an extremely disordered speech pattern, was not only distractible and difficult to discipline but very moody and often gloomily silent as well. After several semesters of therapy, he was able to maintain fair vocal control of speech but only in highly structured tasks such as reading arithmetic problems from flash cards. He was ready for longer self-generated utterances and connected speech practice but balked at "just talking about things." And there was nothing he wanted to work for hard enough to overcome this obstacle. His inventive clinician, however, hit on a procedure which succeeded beyond all expectation. Matthew, who loved to eat, agreed to start with a project devoted to making orange juice. The clinician prepared a handwritten booklet in which each page presented one step of the instructions for producing real orange juice. Matthew read each page aloud properly; then having memorized the steps, he pantomimed the process as he repeated each step aloud employing correct breathing and voicing. After two trial runs, he began again this time actually cutting the fruit, squeezing the juice by hand on a juicer, and pouring the liquid into two glasses for himself and his mother while talking fluently throughout. His mother, who had delightedly brought the fruit and kitchenware, now agreed to furnish supplies for the next project which Matthew chose: hoagie sand-

wiches. In a 5-week program, Matthew listed the ingredients (several kinds of meat, relishes, onion, cheeses, and pickles); dictated the directions for the handwritten booklet; read through the instructions several times; and memorized each step of the way, practicing at home. Fluent productions were the condition for moving ahead. They then conducted several dry runs, and when the big day came, he carried out the process of putting together four enormous hoagies which were then wrapped and taken home for the family's supper. He had described the entire procedure with perfectly fluent, naturally produced speech.

PARENT PARTICIPATION. A therapy session with a child usually includes parent or surrogate parent participation. In innumerable cases parents have served as surrogate clinicians, assuming responsibility and reaping due recognition for their contribution to a well-ordered clinical program.

With adult therapy sessions, on the other hand, the clinician urges the client to invite a spouse, lover, friend, or relative to attend and discuss pertinent issues. These significant others can provide an effective means for extending therapy systematically beyond the clinic and into daily life activity.

PHYSICAL BEHAVIORS

The VCT approach to concomitant behaviors of stuttering is shaped by the fact that most "secondary" motor habits fail to appear when adequate respiratory/phonatory control is exerted. Wingate states, "There is no need to direct attention to whatever accessory features may occur as part of a patient's stuttering, since these features are simply eliminated by the effect of the fluency-producing procedures" (1976). Such activities as eyeblinks, head-turning, and chin elevation occur at a weaker rate than the "core" behaviors of audible or inaudible repetitions, prolongations, and silent blocks (Wingate, 1964). Our working hypothesis that stuttering is a "source" phenomenon, that is, a disruption of the laryngeal sound source system (Freeman and Rosenfield, 1982), would tend to explain why the accessory behaviors disappear when the source is functioning efficiently. It seems that all the learned struggle behaviors dissipate when a new motor program takes over, with those more recently acquired and more distant from the source, going first. VCT, therefore, rarely treats these as problems independently of the need to establish basic vocal control.

What sometimes will persist, however, are certain minor habits ostensibly vocally connected, such as throat-clearing, use of "ums" and "uhs," and of course recourse to circumlocution, which tends to wane, but may not vanish, as phonational proficiency increases.

For throat-clearing, or "coughing" types of behavior, we employ a series of measures which may have to progress from swallowing to a gentle, *voiced* throat-clearing maneuver, and finally to sipping water in order to satisfy the urge to remove phlegm, which often is nonexistent. This last step is a remedy best utilized only briefly, lest it become a "crutch."

Counting the number of unwanted behaviors within a given space of time and then aiming for gradual decrease is a classic approach for developing awareness of the ultimate need to eliminate these ticlike habits. This holds true for the use of "starter" sounds such as "um," "uh," or a chain of "um-er-uh's," as well. A consistent plan of cueing and tallying for both awareness and reduction usually produces the desired effect, and the speaker is glad to get rid of the tiresome overuse of these fillers and stallers.

In the case of persistent circumlocution, we insist that the speaker resume the original wording of an utterance, using good vocal control. Clinicians can become just as adept at detecting highly refined word substitutions as stutterers are at generating them; and we sometimes impose cost response penalties, such as timed periods of silence, on a client immediately after he has committed the "error."

ATTITUDINAL WORK

Every stutterer wants to become easily and effortlessly fluent in as brief a time as possible. He is not usually surprised, however, when told that VCT insists on a goal of normal, lasting fluency and that this goal must be well in view before termination. Thus rehabilitating the vocal system and eliminating associated stress is not a "quickie cure," but is, on the contrary, a thorough and sometimes arduous undertaking. Fortunately, most stutterers agree to accept these terms of treatment, and more than a few appear to understand early on that, while we will show the way, they are the true agents of change and must themselves endeavor to make it all work. These clients are the more likely to complete the program in good time after having achieved a reliably high level of fluency and having agreed to a plan of maintenance and follow-up.

Unfortunately other clients, usually but not always those manifesting severe symptoms, appear to cling to the notion that mere attendance in therapy will result in normal speech. It is difficult to say what distinguishes them from the others, but they seem, in spite of clinicians' efforts, to persist in expecting relief from disfluency as from an illness. At some level, these clients still appear to be counting on success to grow, like Topsy, of its own accord. The resulting conflict between client and clinician expectations invokes the label "problem" stutterer and raises the age-old issue: "Is it the person or the disorder causing the trouble?" Does this person really prefer to stutter, as some schools of therapy have implied? Is there some underlying advantage ("secondary gain") to stuttering that overwhelms even a sincere plea for help? Or is it within the nature of stuttering itself to resist long-term remediation?

Observations stemming from the VCT method and especially from a recent study (Weiner, 1983) may throw light on the problem of motivation and clarify some basic characteristics of the stuttering syndrome. We will bypass the ample literature on the acquisition of learned stuttering behaviors and dwell briefly, instead, on prevailing theories of speech motor control and their possible relevance to the persistence of stuttering in some speakers.

The study of 12 stutterers produced a total of 114 tokens of stuttering which were recorded by electroglottograph and analyzed for patterns of vocal fold vibration. These samples presented the eight types of stuttering that follow: single repetition; multiple repetition, both voiced and unvoiced; prolongations of [s]; prolongations of [z]; phrase repetition; silent block; and strangled voicing. We viewed these behaviors as the core of the stuttering event and not as associated or "secondary" behaviors. In each case we observed the stutterer attempting to initiate and sustain steady state vocal fold oscillation, regardless of the type of disfluency displayed. A common feature of note, both in the study and in the clinical setting, is that stutterers appear to utilize only a few core behaviors from among the many possibilities available to them. Those strategies that are used consistently may be said to constitute his pattern of disfluency, and this limited stock of ritualized devices strongly suggests a certain lack of intention or effort to change course. Stuttering appears to be a habit that reflects a previously "stylized" search for phonational viability, and implies the absence of deliberate struggle to arrive at fluent utterance. From this premise one may deduce that the original disruption of speech flow impels the young speaker to seek some sort of hit-or-miss release from a blocked vocal tract, and the "search," inefficient though it may be, becomes both habituated and largely involuntary. One may infer further that the stutterer is "acting out" a series of old, albeit sadly limited, maneuvers for which there is no longer an original impulse.

Theorists, such as Fowler and associates (1980), have recently suggested a view of coordinative motor activity that may help to explain how the behaviors just described are maintained. These research scientists propose that well-learned motor acts are governed not from central nervous system stations, but are under autonomous control by a system of loosely coupled oscillators within peripheral muscle groups, which are programmed to sustain coordination of skilled movements. Polit and Bizzi, who experimented with deafferented monkeys (1978), produced evidence that central programming may be necessary for new learning to occur. but that muscle mechanisms located in the periphery may provide independent regulation for highly practiced motor tasks.

When applied to abnormal speech behaviors, these theoretical propositions suggest that stuttering patterns may actually be forged through trial and error during a period when the nonfluent child, suddenly aware of his abnormal speech behavior, strives to repress it. Let us assume that for most of these children the original causative conditions will fade with maturation taking with them the associated speech anomalies. For children who become confirmed stutterers, however, the patterns that persist include both the stutterings and the attempts to "fix" them. These are now ingrained in a motor program outside the habitual control of the central nervous system. If our assumption holds true, the motor program for stuttering is now predominantly activated by a peripheral system of involuntary and autonomous control which, by its nature, is resistant to long-term intercession from higher neurologic centers.

If such an hypothesis is considered for argument's sake, it could account for the fact that stutterers, because they are stuttering "mechanically," are equivocal observers of specific attributes of their disfluencies (Bloodstein, 1981), as well as poor predictors of the loci of their stutterings (Wingate, 1976; Shapiro, 1980). The frequent bouts of fluency which all stutterers experience may be viewed, therefore, as periods of "top-down" control when the system is responding to temporarily changed drive levels. The customary patterns of disfluency return inevitably when conditions again resemble the original learning situation.

Stutterers do exhibit notable consistency, however, in the precision with which they perceive details of their social and emotional interactions. Their understandable preoccupation with feelings of distress originates in what may be termed prevailing "ecological" conditions, i.e., the external and internal sources of speech anxiety. We infer that these feelings are strongly bonded through social learning to the faulty speech motor plan, which interacts reciprocally with varying levels of stress. An example of this interaction is the actor or platform speaker who is mellifluously fluent in performance, yet unaccountably nonfluent off-stage. We suggest that when the phonational/respiratory system is under maximum drive, superior voicing is temporarily in force under CNS control. As this condition recedes the customary pattern of stuttering resumes, including habitual and mechanical efforts to "correct" the halting speech (repetitions, prolongations, etc.) A different order of stress may increase speech disruption; an absence of stress may be linked to reduced stuttering depending on an individual's history. But the stereotypical stuttering behavior remains locked into the stutterer's "normal" machinery of communication.

If there is any basis to the idea that what stutterers are really wrestling with is a deeply imbedded habit system acting autonomously, then it can be argued that establishing a new speech motor program may be the most logical and workable recourse. That is what VCT purports to do. Relearning an improved method of vocalization for speech, however, places the task back under central cortical control at a time when the highly plastic learning period of childhood may be long past. Concentrated effort and practice is necessary, therefore, in order for the new habit to succeed in rivaling the power of the old. One result of the hypothesis of a shift in autonomy to the periphery is a deeper respect for the learning tasks faced by the "problem" client and a decline in the temptation to "blame

the victim" for slow, modest, or even no progress. Our heightened awareness marks the difference in philosophy between therapy which says in
effect "You now have the capacity to be fluent; the rest is up to you" and
one such as VCT, which assists the client in achieving not only usable
fluency but a fluency that is gradually and patiently brought into habitual
usage.

> Rod, a severe stutterer, displayed speech blockages with cheek-
> puffing, facial grimaces, and lip and jaw tremors. He has been
> in therapy for 4 years, making slow but steady progress to a point
> of inconsistent but growing fluency in therapy at the conversa-
> tional level. The slow rate of advance has often raised the ques-
> tion, on Rod's part as well as his clinician's, whether at some
> unconscious level he really wanted to be nonfluent. He himself
> cited the fact that he was embarrassed to display fluency with
> anyone but his mother. Clinicians tended to scold and remon-
> strate with him, implying that he was in some fundamental way
> inadequately motivated. On the other hand, the evidence for a
> high degree of dedication and aspiration is undeniable: he waged
> an earnest campaign for entry into therapy when there were few
> openings, and in spite of night work and sometimes two jobs,
> his attendance is exceptional; he even came during a serious ill-
> ness which required debilitating chemotherapy.
>
> Rod is constantly concerned that he will be dropped because
> of inadequate progress, but he clearly and expressly wants to
> change his speech since he feels at a disadvantage in the job
> market and in social intercourse. His major battle, however, ap-
> pears to be with the "programmed-in" nature of a long-standing
> speech motor plan which to him is really the way he "normally"
> speaks. With all its waste of energy, the puffing cheeks, the re-
> petitive glottal closures, and the voice tremors, this way of talking,
> though greatly improved even at its worst, is what to Rod seems
> truly "effortless," undemanding and, above all, known. It has
> taken Rod a long time to tune into the far easier and more logical
> vocal behaviors that make his speech increasingly smooth,
> pleasant, and like other people's. It is the tremendous social pen-
> alty for failing to communicate according to the norms of his
> social and vocational milieu that drove and still drives Rod to
> undertake the difficult task of mastering and internalizing a new
> speech motor program.

SUMMARY OF DESCRIPTION OF THERAPY

A schematic diagram of programming is presented (Figure 6-1) to indicate
roughly the customary sequence and interrelationship of the various segments within the VCT program.

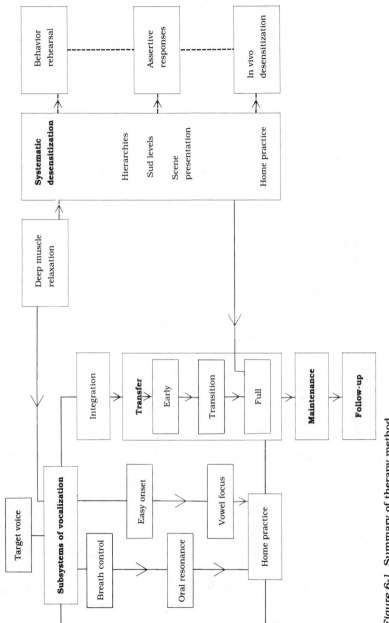

Figure 6-1. Summary of therapy method.

TRANSFER AND MAINTENANCE

Speech-language pathologists are aware that carryover of new behaviors is the crucial test of therapy no matter what the disorder may be. With stutterers, we know only too well that for many fluency develops in the tension-free therapy situation but does not hold up in daily life, a very cruel failure indeed.

When we arrive at the process of transfer, there is often the feeling that we are approaching completion, a mistaken notion. The truth is that the major part of therapy lies ahead, often requiring a long and painstaking period of specifically selected strategies and countless desensitizations. In VCT this period is organized into three phases: early, transitional, and full transfer.

Early Transfer

We have found it expedient to take every new skill as it is acquired in the therapy room and apply it in other settings. For example, when clients have mastered breath duration or easy onset exercises, they demonstrate this accomplishment for visitors, family members, other clinicians, clients, staff. The activity may occur in the hallway, in other rooms, or on intraclinic phones. In addition, clinicians call clients at home between sessions to listen to them do their practice and reduce phone fears at the same time. In this way the typical experience of perfecting fluency in the therapy room only to find it falling apart at the doorway, is replaced by a gradual accretion of successful trials under different discriminative stimuli, thus inducing early generalization.

Transitional Transfer

This phase encompasses communicative situations that remain confined to "safe" environments, i.e., where stress remains low. If such settings arouse anxiety, the clinician will postpone these steps until the client engages in systematic desensitization and other techniques for eliminating negative emotion.

The sequence of contexts for these activities might look like this, with the proviso that the client agree to the choices and the order suggested:

1. Reading and conversing during therapy while observers are present in an observation room.
2. Reading and conversing during therapy while visitors are present in the therapy room.
3. Reading to a visitor; talking; engaging in questions and answers.
4. Adding to the number of visitors.
5. Approaching others outside the room; clinicians, secretarial personnel, guards, librarian, bookstore, lunchroom people, teachers and/or peers.

6. Working with a telephone: Choose a room with a telephone present. Practice exercises with hand on the phone. Hold receiver with button held down. Then do exercises for clinician on intraclinic phones.
7. Making outside calls: Ask operator for information. Call department store for information on an advertisement. Call theater for ticket prices. Call airline for flight information. Use public phone.

Gene, a premed student, was a moderate stutterer who exhibited mainly tense vocal initiation and glottal fry voicing, with frequent repetitions and silent blocks as his dominant pattern of disrupted speech flow. He learned to improve voice production rapidly, adapting to S.D. techniques readily and proceeding in admirable fashion to full transfer operations. His fluency control failed him however when he attempted to apply his skills from the speech tasks in the Center to his tasks of oral classroom participation. An intermediate step was needed, and his clinician, Eve, devised an ingenious stratagem: Gene and she invented a fictitious questionnaire with which to poll students on campus. They would solicit student opinions about TV commercials, with Gene posing as a psychology major. Gene and Eve rehearsed his approach speech, "I'm a psych major, and I have this project to do for my class. It will only take a minute." The questions were typed and attached to a clipboard which Gene carried with him during the polling. As students responded, Gene wrote down the answers, and Eve kept a tally of Gene's vocal behaviors. After several successful outings, Eve arranged to attend one of Gene's regular classes and sit in the rear as he delivered a short oral assignment. From there, with the aid of systematic desensitization and advance behavior rehearsal, Gene was able to carry through the list of speech events drawn up for his transfer program. He has since moved on to become a biocomputer programmer working for a large Baltimore firm where, among other things, he conducts training seminars for other professionals.

Full Transfer
This is the most difficult phase of transfer because the clinician begins to have less and less control over on-going circumstances. Yet, if there is to be success, the process should be as orderly, as thoroughly planned, and as carefully logged as possible. The fact is that the tasks of daily life have been making constant demands for communication all along in encounters with family, peers, strangers, and the phone. We have had to ignore these demands while teaching the client new ways to secure fluent utterance. Now we have arrived at the task of systematically replacing stuttered speech patterns with fluent ones that are to be consciously and

deliberately instated step by step into everyday life until only fluent speech becomes the currency of communicative exchange.

What must be reiterated here is the deleterious effect of speech situation stress: fluency and anxiety at this juncture of therapy are incompatible states. In the VCT program, eliminating stress by methods of desensitization is a prerequisite to full transfer. Setting this aspect of therapy aside, for the moment, however, the transfer program will include steps such as the ones that follow:

For example, assign the client a specified segment of time for focusing on vocal control (VC) daily, starting with an acceptable minimum, such as 5 minutes after dinner or before bedtime; and identify the person chosen as listener, usually a relative in the home. The client keeps a daily calendar record of these events and their success. This schedule of assignments should be accompanied by positive reinforcement or cost response measures suitable in turn to children or adults.

The intervals for VC usage are slowly expanded to larger time periods and extended to other people according to an agreed-upon plan. Assignments include responding in class; telling a joke, first to one person and later to a small group; speaking to the boss; and talking to certain strangers such as waiters, policemen, and clerks.

We approach the task of talking on the telephone in graded steps of difficulty. The client is assigned to make or receive calls, starting with whichever is easier, to or from a range of individuals, such as sister, uncle, dentist, lawyer. The client moves at a pace that allows for a maximum of success. This may mean starting with brief factual exchanges and moving gradually to longer chatty conversations.

Maintenance

When the use of fluent voicing is expanding smoothly into all parts of the client's daily life, he will make a posttherapy videotape for comparison to the pretherapy baseline tape. At this point the person arrives at the "maintenance" phase and typically terminates formal therapy sessions. The client attends a monthly conference to present records of assignments including an account of daily practice of vocal control and desensitization exercises. He reports at monthly meetings for 2 months, then every other month for 3 or 4 months, then only every 6 months.

FOLLOW-UP PROCEDURES

Follow-up is usually a matter of contractual agreement after maintenance sessions are terminated. The contract calls for periodic mail contact (questionnaires) and telephone calls for 3 years or more. Clients are welcome to request "booster" sessions when and if unresolved stress recurs or if there is some slippage in vocal control. Typically, one or two people a year request this service.

EQUIPMENT AND MATERIALS NEEDED

VCT is the kind of therapy for which equipment can run the gamut from paper and pencil to elaborate electronic instrumentation. The public school therapist, for example, requires little more than is needed for any other type of speech problem.

The only need for additional equipment that might arise would be in connection with desensitization when and if a child needs it. In such cases, school clinicians have been known to use the cot in the nurse's office, a friendly administrator's armchair, the gym pads borrowed from the "phys-ed" teacher, or even, in several cases we know of, a lawn chair carried from home in the trunk of the car.

On the other hand, one can find very good use for such aids as audiotape or videotape recorders or the Voice Lite, an electrical contrivance that responds to voice intensity levels. Two electronic devices popular with clinicians at Temple University are delayed auditory feedback (DAF) and portable electromyographic (EMG) machines. DAF has been used, either briefly or extensively, as a method for artificially inducing good vocal resonance. Under settings of high volume and moderate to maximum delay (300 to 500 ms), the speaker can often achieve the vowel sound with the headset on and then off. The use of DAF for obtaining a sample of target voicing for the purpose of identification was discussed earlier. An involuntary fluency response to DAF may sometimes be evoked but that will not in and of itself teach the speaker a readily retrievable behavior. Using stretched speech under DAF in serial forms, such as counting and saying the days of the week, will often help to sustain improved voicing, a product of DAF stimulation. We exploit this instrument to produce the ends for which we will then teach the means, and not the reverse.

The second instrument, a portable EMG set, is used to obtain objective measures of bodily tension. By means of electrode placement, and through either auditory or visual (VU meter) feedback, we have access to three levels of sensitivity response (0–50, 0–500, 0–1000mV). Action potentials of muscle groups, such as the masseter or the frontalis muscles, are tapped to indicate either localized or generalized body tension levels. The portable EMG has thus been useful not only for convincing a client that his subjective reports of felt tension (sud levels) are consistent with that of the machine, but also for reducing stress by the well-proven method of biofeedback therapy. Nevertheless, we still prefer self-monitoring of stress levels in order to facilitate home practice and personal mastery without external aids, except perhaps for the ever-serviceable tape recorder. Spectrographic analysis is rarely used since it requires laboratory assistance for the average clinician. In special cases, however, it can be helpful in indicating the presence of a diphthongal glide or in supplying a graphic representation of an abrupt onset. It may also provide evidence of greater intensity in the high frequency formats when the voice is fully resonant (provided volume is held constant).

CLINICIAN SKILLS AND TRAINING REQUIRED

The ideal background for a VCT clinician is one with training in stuttering, voice, and general therapeutics, especially behavior modification. If familiarity with systematic desensitization were added, there would be little need for a full-dress training program in VCT. For training of graduate students and speech professionals who lack the requisite skills, the main instructional medium is a black-and-white videotape series, the result of 2 years' preparation, which was produced in 1978 with the support of the Temple University Media Learning Center and Office of Television Services. The series is composed of one introductory tape and 10 others, each describing a specific aspect of the program and depicting illustrative scenes from actual therapy sessions. These tapes have the following titles: Overview, Diagnostic Evaluation, Breath Control, Easy Onset, Oral Resonance, Vowel Focus, Systematic Desensitization, Auxiliary Desensitization, Programming and Practice, Transfer (plus Maintenance and Follow-up), and VCT with Children. In addition, apart from the series proper, we have segments of tapes from pretherapy and posttherapy sessions with clients who have completed VCT.

Also available is a mimeographed supplementary manual which contains additional suggestions for remedial techniques as well as stimulus materials, including a sizable store of exercises, word lists, sentence lists, and reading paragraphs arranged according to the topics described in the tapes. In addition, we provide an intensive short course in systematic desensitization with live demonstration and supervised practice by the participants.

For speech professionals, many of whom are public school speech-language pathologists, we regularly conduct workshops (a total of 12 to date) in the Philadelphia and South Jersey areas. We schedule these 3-day workshops in two segments, one of 2 consecutive days and then a third day, a month later. Prior to the initial session, we provide a 6-week reading period for a prescribed list of assignments.

The training of VCT clinicians is really a straightforward process of acquainting practitioners with the theory and techniques of the method in as economical and productive format as possible. A sophisticated clinician interested in pursuing this method could easily structure a similar program of therapy without formal training. Any speech-language pathologist with the right sort of bent and background, whether a graduate student or an experienced professional, can practice successful Vocal Control Therapy.

CLIENT REQUIREMENTS

The VCT program admits stutterers without qualifications as to severity or type of disfluency. In addition, clients are not refused on the basis of age, sex, or the presence of disabilities other than stuttering. The number of people seen at Temple University is limited only by the number of graduate students available for clinical practice in stuttering therapy in a given semester.

Evaluation of the Therapy

PROCEDURES, RESULTS, FOLLOW-UP

Beginning in 1972, even before the treatment program was formulated as Vocal Control Therapy, we adopted the procedure, which still continues, of videotaping clients before and after therapy in five speaking situations: stating place, date, name, and educational level; reading a passage from Gray's *Oral Reading;* talking to two strangers, an authority figure (faculty) and a nonauthority figure (graduate student); addressing a group of five strangers (topic: a typical day); and making a telephone call to get travel information. Two trained observers tally the number of stuttering events occurring during timed segments of speech, and an assessment of severity of stuttering (Riley's SSI, 1972) and a measure of general anxiety (IPAT Self-Analysis Scale) are recorded for each case.

Of the 66 clients enrolled in VCT proper since 1973, 8 have been children whom we, as a matter of policy, do not videotape (except for one 13-year-old boy). Our experience has been that exposure to cameras and strangers is often so traumatic to youngsters that the benefit of recording is not worth the risk of lingering emotional upset. We also have not taped several adults who received private VCT beforehand or, in one case, with whom we observed no overt stuttering. Of the total 66, 12 are currently in therapy, 25 (4 children) have completed the program and 29 have not. Of these last, 13 left because of a change of job or work schedule, a move outside the state, or because they were referred to a school clinician to continue therapy there. Of this group of 13, 8 were judged to be much improved when they left and 5 improved. Two, R.R. (#17) and A.S. (#13) (Table 6-1) replied to the last questionnaire. The remainder of those who failed to complete VCT (16) we consider dropouts. Among them, however, are those (10) who had expressed a positive attitude toward the program and felt they had improved enough to go it alone, their progress reports indicating that all had made much improvement in fluency. The other 6 who dropped out are judged to have been disaffected with the aims, techniques, or demands of VCT and were thought to have made only minimal improvement if any.

Table 6-1 presents the results of replies to questionnaires, but also in some cases to unannounced telephone inquiries and visits to the Center. The most recent questionnaire (1982) reached 27 clients (23 had no forwarding address) of whom 18 replied (66%). It requested information about the percentage of fluency under stress as well as in daily circumstances.

Table 6-1. Follow-up: Percentage Fluency Maintained

Client	Severity[a]	No. of Sessions[b]	Year Terminated	Percent Fluency Maintained				Comments
				1977	1978	1979	1982[c]	
1. B.B.L.	Severe	57	1973	90	87	92		Does not consider self stutterer
2. P.S.	Severe	46	1973	90				Does not consider self stutterer
3. A.H.	Severe	118	1975	80	94	95		
4. N.B.	Moderate	42	1975	95				Does not consider self stutterer
5. J.C.	Severe	64	1975	95	99	90		Does not consider self stutterer
6. G.F.	Mild	39	1975	98		90		Does not consider self stutterer
7. S.M.	Moderate	70	1976	95	Deceased			
8. D.M.	Severe	88	1976	93	90	90		
9. R.P.[d]	Moderate	15	1976				100–100	Does not consider self stutterer
10. J.F.	Mild	30	1977		99	90	98–95	Does not consider self stutterer
11. F.P.	Moderate	52	1977		90	90	80–70	
12. L.T.	Moderate	124	1977		90			
13. A.S.	Severe	33	1977				90–85	Did not complete VCT
14. J.S.	Mild (severe anxiety)	14	1977				100–99	No videotape record
15. D.Y.	Moderate	69	1978		98	98		

						1982	
16. F.N.	Mild	33	1978			95–95	
17. R.R.	Severe	140	1978	95	90	80–60	Did not compete VCT
18. W.I.	Severe	80	1978			95–80	No videotape record
19. R.G.[a]	Severe	156	1979			100–99	
20. T.S.[a]	Moderate	34	1979			92–75	
21. D.M.	Moderate (severe anxiety)	101	1980				
22. S.McD.	Moderate to severe	138	1980			95–90	
23. E.R.	Moderate to severe	112	1980			95–90	
24. E.L.	Mild (severe anxiety)	137	1980			95–85	No videotape record. No overt stuttering
25. G.B.[a]	Moderate	54	1981			98–95	
26. M.H.[a]	Moderate	114	1981			90–85	No videotape record
27. C.C.	Moderate	62	1982			90–90	

[a]Stuttering severity determined by the Stuttering Severity Instrument (Riley, 1972) which includes parameters of frequency, duration of stuttering events, and concomitant physical behaviors.

[b]Therapy sessions are 50 minutes long and are customarily held twice a week during the college semester.

[c]The 1982 column reports two percentages of fluency: a "daily" level (left), and an "under stress" level (right). Occurrences of stuttering are reported to be mild, except for T.S. (#20) (moderate).

[d]Child.

Note: Two other replies were received of which one was incoherent and the other reported that a former client had entered another therapy program.

Part of the information in Table 6-1 was published in 1978 (Weiner) with additional data showing a statistically significant difference between stuttering before and after therapy for each subject. Inasmuch as completion of therapy in VCT is equivalent to having achieved high levels of fluency in a variety of communication settings, we viewed the inclusion of data on fluency for this particular table redundant.

Comments on Table 6-1

It will be noted that of the two people reporting a fluency percentage of only 80 percent for daily situations and less for stressful ones, R.R. (#17) did not complete the program, whereas F.P. (#11) seems to have regressed since his report 3 years ago.

Five respondents report the "under stress" condition to be between 70 percent and 85 percent. A.S. (#13), who notes an "85%" level, was unable to finish S.D. tasks before moving to another state but wrote to say that "VCT gave me the greatest sense of improvement of any therapy tried." Another client, E.L. (#24), also at an "85%" level under stress, may be reflecting her chief complaint, a strong fear of stuttering, rather than overt stuttering itself. In 2½ years of therapy, we observed only two stuttering episodes and E.L. herself reported only two. Her latest questionnaire reads "In 90% of situations, I do not consider myself a stutterer. Occasionally it haunts me, but then I practice my exercises."

As for D.M. (#21), he too writes that although VCT gave him confidence that "I could in fact lead a normal life," he continues to struggle with stress-filled situations which he describes as "answering the telephone and dealing with higher executives in the work environment." His mother, who was asked to forward the questionnaire, wrote to thank us for our assistance to D. She reports that he had just received a promotion with a substantial increase in salary, that he does a great deal of traveling, and when he was home for the holidays, "There wasn't a trace of stutter."

M.H. (#26), now 12 years old, still keeps in touch with the Center. He and his mother are encouraged to return at any time he feels that his speech is slipping back.

R.G. (#19), who had done much of the tedious work of voice and S.D. practice by himself when he was away at law school, now reports an 80 percent fluency level under stress. He says of his self-image as a stutterer, "I am still aware," which of course puts him at some distance from the goal of normal, automatically processed speech flow, but reflects the honest reckoning of a young man who has surmounted severe stuttering to become a successful attorney-at-law, able both to plead in court and teach in a nearby college.

Additional Data from Area Professionals

In addition to contacting the clients at Temple University Speech and Hearing Center, we have conducted periodic surveys through questionnaires mailed to area professionals who practice VCT. A summary of the responses to three questionnaires sent out to some 50 clinicians for each of 3 years (1977, 1978, 1982), shows that an average of 26 responded. They report having treated a mean of 93 cases a year, over 50 percent of whom are children. An average of 40 percent of cases reach completion, with 88 percent of these attaining 90 to 100 percent fluency levels, and almost 10 percent more reported to be much improved. Area clinicians find that in cases they follow their clients maintain an average of 90 percent fluency although their number is few.

The comments of speech-language pathologists indicate some of the problems encountered; those who see clients in hospital, agency, or private practice settings report more favorably on both the feasibility of the program and the results. One clinician wrote "VCT is effective in facilitating fluency for all the clients I've used it with." Another: "Program encompasses all important parameters of fluency control. Patients feel secure in knowing they have internalized these concepts and can resort to them in crisis." One simply commented "I love it." Almost every respondent in this category made a point of the usefulness of systematic desensitization, which "makes it possible to help the stutterer deal with some of his fears (that) ordinarily interfere with his progress" and "S.D. is crucial to transfer effectiveness."

On the other hand, some public school speech-language specialists find the typically brief 20- to 30-minute therapy period and the frequent transfer of pupils and clinicians between schools the main drawbacks to achieving sound results. Among comments on VCT techniques, some sample replies are: "Best program I've discovered; but impossible to use S.D. in the school"; "Felt S.D. most valuable aspect of therapy"; "Good program. Somewhat difficult to carry out in school setting. Client(s) needed more parental support"; "Gives client strategies and controls, a *way* of speaking fluently. Sometimes difficult to implement in school setting because of time constraints." The discrepancies among this group of responses call, at the very least, for closer attention to training procedures for school clinicians.

Discussion

Evaluation of the VCT program at Temple should include an account of the circumstances under which it is tested. The clinicians are second-year graduate students who have satisfied the requisite academic course of study in the disorder of stuttering and received training in the VCT method from me directly. The fact that practice of this therapy is accessible even to inexperienced clinicians reflects positively on its general usefulness. On the other hand, much time is lost to such relative want of skill; and from the client's standpoint, the turnover of personnel every 4 months is not conducive to a feeling of continuity, nor to the efficient use of therapy time. Nonetheless, the enthusiasm and creativity of our student clinicians may well cancel out the negative factors. Moreover, stutterers more than likely gain as much as they lose from being required to talk and work with new people at regular intervals.

Another factor that should be considered is the limitation in the number of stutterers that can be admitted to the program. Admissions are based on the number of clients required for student's practicum training hours in order to fulfill ASHA standards. At any given time, the group of graduate student clinicians carries a case load of between 9 and 12 stuttering clients, which permits an average of 8.3 admissions per year. These restrictions have resulted in a continual stream of requests for therapy that we must turn away and refer to other agencies and programs.

Thus, the small numbers in this report do not reflect the general interest and the demand for Vocal Control Therapy from among the local population.

We must acknowledge that client reports of their own fluency status do not constitute unassailable data. Although we are in direct communication with many of these reportees by phone and by visit, the lack of objectivity in these informal assessments does not meet the stringent demands of controlled and reliable standards of measurement. Failing these, which we simply cannot meet, there still seems to be sufficient evidence to warrant continuation of the program, though preferably with better evaluation procedures. VCT programming for stutterers supports the major goals of therapy: a high level of normal, stable fluency which meets the criteria of natural speech rate, unaffected prosody, and continuity of speech flow. If these are not always perfectly in hand, they do seem to be firmly within the grasp of VCT participants who have learned a better and calmer way to talk based on a more efficiently managed system of vocalization.

Clients who early in the therapy express concern about the mental and physical effort needed to acquire the skills of "fluent" vocalization later agree that these eventually converge with a single focus that is represented by a sensory image such as "good voice" or "sound the vowel." Such a simple "tag" has the power to call up a cluster of breathing and vocal behaviors that act as an immediate signal for "fluent" voicing until even this minimal cueing effort becomes unnecessary and fades altogether, as it already has in several cases. In the meantime, VCT speakers inform us that the need for attentiveness and self-monitoring gradually, but consistently, diminishes.

Reasons for Therapeutic Effectiveness

These are exciting times for those of us who are engaged in stuttering research and therapy. The last decade's record of experimentation has opened minds and imaginations to bold, unconventional views of stuttering which at their best suggest new avenues of investigation, both theoretical and applied.

One of these, we hope, is the VCT program which in my view, owes its reparative effect to a cohesive, internally consistent theoretical model. To recapitulate briefly, this model suggests that stuttering consists, not in its origin but in its legacy, in the failure of reciprocal interaction between adductory and abductory laryngeal forces (Freeman and Ushijima, 1978; Shapiro, 1980). The task of remediation, as we see it, is to assure a continuous equilibrium of steady-state vocal fold movement during vowel phonation thereby counteracting chronic, intermittent hyperadduction at the glottis. For this purpose, VCT provides the speaker with a natural method for inducing vigorous vocal fold vibration: strong, open oral resonance for which breath control, smooth initiation of voicing, and focus on the vowel elements of speech are essential expedients. Removal of excessive constriction which arises within the vocal tract as a result of emotional tension, becomes a logical necessity as well.

We selected the repertory of skills and corollary techniques of VCT to meet the conditions for generating dependable, stable vocalization. If other, better strategies can be found, there is no hindrance to their immediate use. We hope, even if present procedures should some day be superseded, that the thrust of the VCT method will be judged a creditable approach to genuine fluency and a useful source of new perceptions about stuttering.

Advantages of the Therapy

ADVANTAGES FOR THE CLIENT

In our view, the dominant advantage of VCT is its high rate of applicability and success with all types of stutterers. Other beneficial aspects of note are that VCT assumes an holistic approach to the rehabilitation of the speech system rather than a segment-by-segment attack on discrete faulty productions.

In addition, speech at the completion of therapy is free of distortions of rate, airflow, continuity, and prosody. Further, effort expended to maintain fluency is roughly equivalent to that needed for effective speaking by teachers, lawyers, broadcasters and others engaged in active oral communication. The energy and attention required diminishes as use becomes habitual. Fluency has every chance of becoming a customary way of talking.

When stress arises, as it surely will in this imperfect world, the client who has mastered the therapy skills has the means to reinstate calm vocal control and the know-how to prevent recurrence. The procedures of therapy are straightforward, and knowable, and they become the property of the client.

"Belief" in VCT is not a prerequisite for a favorable outcome, provided the program gets an honest trial. Since improvement results from a set of clinical techniques which produce consistent rather than haphazard success, the understandably skeptical stutterer is free to withhold judgment for a while without jeopardizing immediate gains.

ADVANTAGES FOR THE CLINICIAN

The main attraction of VCT reported by speech-language pathologists is its concrete, effective "systems" approach, which evokes a confident response to stuttering therapy that is in direct contrast to that expressed by the clinicians' survey cited at the beginning of this chapter (Ragsdale and Ashby, 1982). Well-trained clinicians in our profession generally possess the major skills needed for VCT with the possible exception of systematic desensitization. The latter is worth acquiring for those types of cases where tension may be a complicating factor, such as in voice cases or aphasia, to name only two examples.

Clinical style and choice of stimuli are free of prescription and, therefore, open to clinically creative invention, as is the amount and elaboration of equipment.

The clinician need not "believe" in VCT any more than the client although confidence in the method is admittedly useful. The uncommitted clinician typically develops favorable feelings toward VCT as she experiences consistent, plausible success.

Professional speech-language specialists who apply for VCT training frequently evince a special brand of enthusiasm toward the program which contrasts sharply with methods requiring pseudostuttering and public displays of disfluency. These professionals cannot ordinarily refer their clients to full-time remedial programs, usually for financial reasons. And the mass-produced operant-conditioning projects, if available, are considered by many to show declining fluency when subjects are no longer in the presence of the clinician. So clinicians are drawn to the program for these reasons as well as for their appreciation of VCT's overall efficacy.

References

Adams, M. R. A physiological and aerodynamic interpretation of fluent and stuttered speech. *J. Fluency Disord.* 1:35–37, 1974.

Adams, M. R., and Hayden, P. The ability of stutterers and nonstutterers to initiate and terminate phonation during production of an isolated vowel. *J. Speech Hear. Res.* 19:290–296, 1976.

Adams, M. R., and Hutchinson, J. The effects of three levels of auditory masking on selected vocal characteristics and the frequency of disfluency of adult stutterers. *J. Speech Hear. Res.* 17:682–688, 1974.

Adams, M. R., and Moore, W. H., Jr. The effects of auditory masking on the anxiety level, frequency of dysfluency and selected vocal characteristics of stutterers. *J. Speech Hear. Res.* 15:572–578, 1972.

Adams, M. R., and Reis, R. The influence of onset of phonation on the frequency of stuttering. *J. Speech Hear. Res.* 14:639–644, 1971.

Aronson, A. E. *Clinical Voice Disorders: An Interdisciplinary Approach.* New York: Thieme, 1980.

Bernstein, N. *The Coordination and Regulation of Movements.* London: Pergamon, 1967.

Bloodstein, O. *Handbook of Stuttering.* Chicago: Easter Seal Society, 1981.

Boone, D. *Voice and Voice Therapy* (2nd ed.). Englewood Cliffs, N.J.: Prentice-Hall, 1977.

Borden, G. J., and Harris, K. S. *Speech Science Primer: Physiology, Acoustics and Perception of Speech.* Baltimore: Williams & Wilkins, 1980.

Brady, J. P. Metronome conditioned speech retraining for stuttering. *Behav. Ther.* 2:129–150, 1971.

Bruce, M. C., and Adams, M. R. Effects of two types of motor practice on stuttering and adaptation. *J. Speech Hear. Res.* 21:421–428, 1978.

Conture, E. G., McCall, G. N., and Brewer, D. W. Laryngeal behavior during stuttering. *J. Speech Hear. Res.* 20:661–668, 1977.

Fowler, S. A., Rubin, P., Remez, R. E. and Turvey, M. T. Implications for Speech Production of a General Theory of Action. In B. Butterworth (ed.), *Language Production.* London: Academic, 1980.

Freeman, F. J., and Rosenfield, D. "Source" in dysfluency. *J. Fluency Disord.* 7:295–296, 1982.

Freeman, F. J., and Ushijima, T. Laryngeal activity accompanying the moment of stuttering: A preliminary report of EMG investigations. *J. Fluency Disord.* 1:36–45, 1975.

Freeman, F. J., and Ushijima, T. Laryngeal muscle activity during stuttering, *J. Speech Hear. Res.* 21:538–562, 1978.

Gray, B., and England, G. Some effects of anxiety de-conditioning upon stuttering frequency. *J. Speech Hear. Res.* 15:114–123, 1972.

Heuer, R. J. The frequency of occurrence of harsh glottal attack in vocal nodule subjects and normal control subjects. Paper presented at the annual convention of the American-Speech-Language Hearing Association, Houston, 1976.

Jacobson, E. *Progressive Relaxation.* Chicago: University of Chicago Press, 1938.

Johnson, W., Darley, F., and Spreistersbach, D. C. *Diagnostic Methods in Speech Pathology.* New York: Harper & Row, 1963.

Kelso, J. A. Contrasting Perspective on Order and Regulation in Movement. In J. Long and A. Baddeley (eds.), *Attention and Performance,* vol. IX. Hillsdale, N.J.: Lawrence Erlbaum and Associates, Inc., 1981.

Leith, W. R. Clinical training in stuttering therapy: A survey. *ASHA* 13:6–8, 1971.

Moncur, J. P., and Brackett, I. P. *Modifying Vocal Behavior.* New York: Harper & Row, 1974.

Perkins, W. *Speech Pathology: An Applied Behavioral Science* (2nd ed.). St. Louis: Mosby, 1977.

Polit, A., and Bizzi, E. Processes controlling arm movements in monkeys. *Science* 201:1235–1237, 1978.

Ragsdale, J. D., and Ashby, J. K. Speech-language pathologists' connotations of stuttering. *J. Speech Hear. Res.* 25:75–81, 1982.

Riley, G. D. A stuttering severity instrument for children and adults. *J. Speech Hear. Disord.* 37:314–322, 1972.

Schwartz, M. F. The core of the stuttering block. *J. Speech Hear. Disord.* 39:169–177, 1974.

Schwartz, M. F. *Stuttering Solved.* Philadelphia: J. B. Lippincott, 1976.

Shapiro, A. I. An electromyographic analysis of the fluent and dysfluent utterances of several types of stutterers. *J. Fluency Disord.* 5:203–231, 1980.

Starkweather, C. W. A multiprocess behavioral approach to stuttering therapy. *Semin. Speech Lang. Hear.* 9:327–338, 1980.

Sundberg, H. Format Structures and Articulation of Spoken and Sung Syllables. In J. Large (ed.), *Contributions of Voice Research to Singing.* Houston: College Hill Press, 1980.

Vennard, W. *Singing: The Mechanism and the Technic.* New York: Fisher, 1967.

Webster, R. L. An operant response shaping program for the establishment of fluency in stutterers. *ASHA Abstracts* 15:136, 1975.

Weiner, A. E. Speech therapy and behavior modification: A conspectus. *J. Spec. Educ.* 3:285–293, 1969.

Weiner, A. E. Vocal control therapy for stutterers: A trial program. *J. Fluency Disord.* 3:115–126, 1978.

Weiner, A. E. A case of adult onset of stuttering. *J. Fluency Disord.* 6:181–186, 1981.

Weiner, A. E. Patterns of vocal fold movement during stuttering. *J. Fluency Disord.* (in press).

Wilson, D. K. *Voice Problems of Children* (2nd ed.). Baltimore: Williams & Wilkins, 1979.

Wingate, M. E. A standard definition of stuttering. *J. Speech Hear. Disord.* 29:484–489, 1964.

Wingate, M. E. Sound and pattern in "artificial" fluency. *J. Speech Hear. Res.* 12:677–686, 1969.

Wingate, M. E. Effect on stuttering of changes in audition. *J. Speech Hear. Res.* 13:861–873, 1970.

Wingate, M. E. The fear of stuttering. *ASHA* 13:3–5, 1971.

Wingate, M. E. *Stuttering: Theory and Treatment.* New York: Irvington, 1976.

Wolpe, J. *Psychotherapy by Reciprocal Inhibition.* Stanford, Calif. Stanford University Press, 1958.

Wolpe, J. *Practice of Behavior Therapy* (2nd ed.). New York: Pergamon, 1973.

Wolpe, J. with Wolpe, D. *Our Useless Fears.* Boston: Houghton Mifflin, 1981.

Zemlin, W. R. *Speech and Hearing Science, Anatomy and Physiology.* Englewood Cliffs, N.J.: Prentice-Hall, 1968.

SELECTED SOURCES OF VOICE THERAPY TECHNIQUES

Aronson, A. E. *Clinical Voice Disorders: An Interdisciplinary Approach.* New York: Thieme, 1980.

Anderson, V. *Training the Speaking Voice.* New York: Oxford University Press, 1977.

Boone, D. *The Voice and Voice Therapy.* Englewood Cliffs, N.J.: Prentice-Hall, 1977.

Eisenson, J. *The Improvement of Voice and Diction.* New York: Macmillan, 1958.

Fairbanks, G. *Voice and Articulation Drillbook.* New York: Harper & Brothers, 1960.

Greene, M. C. L. *The Voice and Its Disorders.* New York: Macmillan, 1957.

Lessac, A. *The Use and Training of the Human Voice.* New York: DBS Publishers, 1967.

Moncur, J. P., and Brackett, I. P. *Modifying Vocal Behavior.* New York: Harper & Row, 1974.

Vennard, W. *Singing: The Mechanism and the Technic.* New York: Fischer, 1967.

SELECTED SOURCES OF APHASIA THERAPY WORKBOOKS
Brubaker, S. H. *Workbook for Aphasia*. Detroit: Wayne State University Press, 1978.
Keith, R. L. *Speech and Language Rehabilitation: A Workbook for the Neurologically Impaired*, Vols. 1 and 2. Danville, Ill.: Interstate, 1977.
Kilpatrick, K., and Jones, C. L. *Therapy Guide for the Adult with Language and Speech Disorders. A Selection of Stimulus Materials*. Akron: Visiting Nurse Service, 1977.

7. A Rational Management of Stuttering

Marcel E. Wingate

Overview

This approach to the management of stuttering focuses on the generation and maintenance of fluent speech and contrasts most directly with approaches that focus on stuttering in respect to the stutter events themselves and/or the stutterer's presumed reactions to his stuttering.

The approach has a didactic dimension and an experiential dimension which are interrelated in the course of the treatment program. The intent of the didactic dimension is to lead the patient to the appreciation of the nature of normal speech, particularly those aspects of it that seem to be primarily involved in stuttering. The experiential dimension endeavors to guide the patient through experiences that implement and demonstrate the principles of the didactic dimension. The experiential dimension is not a "method"; rather, it makes flexible use of a variety of techniques. These techniques, although apparently quite different, evidently share certain core features that are common to speaking conditions known to have a beneficial effect on stuttering.

History of the Therapy

This approach to stuttering management evolved gradually over a period of approximately 16 years from both research and clinical experience. The development progressed in roughly two stages. In the first stage the major contributions came from clinical work and activities related to clinical practice. In the second stage the major contribution came from research, both experimental and descriptive/analytic research.

STAGE 1

My original involvement and interest in stuttering developed quite adventitiously. My undergraduate major was in psychology and at the graduate level I specialized in clinical psychology. During my graduate years I was advised that speech pathology would be a suitable minor area of preparation for a clinical psychologist, and largely through matters of convenience in academic scheduling, I elected to accept speech pathology as my minor field. It was quite natural that stuttering should attract the interest of someone preparing to be a clinical psychologist since the disorder has been considered a psychological problem for a very long time.

There are many ways in which stuttering has been explained as a psychological problem; most often such explanations have taken one of two somewhat different forms. The most dramatic, and the most fascinating and appealing, kind of explanation is to interpret stuttering as a symptom of an underlying dynamic psychological disturbance. In such accounts the stutter is seen as a symptom of some hidden conflicts deep within the individual's nonconscious mind, and the stutter as a symptom is supposedly related in some unique way to the underlying conflicts. In such conceptions the objective of therapy is to resolve the inner conflicts which the individual is assumed to have, after which, it is further assumed, the symptoms of that conflict (the stutter) will no longer serve their purpose and will therefore dissipate. This psychodynamic orientation makes the assumption that working with the stuttering itself (the symptoms), or even with the individual's speech, is working only with surface features and that such management does not get at the root of the problem.

The other type of psychological explanation of stuttering views the disorder as somehow having developed through the agency of fear. The presumed source of the fear varies from one account to another, for example, fear of stuttering, fear of disfluency, fear of disapproval of speech performance, fear of speech as difficult, or fear of speaking. These explanations assume that the person would not stutter if he did not have such fears and that stuttering would not be manifest if he did not struggle with his speech as a result of the fear. Treatment methods centered in this orientation do deal directly with the stuttering but they also have traditionally placed heavy emphasis on the modification of attitude, proceeding from the belief that if attitude is adequately modified, the fear will diminish and the struggle thereby subside.

My direct and vicarious experiences in working from both of these orientations were illuminating but also discouraging. To be sure, there were some stutterers who had inner personality conflicts of which they were unaware and which affected at least some areas of their personal adjustment, just as there are some people who are free of any kind of symptom who have problems which in some way affect some of their adjustments. Most of the stutterers with whom I worked were able to resolve their personal problems, but such resolution did not have the expected effect on the presence of the stuttering itself. Reports I found in the literature corroborated my personal experiences.

Approaching the management of stuttering with the explanation that it reflects fear and struggle also proved disappointing for a number of reasons. Basically, there is something very superficial about the fear explanations. As off-handed, gloss explanations they have a certain appeal, and this appeal has had a wide-spread following for many years. However, if one attempts to find evidence for such explanations among individual clients, the search yields disconcerting inconsistencies[1]. Many stutterers accepted a fear explanation, some from their own reflections and others who heard it from another source, but a number of stutterers insisted that they did not fear their stuttering, or speaking, and still others pointed out (quite reasonably) that fear was a plausible explanation only for certain circumstances. Additionally, in my experience, a change in attitude alone yielded only a modest change in stuttering. In the long run what did make a difference was working on the person's speech. Once some improvement was made in that direction it was easier to incorporate into therapy any contribution to be realized from a change in attitude, and that was a sequence that made sense.

Other clinical experiences further contradicted the supposed role of fear; for instance, my contact with little children who evidently did not realize they stuttered, and with other youngsters who knew they stuttered, but were clearly indifferent to, or casual about, it. Then there were those children whose stuttering was intermittent, appearing for weeks or months at a time and then absent for perhaps comparable periods; it was very difficult to discern or explain how fear or reaction could be centrally involved in these episodes.

My clinical experience led to disillusionment with psychological explanations of stuttering and with their related treatments. This disenchantment was increased by what I found in the results of research pertinent to psychological explanations of stuttering. For example, an extensive review of relevant literature by Goodstein (1958) yielded very little evidence of personality problems in stutterers and, in fact, little evidence that stutterers are particularly maladjusted relative to persons who do not stutter. Comparable reviews by Sheehan (1958, 1970) and Van Riper (1982) yielded the same findings and conclusions. In addition many sources in the literature, representing various viewpoints, clearly contradicted the simpler psychological explanation that relates stuttering to fear (for an extensive review of this material, see Wingate, 1976).

It is pertinent to note here in recent years that explanations and treatments for stuttering have shown an increased emphasis on learning theory terms and concepts, particularly on "operant" terminology and beliefs. It seems that this emphasis has been presented, and accepted, as a new and different orientation to stuttering. However, one should recognize clearly that all psychological interpretations of stuttering incorporate concepts and ideas of learning theory in their formulations even though such dimensions are not featured, nor in some cases made very evident, in the statements of the various positions. For instance, psychodynamic explanations of stuttering and the "caused-by-fear" accounts are not identified, nor ordinarily thought of, as learning interpretations of stuttering. Actually, however, all of these explanations rely heavily on learning concepts, and all of them invoke affective (emotional) factors as an important dimension in the formulation. The essential difference among the several types of explanation (psychodynamic; fear-generated; learning theory) lies in whether they emphasize the emotional factors or prefer an emphasis on the concepts of learning.

The point of the foregoing discussion is simply this: faults in any one of the different psychological explanations of stuttering have serious implications for the credibility of any of the others. This point can be exemplified at even a very general level: the substantial evidence contradicts the central role of affective factors in stuttering, immediately giving reason to doubt psychodynamic interpretations and those accounts that emphasize fear and reaction. What is more, such findings compromise learning explanations as well, because these explanations also rely heavily on the supposed importance of affective factors. Beyond this, learning theory explanations, as applied to stuttering, have their own sets of serious contradictions and inconsistencies[2].

STAGE 2

The second stage in the development of the stuttering management described in this chapter was shaped more by the results of research, my own and that of others, and by analysis of these results relative to the existing literature and my clinical experience.

One observation about stuttering which had impressed me increasingly was the extent of variability among stutterers, beyond the matter of the speech defect itself. Of course, psychological explanations contain within them marvelous ways of accounting for variation, but it seemed to me that individualization could be taken too far and that the adaptiveness of such explanation was more facile than flexible. It occurred to me that the focus on variability, and ways of accounting for it, led to an expanding set of circular reasonings reminiscent of the Ptolemaic explanation of the movements of heavenly bodies. It seemed to me that a much more worthwhile approach would be to look for and investigate similarities among stutterers: what I began to think of as "universals" of stuttering. By "universals" I had in mind those features about stuttering which could be honestly claimed to be characteristic of, or true for, the vast majority of stutterers, if not all of them.

Some of the features that qualified as "universals" had been known about for a long time but had been ignored or dismissed in one way or another. Chief among these was the frequent report that stutterers do not stutter when they sing. Another observation widely reported for a long time was that stutterers do not stutter, or stutter very little, when speaking to rhythm. A third circumstance known to have a markedly beneficial effect on stuttering is the influence of choral, or unison, speaking. This effect has been observed casually in circumstances such as responsive readings in church or similar situations that call for group recitations of one kind or another. Furthermore, a number of studies conducted during the 1930s and 1940s corroborated the ameliorative effect of all these circumstances.

Now, these impressive effects have been explained away over a period of many years with the contention that they are the result of distraction.

Such an account, however, is a classic example of a glib and superficial explanation impeding progress toward a scientific and rational understanding of stuttering. The distraction account is never elaborated; one never hears how a condition is distracting or why it should be distracting. Actually the concept of distraction is completely illogical in this context. The meaning of distraction is that one's thoughts are *diverted* from some particular focus to something different; the essential point here is that the person is now preoccupied with the distraction and is no longer thinking about that from which he was distracted. But how does singing, speaking to rhythm, or speaking in chorus divert the stutterer's thoughts from his stuttering or the fact that he stutters? If he thinks about what he is doing in these circumstances, which he must, he should be aware that he is not stuttering, which should certainly remind him that he stutters. Also, one can have a stutterer sing about his stuttering, or speak about it in rhythm or in chorus, and the salutary effect of these conditions will nonetheless be manifest. (Other difficulties with this concept are discussed in Wingate, 1976.)

Several other conditions, "shadowing," auditory masking, and delayed auditory feedback, have also been reported to result in substantial reductions in stuttering. These conditions were discovered more recently than the others and were not as widely known, but the reported extent of their ameliorative effect was impressive.

These varied circumstances were reported to have a regularly remarkable effect on stuttering. Their consistent influence met the criterion of "universality"; the next step was to determine whether there might be some feature, or features, common to them which could logically account for the reduced stuttering in each of them.

I was struck by the fact that, in the literature describing each condition and its effect, the discussion always centered on the stuttering, specifically on the marked reduction in frequency of stuttering evidently occasioned by the condition. This preoccupation with the fact that stuttering was minimized left the implication that the resulting speech was otherwise unaffected. It was as though the sole effect of the ameliorative condition was to eradicate stutters, leaving (or revealing) ordinary normal speech as the result. It was rare to find mention of any other changes in the stutterers' speech (or "oral performance"), even for those conditions which produce other changes that are quite dramatic. For example, at least the superficial difference between speaking and singing should be obvious; stuttering eliminated by singing leaves song, not ordinary speech. Similarly, stuttering eliminated by speaking to rhythm leaves speech marked by unnatural cadence (and related changes), not the kind of speech one usually hears. In like vein, reduced stuttering is not the only effect produced by choral speaking, shadowing, auditory masking, or delayed feedback. All of these conditions result in speech that is unlike ordinary spontaneous speech. But the differences in stutterers' speech other than the reduction or elimination of stuttering either went unnoticed or were not considered important.

The singular focus of attention on stuttering also obscured the fact that these conditions effect changes in the speech of normal speakers as well and that, excluding stuttering, the changes are the same for normal speakers as for stutterers. At base, then, these conditions induce certain changes in anyone's speech. In the case of stutterers such changes are accompanied by at least a marked reduction in stuttering.

So, the first stage in the search for commonality among these conditions was recognizing that they all induce change in manner of speaking, change which extends considerably beyond the matter of "eliminating" stuttering. It seemed plausible, then, that their common effect of reducing stuttering might reflect features common to the changes in manner of speaking which they induce. The next step, therefore, was to inquire what those common features might be.

The development of this step took a long time. Fortunately, the procedure and essential results of the inquiry can be reviewed rather succinctly. A careful extensive analysis was made of each of the major ameliorative conditions, and a number of other circumstances also known to have a beneficial effect on stuttering, relative to the evident nature of their effect on speech[3]. These analyses indicated that the major common features involved changes that emphasized the prosody, or melody, of speech, those aspects of spoken language that are expressed through variations in pitch, loudness and duration.

Assessment Procedures

The objectives of assessment are much the same regardless of the age of the patient, although the method and techniques for obtaining the desired information must be adjusted to patient age and related circumstances, such as the presence of an accompanying adult, usually a parent.

The principal objective of the assessment is to obtain an adequate and representative sample of the patient's spontaneous speech. (Use of oral reading in a diagnostic evaluation should be considered only as a last resort or for purposes of special interest.) The patient's performance in spontaneous connected speech is the focus of the assessment. In particular, the sample must be representative relative to the reason for referral, that is, whether the stuttering that occurs during the examination is typical of the patient's speech in most other circumstances. This determination can be made by direct questioning of the patient or, when appropriate, of the accompanying adult. Infrequently, a young child may not stutter during the evaluation; one must not then assume that the child does not stutter (and therefore that the parent is in error). Most often the accompanying parent will partially resolve the issue by spontaneously expressing embarrassment that the child's speech does not, on that occasion, contain clear examples of the cause of the parents' concern. In almost all cases the examiner can fully resolve any uncertainty about whether the child stutters by asking the parent to describe or imitate the speech features that were the reason for referral.

Accurate diagnosis is important, of course, but it is not as difficult as some writers have contended, even with young children. The essential criteria of stuttering, established through repeated observation over many years, are elemental repetitions and prolongations occurring as the distinctive "markers" of inability to move forward in the speech sequence. The distinctiveness of these criteria has been corroborated repeatedly by pertinent research. (For a full discussion of the identification of stuttering, see Wingate, 1976; for special reference to these features in the speech of young children, see Wingate, 1962. Very recently Yairi and Lewis [1984] report corroborative evidence gathered on very young children within a few weeks of reported stuttering onset.)

Several subsequent dimensions of assessment are of value for counseling patient and parent and as contributions to some aspects of direct therapy. The examiner should note certain qualitative features relative to the stuttering: the nature of the stutter events; their frequency of occurrence; and the amount of "involvement," particularly the degree of apparent effort exerted. One should also explore the extent to which the patient is familiar with his stutter. Contrary to popular belief, stutterers often have only a generalized awareness of their inability to move on in speaking and have limited recognition of the details of the stutter events. Often, too, they are not aware of all instances of stutter.

One should inquire about how the client perceives variability in his stuttering and note as well circumstances of stuttering commonly reported by stutterers. Circumstances of stutter occurrence relatively unique to the client, such as substantial increase or decrease in stuttering in the presence of a certain individual, will require special attention in management. On the other hand, typical findings, such as that the patient does not stutter when singing or is likely to stutter more when speaking on the telephone, have multiple value. For instance, it is instructive, and sometimes comforting, to the stutterer to know that many aspects of his disability are shared with other stutterers. Moreover, this information can be used later to help him better understand his disability and to appreciate certain aspects of treatment.

It is worthwhile to obtain, where possible, pertinent case history information such as family history of stuttering, the nature of stuttering at inception, and changes of any kind noted subsequently. Inquiry about family history of stuttering has value even if the respondent can report none; this inquiry broaches the topic of the probable physiological basis of stuttering. In regard to history of stuttering onset, one must be circumspect about those reports in which a definite date or place of onset is attributed to specific events or circumstances. There is a tendency, by no means limited to stuttering, for retrospection to link events which in reality were not so closely associated. Inquiry in this area also generally provides an appropriate opportunity for the examiner to impart some well-founded information about stuttering. It is helpful to parents and patient alike to learn that stuttering is not known to be causally related to external events; that it is typically gradual in onset; that stuttering seldom gets worse; that almost half of stuttering youngsters will recover before puberty; that improvement can be achieved by older stutterers; and that recovery, too, is typically gradual.

One should always explore carefully the attitudes of the patient, and of the parents when appropriate, including the beliefs they may have about the nature and cause of stuttering. Clinician awareness of these matters is important to both counseling and direct therapy. Assessment of attitudes may require a lengthier period than is available during the initial evaluation, but most often the major outlines of attitude will be at least fairly clear. Clients' beliefs about the nature and cause of stuttering should be countered by pertinent established facts, principal among which is the fact that we do not know what causes the disorder.

Overall, an adequate assessment requires that the clinician be knowledgeable about stuttering and be able to pursue relevant inquiry without preconceptions. Equally important is the clinician's sensitivity to recognize individuality among stutterers.

Description of the Therapy

THERAPY GOALS

The goal of this treatment approach is to help the patient develop, to the extent of his capabilities, the skills necessary to generate fluent-sounding speech. In other words, the goal is to help the stutterer develop improved speech, speech which is more fluent than his present speech and which is also closer to the kind of speech that is typical of normally fluent speakers.

Note that the goal is not "stutter-free" speech or speech with less stuttering. Some methods and techniques can produce speech with fewer stutters, but the resultant speech is discriminably odd in some other way. Speaking to a strict rhythm and speaking in a monotone are two good examples. The approach described in this chapter anticipates speech with less stuttering, but as a by-product of treatment, not as its focus.

Note also that the goal is not "normal fluency" or "normal speech." We cannot honestly encourage any individual stutterer to anticipate achievement of fluent speech in the sense that normally fluent speakers experience it; that is, speech which appears to flow smoothly and which seems to be produced without a sense of conscious control. All too frequently the literature on stuttering therapy conveys the belief and aspiration that a stutterer's speech can be modified to the point that it ("once again")[4] will become automatic. This implies a goal that with treatment all the stutterer need do is think a thought, open his mouth, and the rest will come naturally. Speech pathologists who accept the belief in "returning speech to the automatic level" evidence disregard for the well-established professional recognition that speech at the automatic level is a very low level of utterance. Even phatic expressions (e.g., "How are ya?", "See ya.") though very simple and highly routinized are not automatic. The typical speech of a normal person is not "at the automatic level." It is therefore incorrect, and improper as well, to lead anyone to expect his ordinary speech will eventually be of this nature.

We still do not understand very well the processes by which speech is generated and uttered, but we do know enough to realize that those processes are by no means simple. However, such realization is too infrequently in evidence. Generally speech is regarded quite casually; certainly the lay attitude takes speech very much for granted.

In his delightfully pithy book about the misuse of language, *Strictly Speaking*, Edwin Newman devotes one section to criticism of excessive and banal use of certain words whose very good descriptive value has thereby been eroded seriously. One of the words he chose in example was the word "wonderful," which should have the meaning of eliciting wonder, marvel, awe, or amazement. Newman made the point that, in contrast to what one should expect from the glib vernacular use of the word, few events in our experience truly are "wonderful." My reason for using this one of Newman's examples is to make the point that, in contrast to the way in which it is typically regarded, speech is a prime example of those few events in our experience which are truly "wonderful," that is, worthy of eliciting wonder or awe.

Strangely, speech pathologists seem to maintain an attitude toward speech which belies the professional education they must have received[5]. It seems as though their life-long experience in producing and hearing spoken language has made it difficult for them to set aside their lay attitude toward speech that takes it so much for granted.

It is easy to appreciate the potency of the lay attitude. Not only does it develop quietly, persistently, and thoroughly over a period of many years, it also is firmly based in an awareness of the essential ubiquity of speech in humans. The standard experience of almost all of us is that everyone of our acquaintance speaks, and although we may be well aware of certain varieties of speech in various individuals, this does not alter our implicit understanding that they are all one with us in the fact that we all speak. Speech is all around us, and "everybody" does it. We are puzzled by those few who do not speak, or who do not speak as we expect them to; and for these individuals we persistently assume that the ability to speak and to speak as we do, is in there somewhere.

The apparent assumption that speech, as we know it personally, is a "given" of the human condition probably is enhanced in many ways: for instance, our awareness that people can learn to speak one or more other languages; or our experience that some people talk a lot but don't really say much that is worthwhile, and vice versa. Unfortunately for the speech pathologist, the casual lay attitude is reinforced by widely accepted professional views which conceive speech simplistically as "learned behavior" and stuttering as simply another form of "learned behavior."

The foregoing discussion is highly germane to a statement of goals for stuttering therapy which should convey not only an adequate appreciation of the nature of speech but an awareness that the speech of stutterers differs from that of normally fluent persons. There are, of course, those features of stuttered speech that are the long-standing basis for deciding which speakers among us should undertake stuttering therapy. Beyond that, a growing fund of evidence suggests that the speech of stutterers differs in subtle and arcane ways from the speech of the normally fluent. These data provide additional support for a treatment approach for which the goals are neither to simply eliminate stutter events nor to "return" a patient's speech to the normal fluency that supposedly exists within.

I believe that the treatment of stuttering is conceived most appropriately as a system of helping a stutterer learn certain skills sufficient for producing speech with a type and level of fluency that approaches normal speech as closely as possible. Learning of these skills should be based on principles which, to the best of our current knowledge, reflect what appears to underly normal speech. The stutterer should also understand that improvement, that is, his progress toward normal-sounding speech, will occur as he refines his understanding and use of the skills involved.

It is not realistic to lead a stutterer to expect speech devoid of actual stutters such as he has experienced before, or of incipient stutters (which he can sense and modify or overcome). Some stutterers may be able to attain speech which has neither actual nor incipient stutters, and many can aspire to this as an eventual goal, but it is unlikely that most stutterers will achieve it.

Stutterers show considerable individual difference in the nature and extent of their stuttering. In addition to these differences, stutterers, like normal speakers, differ from one another in terms of motivation, docility[6], personal commitment, and native abilities. These native abilities include whatever abilities are requisite to gain better command over one's speech. To cast the matter into practical terms: Stutterers differ widely in their prospects for benefitting from stuttering therapy; this suggests that "the answer" in stuttering therapy does not lie in a therapy method or a therapist.

No approach to stuttering treatment can honestly identify for an individual stutterer what his level of speech improvement will be. We have only crude, casual, and largely impressionistic means of forecasting improvement in stuttering, and no predictive capability whatsoever for identifying which stutterers will attain improvement that is stable. The substantial amount of information on recovery from stuttering, both from research (see Wingate, 1976) and personal testimonials from "recovered" stutterers within the profession, (see p.282) tell us a great deal about variables likely to be of significance in the improvement of a stutterer's speech. In the end, however, it is an individual matter, and the focal point is the individual stutterer, not the therapist or his method.

One cannot expect treatment to result routinely, even for a majority of cases, in seemingly normal fluent speech. Many stutterers can learn to produce speech that sounds reasonably fluent much of the time. Some can learn to achieve such performance most of the time. A few may even achieve a level of fluency that would pass easily as normal fluent speech. The clinician must face the fact, however, that for most stutterers (particularly older children to adult) the prospects for major, stable, and enduring gains in fluency are not particularly good.

This statement may strike the reader as unduly pessimistic for it almost certainly will seem contradictory to the attitude toward stuttering that has developed in recent years and pervades the many "new" methods of stuttering therapy which at least imply great promise. Several very impressive facts about stuttering testify, however, to an essential pessimism, or at least serious reservation, about "getting over" stuttering.

First of all, the history of the treatment of stuttering does not provide much encouragement. Stuttering has been treated extensively, and in a number of different ways, over a period of many years, without commendably consistent or impressive results. Particularly during the 19th century many different techniques and methods were employed which, on the whole, did not yield particularly remarkable, consistent results. Very often these methods raised great hopes initially but within a relatively short time were recognized to lack the potency they originally seemed to have. It is especially relevant to note that many of these techniques (e.g., rhythm, easy onset, controlled breathing) have reappeared in recent-day "new" methods of stuttering therapy.

Another dimension of pessimism, closely related to the first, is the fact that claims for the efficacy of any "new" method of managing stuttering always arouse skepticism within the profession. The prevailing attitude among those who are knowledgeable about stuttering is laden with doubt that any particular system "really works"; and the more positive and certain the claims for a method the more rigorous the skepticism and the doubt.

A third dimension of skepticism rests implicitly in the attitudes that professionals convey toward the speech problems of individuals aspiring to enter the profession. For instance, a person who has an articulation defect or a voice problem most likely will be counseled to resolve the problem before seriously planning to enter the profession. In contrast, individuals who stutter do not encounter such restrictions, and in fact there are many active stutterers in the profession. The significance of this professional "favoritism" is the implicit recognition that persons who stutter cannot realistically be expected to resolve their problem, at least not within a reasonable length of time.

A fourth dimension of pessimism is to be found in the records of speech improvement among the stutterers one finds within the professional ranks. I know of 52 stutterers in the profession (though I am sure there are many more) and only 5 of these individuals evidence speech I find difficult to discriminate from normal speech. In 1957, and again in 1977, the convention of the American Speech and Hearing Association included a program featuring a panel of "recovered" stutterers from within the profession who gave personal testimonials to their efforts and success in managing their own stuttering[7]. The word "recovered" was deliberately placed in quotation marks on the program because the participants themselves recognized that technically they were not recovered although they had achieved considerable (but varying) levels of achievement[8]. Further, although most of them believed they would continue to improve, there was no serious expectation of cure. In fact, Van Riper, who undoubtedly had worked on his speech longer than any of those participating in either the 1957 or 1977 program, pointedly remarked that he did not believe he would ever be cured.

In respect to the general population, those recovered stutterers within the profession must be considered highly capable individuals, even if one takes account only of the level of their academic achievement (most of them have a doctoral degree). Moreover, most of them have been well motivated to do something about their speech; in fact, at least among the participants in the 1977 ASHA convention program, motivation was the factor repeatedly emphasized in the individual testimonials. One could expect that these individuals should be exemplars of success in overcoming stuttering; yet, for most of them stuttering persists, and it is more obvious in some than in others. Most of the stutterers in the profession with whom I have been acquainted at least reasonably well over a number of years have shown gradual and continuing improvement in speech. However, in none has the course of improvement led to truly normal speech.

Any therapist who has a sincerely professional attitude toward the management of stuttering should be knowledgeable about information that bears on the recovery of stuttering. Certainly, this is a topic which is very relevant to the matter of treatment, but it has received inadequate attention in the professional literature. Articles reporting recovery of stuttering appeared from time to time throughout the first half of this century but the subject was ignored, evidently because the prevailing conceptions of stuttering centered in the belief that stuttering typically gets worse. Then, early in the 1960s several publications evidently forced attention to the evidence that stuttering subsides much more often than it is exacerbated.

The fact of recovery is important in and of itself for its value in understanding the nature of stuttering. Moreover, the statistics of recovery have at least actuarial value for general prognostic purposes. For instance, a cardinal feature of the data on recovery is the evidence that spontaneous remission occurs in approximately 45 percent of youngsters who stutter prior to the age of 8 years. Among other implications of these data they suggest that any treatment method utilized with children under 9 years of age should discount its improvement rate by approximately 50 percent[9]. The recovery data also indicate that after the age of 8 what the individual does in trying to overcome his stuttering evidently plays more of a role in recovery. The following are additional implications for at least prepubertal to adult stutterers: (1) Improvement in fluency is possible. (2) In most cases it will take a long time. (3) One can expect considerable individual differences in range and level of improvement. (4) The stutterer's motivation is a significant element in improvement. (5) The role of the therapist or his methods are not the critically determining features in success[10].

Given these contributing factors the goal of this approach to the management of stuttering is improved speech. In a broad sense the goal of treatment is to improve the overall quality of the individual's speech, with a resultant reduction in instances of stuttering. Improved speech is a realistic goal, one that affords flexible and individualized treatment, defined in each case by the limits of the individual stutterer's capabilities. Moreover, one must recognize that these capabilities (and limits thereof) may become evident only after fairly extended treatment efforts have been made.

Therapy Method

OBJECTIVES, TECHNIQUES, PROCEDURES

It is not appropriate to speak of this approach as being a therapy method or as having a method in the usual sense of the term. "Method" indicates that a certain regimen is specified or outlined and that implementation of treatment is expected to adhere to a rather strict regimen. The approach to stuttering management described in this chapter, however, allows, in fact encourages, rationalized use of a number of procedures and separate techniques.

The central objective of this therapy approach is to educate the stutterer in speech expression. In the long run, the experience of monitoring and managing one's speech is the major substance of the approach, yet this experience must be interwoven, particularly in the early stages, with instruction and demonstration.

The "education" of the stutterer includes didactic as well as experiential teaching. The relative amounts of these two dimensions are determined individually with consideration given to the stutterer's age and ability to understand what is being presented and what can be expected of him. The didactic dimension emerges in dialogue that (1) presents an appropriate level of explanation about the nature of speech, particularly in its peripheral aspects; (2) offers an account of what seems to go wrong when stuttering occurs; and (3) explains why certain speaking conditions ameliorate stuttering so readily, and how this relates to (1) and (2). The experiential dimension pursues a course which (1) leads the stutterer through the experience of a variety of procedures and techniques that can be expected to induce more fluent speech; (2) helps him appreciate the evident principles involved; and (3) guides him in extracting from these experiences his own best system for implementing an improved mode of speaking.

This approach to the management of stuttering is not limited to a particular method or technique, but rather, makes use of a number of different techniques and procedures to induce the patient to speak in a manner different from his usual pattern, exemplify certain qualities inherent to good speech, and provide the patient the opportunity to appreciate and express the qualities of good speech.

The techniques and procedures employed in this management approach all conform to or express a set of principles that are the conceptual core of the approach. These principles were derived from an analysis of a number of conditions which for a long time have been known for their beneficial effect of the speech of stutterers. Most notable among these conditions are: singing, speaking to rhythm, and choral (or unison) speaking. Other less well-known conditions having comparable effects are auditory masking and delayed auditory feedback.

A careful analysis[11] of the various speaking conditions having a notably beneficial effect on the fluency of stutterers revealed that the principal change effected by each condition was some modification of the prosodic (melodic) aspects of speech. Such change evidently is occasioned by inducing the stutterer to emphasize the "tune" in speech, the variations in pitch, volume, and duration carried on vocal resonance. Evidently, intentionally reducing the rate of speech provides an excellent vehicle through which an appreciation and sense of the prosody of speech can be realized.

Sometimes distinctions between the terms *method, procedure,* and *technique* become obscure both in the literature and in discussions between individuals. *Method* refers to an established process, a way of going about doing something which ordinarily involves a set of *procedures* or several more specific kinds of activities usually identified as *techniques.* In the discussion that follows, for example, such activities as voice chewing, poetry reading, and speaking in rhythm approximate a procedure; whereas easy onset, prolongation, and slowing down seem to be more of the nature of techniques. In addition certain other activities of varying value to the therapist are neither procedure nor technique but serve simply and appropriately as demonstrations. These, which include singing, masking, and delayed auditory feedback, can assist the patient to understand how fluency is affected by changes in manner of speaking. They do not, however, give the patient a realistic sense of control over the modulation of his speech: the effect of these conditions is not readily sensed directly by the patient and usually the speech induced is quite unlike speech as one produces or hears it routinely.

Following is a list and brief description of a variety of procedures and techniques for the therapist to utilize in the treatment approach presented in this chapter. These procedures and techniques serve one or more of three different functions: (1) *Basic training*—those activities which typically are presented early in the course of treatment to convey the principles underlying the treatment approach. Often it is necessary to reintroduce them later in therapy and assign the patient exercises that emphasize these activities or bring them into prominence. (2) *Demonstration/instruction*—activities useful primarily for demonstrating important points in the therapy. Frequently some of them are presented early in the treatment but they are typically useful later in therapy as well. (3) *Therapy substance*—procedures and techniques that focus on or implement coordinative control of the speech production system in ways that emphasize the prosodic dimensions of speech.

Voicing, in its simplest form, is phonation, the act of making a sound with the vocal folds. This activity can be elaborated or modified in order to elicit variations in the intensity, pitch, and duration of sound, as well as any of the various combinations of these. An especially important variation focuses on effecting a contrast between easy and hard "attacks" in initiating sound and in making changes in sound production (basic training).

Easy onset is essentially an elaboration of the exercise above. Easy onset refers to making a gentle "attack" on words (and longer units of utterance) with varying forms of sound (vowel, consonant, combinations) in the initial (attack) position (basic training).

Singing, an obvious activity, refers not only to the singing of familiar songs, but also to the substitution of new words as lyrics for familiar tunes or to the invention of tunes with which to sing any particular phrase or expression (demonstration/instruction).

Sounding, a technique in which the tune of a spoken utterance is extracted from the utterance and reproduced alone, emphasizes the prosodic dimension of ordinary speech. "Sounding" relates to speech as humming does to singing, and demonstration as well as explanation to the patient is usually necessary (therapy substance).

Monotone is an activity that calls for speaking without the usual prosodic variation (therapy substance).

Chanting is a form of expression that combines elements of singing and monotone to produce an utterance intoned with sequential changes in pitch levels that are maintained for varying lengths of time (therapy substance).

Rhythm is speaking intentionally with some regular pattern of stress. The pattern may be varied from time to time at the discretion of the therapist; but the basic pattern, and the one used most often, is a rhythm of one syllable per beat. Typically, speaking to rhythm results in a certain amount of monotone (therapy substance).

Prolongation is intentionally lengthening an utterance by extending the duration of syllables in the utterance. Typically this effect is achieved through the syllable nuclei (i.e., the syllabics, most often vowels) (therapy substance).

Slowing down emphasizes reducing rate of utterance by intentionally speaking more slowly. It is similar to prolongation except that the effort is not addressed to specific syllables in words (therapy substance).

Dialect speech involves attempting to speak in a dialect that is not one's own, for instance an Irish brogue or an Italian accent, or for Northerners in the United States, a Southern drawl. This also includes, especially for children, speaking in a stylized voice appropriately associated with certain animals or other nonhuman forms (therapy substance).

Choral speaking refers to reading aloud in unison with one or more other speakers, who may be saying the same thing or something different (demonstration/instruction).

Auditory masking calls for speaking under conditions in which the person's ability to hear himself is artificially reduced, usually through headphones bearing a generated noise, typically "white" noise (demonstration/instruction).

Delayed auditory feedback requires speaking while hearing one's current speech played back at increased volume, through earphones, with a delay of approximately 180 milliseconds (demonstration/instruction).

Voice chewing (also called "breath chewing") produces sequences of articulatory gestures while varying the range of voiced sound[12]. Typically this is done slowly and with great attention to all activities involved (therapy substance).

Ventriloquism is speaking with the intention to reproduce the achievements of a ventriloquist: The objective is to produce reasonably intelligible speech with minimum activity of the oral musculature (therapy substance).

Poetry/prose reading calls for reading poetry, beginning with poems having a clear and simple meter and progressing to blank verse and various kinds of prose. The objective in all of this reading is to read aloud with expression and with the intention of emphasizing the prosodic aspects of the material (therapy substance).

MANAGEMENT STRATEGIES

The early part of the treatment program emphasizes direct instruction through explanation, demonstration, and experiences in order to lay the groundwork for the major dimensions of the treatment approach. The instructions to be described here can be presented in a straightforward manner, at varying levels of sophistication, by anyone knowledgeable about speech; they can be made comprehensible for youngsters as well as for educated adults. In the following synopsis it is assumed that the clinician will know how to adjust the specific content and manner of explanation to the individual being worked with at the time.

Treatment begins by teaching the patient something about the peripheral aspects of speech production and follows by leading him through certain exercises that elucidate what he is being taught. The patient is apprised of the fact that speech does not just happen, as it may seem, but that speech is an activity which a person not only initiates but also guides all the while he is speaking. It is useful to point up a broad description of the process in terms which the patient can readily appreciate. Usually he is aware from his own experience that when speaking he has a "thought" for which he selects appropriate words that he must then utter in the right way so that a listener understands what he had in mind. He also may be aware that sometimes the entire process seems to occur effortlessly but that at other times it proceeds much less smoothly as, for instance, when a thought may be hazy, the right words are hard to find, or pronunciation of the chosen word is inaccurate.

Patients find the emphasis on speech as a skill meaningful for it enables them to liken speech to other skills and, thereby, align the explanation with a broad spectrum of understanding which most patients have acquired or are rapidly acquiring. Specific analogies between speech skills and the skills that patients acquire from an avocation or vocation make emphatic comparisons for them. Moreover, other benefits derive from identifying speech as a skill. One can point to individual differences as the important and relevant factors which surface as variations in native ability and in the ease with which individuals learn various skills. The comparison also serves to identify the need to practice in order to improve aspects of a skill sequence, to apply oneself if one wishes to do well, to be patient with one's efforts and progress, and to move slowly, steadily, and systematically, building on prior achievements. All of these points need not be introduced in the beginning; in fact, it seems to be more effective to introduce (and repeat) them as seems appropriate during the course of treatment.

In describing the speech process particular attention is given to the peripheral aspects: voicing and articulation. The coordinated action of these two functions is emphasized although, of course, each one is discussed separately. Emphasis centers around laryngeal function, identifying it as the immediate source of speech which is modified and shaped at points above the larynx in the vocal tract. Control of voice is described and demonstrated; this includes making clear the reflexive as well as voluntary functions of the vocal folds, their role in changes of pitch and loudness, and the nature of the "hard" and "easy" initiations of sound.

At this point in the initial instructional period of treatment, the patient will have experienced the "basic training" procedures relevant to control of voicing. One should be certain that the patient understands what is presented here before moving on to what is the high point of this early phase of the treatment. The "high point," for which the other instruction has been preliminary and which at this time the patient should be ready to appreciate, is that ordinary speech has a melody which varies with what is being said and that this melody is expressed largely through variations in control of voicing.

The treatment then proceeds through a relatively lengthy period of instruction and demonstration to provide the patient with a broad base of experience and understanding of the melody in speech. This period of the treatment underscores the relationship between melody and linguistic stress, the connection of these two features with stutter events, and the contribution of melody in those conditions under which stuttering is maximally reduced. The activities in this period are designed to help the patient fully appreciate the importance of speech prosody and to acquire a basis for developing his skill in controlling it readily and well.

The most literal procedure for bringing speech melody into focus is "sounding." A few demonstrations, proceeding from several brief utterances to sentences of approximately 10 words in length, are usually adequate, but the patient must be required to do a fair amount of sounding so the clinician can be satisfied that the patient has the "feel" of it. Sometimes choral sounding is indicated as a training technique.

Speaking in a monotone and chanting are rather natural subsequent procedures, but one need not spend a long time with either one. Practice with these activities is necessary only until the patient gives clear evidence that he can do them at will and that he understands what he is doing. Although it is suitable to use reading material when first attempting these procedures, reading from print should be abandoned as soon as possible and the procedures should be implemented in spontaneous speech. During use of all these procedures which induce speech free of stuttering, the clinician should make sure the patient appreciates not only the beneficial effect of the procedures but also the relationship of each procedure to the central objective of the treatment, which is improved speech through control of speech melody.

Procedures ordinarily employed subsequent to sounding are voice chewing, speaking in dialect, ventriloquism, and rhythm, and preferably in that order. The order of their introduction is not rigid, however, and there are occasions when changing their order seems worthwhile. In actuality the procedures of ventriloquism and speaking in dialect are used in some instances for demonstration purposes only. Children are particularly amenable to the dialect procedure, especially "dialects" that represent the voice of animals or imaginary creatures.

Each of these procedures should be accorded its own period of time, with individual needs determining the length as well as the appropriate explanation, demonstration, and practice. The patient must develop a feel for what he is doing, showing that he not only understands each of the assignments but that he also is able to execute each one effectively and comfortably thereby giving evidence that he is developing an adequate level of skill.

Of the four procedures just identified, voice chewing is most similar to the procedure of "sounding" and therefore is a most sensible transition from the early period of treatment efforts to the phase in which ordinary speech is more closely approximated. Whether or not it is introduced right after sounding, some amount of voice chewing should always be included in the treatment for it seems to have great value in focusing on control of voicing while coordinating this function with efforts to change the variety and extent of articulatory movements. Through it the patient can move, in managed sequences, from (controlled) gibberish to slowly and carefully articulated spontaneous speech that retains an emphasis on voicing and highlights its variable coordination with articulation.

Speaking to rhythm ordinarily is introduced last in this sequence mainly because speaking to certain rhythm patterns can be very much like the sequences of stressing-unstressing found in ordinary speech. In fact, the reading of poetry is planned as the next stage in the treatment because poetry emphasizes rhythm patterns inherent in ordinary speech.

Speaking to rhythm turns out to be a rather pivotal procedure in the treatment approach, principally because it does resemble ordinary speech, but also because rhythm is so dramatically effective in inducing speech without stuttering. In addition, rhythm may be "fitted" or applied to any spontaneous speech the patient may attempt; the rhythm pattern can be varied but the effect will still be evident, providing additionally impressive demonstration of what is evidently the effective agent in the therapy procedures.

I have found it advisable to always begin with the most simple rhythm, one syllable per beat. This kind of pattern ordinarily results in a sort of monotone but almost always this effect is soon modified as the speaker develops a sense of the actual stress pattern of the utterance being expressed (in fact, this sense frequently develops spontaneously). The complexity of the rhythm pattern can then be increased for purposes of broadening the range of experience, but the value of complex rhythms lies mostly in their use as demonstrations. The essential objective in using rhythm is to have the patient develop a comfortable sense of command over stress pattern change which is facilitated by speaking to a definite rhythm.

Reading poetry aloud is a form of oral expression that provides a transition between speaking to a definite rhythm and expressing the prosody, or melody, of ordinary speech. The transition to reading poetry begins first with poems that have a clear and simple meter (rhythm) and then progresses gradually from poems with a less regular meter to poetic works with a prosodic structure that is not discriminable from prose or to poems in which a regular meter is at times obvious and at other times absent.

Examples of suitable poems are listed at the end of the chapter; other comparable poems are available in a number of sources. The clinician should collect sets of appropriate poems to use in direct therapy and in homework assignments, but as soon as the stutterer understands the objective of poetry reading, he should be required to supply some of his own poems as well. One should take care to select poems that have an appropriate vocabulary, not only in terms of the age and education level of the patient, but also with consideration for a verbal expression that is straightforward and meaningful. (Avoid poetry that includes too much poetic license or obscurity in either reference or meaning.)

One virtue of many poems with a clear and simple rhythm is that they can be read with full expression of the regular meter or as a more ordinary statement (try for example, Longfellow's "Village Blacksmith" read in both manners). Having the patient read the poem in both ways can highlight the relationships among rhythm, stress, and melody in speech.

The final level of directed exercise using "prepared" materials is to read prose material from various sources. Newspapers, different kinds of magazines, quasi-technical materials, and novels exemplify the sources of prose material that provide a range of prosodic variety. In addition, the scripts of selected plays offer a unique kind of reading material which most closely approximates the speech patterns of ordinary conversation. Moreover, all these materials can be used again as sources for an exercise most like having the patient speak his own thoughts. In this particular assignment the objective is to paraphrase the content of material he has just read aloud.

By this time the patient should be ready to express his own thoughts in his own words while monitoring his performance for the melody of what he intends to say. Actually, as this approach to treatment typically unfolds through the levels described, many patients will already have a certain amount of opportunity to apply the principles of the various procedures to spontaneous speech. These opportunities usually arise naturally in the course of progressing through the various procedures, and the patient is not discouraged from trying to develop these new skills in his ordinary speech when he is interested in doing so. Sometimes, in fact, clinical judgment suggests that he should be encouraged to try before the full range of procedures has been covered.

Two techniques that should be utilized throughout the treatment process whenever appropriate and that articulate well with the focal procedures are prolongation and speaking slowly. Actually, slowing of rate occurs quite naturally as an aspect of many of the procedures, and the clinician should direct attention to this when it occurs under such circumstances. When the patient reaches the level of spontaneous speech, the value of slowing down may need additional emphasis, and monitoring the rate of speech may be necessary. The technique of prolongation, essentially a slowing of rate at the syllable level, is a good means of highlighting these processes and coordinations, and it should be used liberally.

In the course of progressing through the various treatment procedures one must attempt to judge the length of time suitable for developing a particular procedure and when it is appropriate to introduce or to reintroduce another. One should always be ready to repeat some "basic training" exercise for often it is necessary to do so.

As implied earlier, homework assignments are a regular part of the treatment process and should relate to what is being done at each level of the progression. Sometimes a friend, roommate, spouse, or parent can participate in the homework assignments; the clinician should always be ready to make use of such assistance when possible. Of course, the person assisting must be capable of productive participation and would have to attend some of the therapy sessions relevant to such participation to receive appropriate explanation and instruction.

Once the patient shows a reasonable level of success in applying the skills to his regular speech within the clinic, the therapy is carried to external settings, initially in the company of the clinician. The patient and clinician should agree on appropriate situations and these should be ones that reproduce the range of situations in which the patient ordinarily will find himself when he is functioning independently. The objective is to move the patient out of the clinic into circumstances like those (or even actually those) he will experience once he has left therapy. There is no intent to create or seek artificially stressful situations; however, if the patient reports having felt particular stress in certain situations, a special effort should be made to have him practice his new skills in such circumstances.

The therapist's presence in the "external" speaking experiences is phased out as soon as possible, and further such experiences are assigned as "homework" to support the transition to full independence. During the latter period actual contacts with the therapist, though regular, are less frequent and the patient is asked to keep a log to review his achievement with the clinician. A therapist surrogate (friend, parent or other relative, spouse, etc.), if available, may accompany the patient from time to time as indirect assistants, but the emphasis remains on developing the patient's independence.

Therapy is usually terminated gradually as an extension of this period of independent assignments, but with the provision that the patient is free to return for review and possibly further assistance if necessary.

PHYSICAL BEHAVIORS

One of the major values of the procedures utilized in this approach is that the physical behaviors accompanying stutter events subside along with the events themselves, which eliminates the need to direct special attention to any accessory features that may be present. While this treatment approach does not focus on stutter events themselves, there are times, especially when the patient has advanced to the level of spontaneous speech, that stutters do occur. The preferred management of these events is to have the stutterer re-do the word, especially the site of the stutter, utilizing the principles he should know by this time. We encourage the patient to prepare himself for this kind of recovery from actual stutters and from incipient stutters he may sense. The rationale for this facet of the therapy is that the solution, although expedient, nevertheless conforms directly to the overall management the patient should exercise.

ATTITUDINAL WORK

The stutterer's attitude toward his stuttering and himself should always be appraised carefully. I do not mean that the clinician should attempt a thorough assessment of the individual for that is the province of someone, such as a psychologist, who is prepared to undertake that kind and extent of analysis. The kind of assessment I have in mind is one that is free of preconceived notions about what "a stutterer" feels or believes. Each stutterer should be allowed to tell his own story without anyone (theorists, clinicians, or parents) coloring or embellishing the story. One will find that attitudes vary considerably among individuals and are not regularly of the kind claimed in so many literature sources. Even when one does find "negative" attitudes the clinician should address them circumspectly. These personal attitudes are more amenable to change once the patient has clear prospects of improving his speech.

Of course, there are times when attitudes surrounding the speech problem are sufficiently intense or unique enough to require special attention. Various sources in the literature adequately discuss how to deal with such attitudes, and there is no need to repeat the information here. However, one matter deserves mention: the extent to which the stutterer is not open or candid with other people about his stuttering. Stutterers who have difficulty acknowledging their stuttering are likely to compound their problem by increasing the pressure they experience. If a stutterer can be reasonably objective about his stuttering he is more likely to experience less emotional tension and therefore be better able to acquire the necessary speech skills.

In the larger picture, however, one should not be swept away by a concern with attitude except as it pertains to the patient's expectations of therapy, a consideration too infrequently addressed in the literature. The clinician should attempt to help the patient develop a realistic perspective of treatment results drawing from the clinician's knowledge of the prospects for recovery, the amount of time improvement will likely take, the sort of application necessary on the part of the patient, and how the responsibilities of the patient contrast with those of the therapist.

TRANSFER, MAINTENANCE, AND FOLLOW-UP PROCEDURES
With regard to "carry-over," maintenance and follow-up are built into the treatment approach since this approach prepares the patient with a basis for conducting and extending his treatment beyond the sessions and beyond the time when he is formally in therapy. At the same time, the patients are encouraged to return, should they feel the need to reinforce or polish their skills. Just as even good golfers, skiers, and those who play other sports occasionally return to a professional for "brushing up" or a check on their performance, some stutterers may find their skills are refined by an occasional return to the speech therapist.

EQUIPMENT AND MATERIALS NEEDED
The only equipment considered necessary in implementing this treatment approach is a cassette tape recorder of reasonably good quality. The previous discussion of treatment procedures did not describe the use of recorder simply to avoid redundancy. However, a recorder should be used routinely as a means of logging what the patient does in a therapy session, primarily for purposes of immediate review, but also for a record of particular problems and achievements. It is not necessary to keep all tapes but some sort of periodic or systematic sampling should be retained, particularly for the patient's benefit. The patient should have his own cassette recorder for use in fulfilling homework assignments, and as a means for continuing his self-help once he has left therapy.

There are certain other items of equipment one should consider. Although speaking to rhythm can be achieved in many ways without instrumental support, a metronome is very useful, particularly when first beginning work with rhythm. The standard wind-up desk type metronome is adequate and highly serviceable. In addition the little Pacemaster[13] electronic metronomes which can be worn like a hearing aid work well and are especially suited for use outside the clinic. Some patients clearly prefer using the small instrument at all times. We have found it particularly suited to use with children.

An endless tape cassette bearing a white noise signal is an inexpensive item to acquire. Blank endless cassettes are easy to obtain and the recording of the white noise signal can be arranged through a number of sources (a college or university clinic or merchants who sell audio equipment should be able to provide the service). Use of the white noise tape also requires a pair of headphones, which need not be expensive but should adequately block external sounds. This equipment is needed to demonstrate the effect of auditory masking, but since this procedure is optional in this treatment approach, possession of the necessary equipment is also optional.

CLINICIAN SKILLS AND TRAINING REQUIRED
There are three important requirements for successful use of this approach: The clinician (1) must understand the speech process; (2) must have true clinical skill, which implies flexibility, adaptiveness, and a certain amount of creativity; and (3) must not be constrained by a set of beliefs about stuttering that obstruct appropriate use of the procedures as discussed.

Although any clinician would benefit from direct training in the approach, it is entirely possible for anyone having the intelligence and level of training expected of a speech therapist to understand the approach and develop the ability to use it constructively.

CLIENT REQUIREMENTS
As indicated earlier, this approach is adaptable as direct therapy to persons of normal intelligence from kindergarten through adult levels. In fact, most of the procedures and techniques are adaptable for both direct and indirect use with children at the preschool level. The adequately prepared clinician should be able to enlist the cooperation of parents, especially those of younger children, to extend treatment with a complementary program in the home.

Evaluation of the Therapy
Almost all of the patients who have experienced the treatment described here[14] have utilized the clinical services of the Communications Disorders Program at Washington State University. Washington State is located in a rural-remote area where most of the stutterers are students at the university; a few have been adults living in immediate or nearby communities, and even fewer have been children in schools within the radius covered by a practicum program. Almost all patients have been seen by student therapists, functioning under ASHA requirements for supervision, on a semester-by-semester basis. Patients do not regularly work with the same student clinician for more than one semester. Sometimes this is a result of the clinician's required assignment; sometimes it is because a patient does not continue for two consecutive semesters; and sometimes it is due to some combination of circumstances. Therapy ap-

pointments are typically set at no more than two sessions per week for approximately 45 minutes each session, but occasionally a schedule with more frequent appointments is arranged, although this generally amounts to no more than three weekly sessions. Patient attendance is completely voluntary, of course, and only minimal efforts are made to pressure the patient into regular therapy attendance. Actually, attendance has generally been quite good except when academic concerns (and sometimes extra-curricular interests) have affected not only attendance at individual sessions but enrollment in therapy for consecutive semesters.

These circumstances for providing therapy interfere with efforts to conduct a serious, formal evaluation of the treatment because conditions vary so from patient to patient. Moreover, follow-up is not routinely available since students leave school, transfer, or graduate whereupon they no longer are accessible. Only a few patients dismissed from therapy are local residents and only on rare occasions does a former student patient return to visit the campus and report to us at that time.

The result of these circumstances is that the evaluation of the treatment approach has been as qualitative as the administration of the treatment itself. However, we do have two general measures of the effectiveness of the treatment: one addresses the "short-term effect" and includes both a qualitative assessment of how well the patient follows instructions and carries out assignments and a quantitative measure of the percent of reduction in actual stutter events per unit of time and unit of expression (number of words). The second measure is more long-term and is based on assessment of how the patient continues to understand what he is doing as he progresses through the various procedures. This measure considers to some degree how often the patient needs to review "basic" training features, how consistently he progresses with the various procedures, and how easily he applies his skills to new materials and situations.

Short-term assessments of the effects of a therapy are very likely to be misleading, generally inflating the patient's apparent achievement. Stable gains require a lengthy period of application by the patient, utilizing controls that he can understand and manage on his own.

Reasons for Therapeutic Effectiveness

The effectiveness of this treatment stems from several factors. First, the approach utilizes certain procedures which either reproduce or are logically consistent with conditions that for many years have been known to induce more fluent speech in stutterers. Second, these procedures evidently embody principles of speech production and control which are central to good speech. Third, the treatment has a broad base and a range of procedures which are interrelated and contribute to the effectiveness at various levels. Fourth, the patient learns to appreciate how and why the treatment "works" as he learns general "rules" of speech production that he can apply to all kinds of utterances in a variety of circumstances. Finally, we emphasize the patient's responsibility and essential independence in the implementation of treatment and this enables him to recognize that improvement in speech is something he can and must learn to effect and not something that results simply from a particular technique or method that the therapist provides for him.

Advantages of the Therapy

The advantages of this approach exist for both the clinician and the stutterer and include flexibility, the accessibility of a number of procedures, and the adaptability of the approach to different patients and circumstances that develop in therapy. The approach does not rely on one or even a few techniques, but is broadly based in terms of procedures and rationale. Except for the valuable use of a small tape recorder, no equipment is necessary, and the approach is therefore highly "portable." Beginning quite early in therapy the patient undertakes assignments which he is expected to do on his own in the intervals between therapy visits. Preparation for self-help is a major feature and advantage of this approach. We arrange for and encourage the assistance of individuals close to the patient which not only extends the scope of therapy activities, but also broadens the base of the patient's involvement in his own therapy.

References

Goodstein, L. D. Functional speech disorders and personality: A survey of the research. *J. Speech Hear. Res.* 1: 358–377, 1958.

Newman, E. *Strictly Speaking.* New York: Bobbs-Merrill, 1974.

Sheehan, J. G. Projective studies of stuttering. *J. Speech Hear. Disord.* 23: 18–25, 1958.

Sheehan, J. G. Personality Approaches. In Sheehan, J. G. (ed.), *Stuttering: Research and Therapy.* New York: Harper & Row, 1970. Chapter 3.

Van Riper, C. *The Nature of Stuttering.* Englewood Cliffs, N.J.: Prentice-Hall, 1982.

Wingate, M. E. Stuttering adaptation and learning: I. The relevance of adaptation studies to stuttering as 'learned behavior.' *J. Speech Hear. Disord.* 31: 148–156, 1966.

Wingate, M. E. Stuttering adaptation and learning: II. The adequacy of learning principles in the interpretation of stuttering. *J. Speech Hear. Disord.* 31: 211–218, 1966.

Wingate, M. E. Stuttering 1970: Where do we stand? *J. Speech Hear. Res.* 13: 5–8, 1970.

Wingate, M. E. The fear of stuttering. *ASHA* 13: 3–5, 1971.

Wingate, M. E. *Stuttering: Theory and Treatment.* New York: Irvington-Wiley, 1976.

Wingate, M. E. The relationship of theory to therapy in stuttering. *J. Commun. Disord.* 10: 37–44, 1977.

Yairi, E. and Lewis, B. Disfluencies at the onset of stuttering. *J. Speech Hear. Res.* 27: in press, 1984.

Endnotes

1. The interested reader is referred to Chapter 3 in *Stuttering: Theory and Treatment*, and "The Fear of Stuttering," *ASHA*, 1971.
2. See Wingate, 1966, 1970, 1976, and 1977.
3. Readers interested in the details of these analyses are referred to Chapters 7 and 8 in *Stuttering: Theory and Treatment*.
4. The idea of "returning to" this level implies that, except for the instances of stuttering, the speech of the stutterer is basically normal. There is mounting evidence of differences between even the "fluent" speech of stutterers and normally fluent speech.
5. Perhaps there is need for more coursework in linguistics, psycholinguistics and speech science.
6. Teachability: readiness and amenability to being taught.
7. In 1957: C. S. Bluemel, W. Coleman, J. Clancy, J. Frick, W. Johnson, J. Sheehan, C. Van Riper, D. E. Williams. In 1977: J. Aten, R. Barrett, H. Luper, G. Moses, F. Murray, T. Peters, J. Sheehan, M. Tebb, D. E. Williams.
8. The quotation marks were erroneously omitted in the printing of the 1957 program. However, J. Sheehan, who served as chairman of the panel, corrected the error in his opening remarks of introduction.
9. The true percentage value may be considerably higher. At least two sources in the literature indicate that the prevalence of stuttering among preschool-age children is as high as 15 percent; in contrast, there is extensive documentation that prevalence among school-age children is slightly less than 1 percent. The difference between these two values is substantial.
10. See Chapter 5 in *Stuttering: Theory and Treatment* for a review of the recovery findings.
11. An extended discussion of the analysis which led to identification of these principles is presented in Chapters 7, 8, and 9 of *Stuttering: Theory and Treatment*.
12. The interested reader will find a fuller description of voice chewing, and references, in *Stuttering: Theory and Treatment*, pp. 275–277.
13. The Pacemaster is available from Associated Auditory Instruments, 6796 Market Street, Upper Darby, PA 19082.
14. Certain other treatments are based on, or make considerable use of, the concepts underlying this approach. Probably the one most similar, and oriented more toward children, is that of Adeline Weiner (see Chapter 6 in this volume).

Appendix 7-A. Example Poems

The list is ordered in respect to meter; the earlier poems have the simplest and most obvious meter.

The Village Blacksmith	Henry Wadsworth Longfellow
The Owl and the Pussycat	Edward Lear
Father William	Lewis Carroll
Jabberwocky	Lewis Carroll
Annabel Lee	Edgar Allan Poe
Invictus	William Ernest Henley
Stopping by Woods on a Snowy Evening	Robert Frost
Sea Fever	John Masefield
The West Wind	John Masefield
To Autumn	John Keats
The Rubaiyat of Omar Khayyam	Edward Fitzgerald
Ozymandias	Percy Bysshe Shelley
Mending Wall	Robert Frost
Birches	Robert Frost

Epilogue

This book has provided a range of contemporary therapies for stutterers, which I hope has widened your horizons about effective management strategies. Compare your method with those presented. If the therapy you are presently using with stutterers is not always effective, you may find that one or more therapies in this book are more compatible with your clients' needs and your own.

Considering a change from the therapy that we have grown accustomed to using to one that is new and different may cause us to hesitate because it presents a choice: to remain where we are or to alter our course and move ahead in a different direction. Making such a choice can be difficult. Yet change can make an essential difference in our lives, and a wise decision can lead to inner growth, enhanced creativity, and unanticipated benefits. We sometimes travel the rutted road for so long that veering off in another direction may seem too risky. But often by choosing to take the less-traveled road, we find new vistas. Each of the authors in this book at some point chose to take the less-traveled road, and that decision made all the difference. I invite you now to join us on our journey and discover new ways of treating stutterers effectively.

Maryann Peins

Index

Accessory behaviors and features, 127–128, 129, 140–144
Accountability, 73, 109
Adjunct therapy, 91, 95–96, 102–103, 109, 110
Air flow, 81, 82
Arizona Articulation Proficiency Scale, 188
Articulatory movements, 81, 82
Assignment and Evaluation Worksheet, 21, 28
self-assignments, 80, 90
Attending disorders, 124, 132–133, 146, 147, 151–153, 164, 166
Attenuation. *See* Auditory masking
Attitude
change and stuttering therapy, 99–100, 146–147, 150–151
Iowa Scale of Attitude Toward Stuttering, 96, 99–100
Parent Attitudes Toward Stuttering Checklist, 7–8
Auditory awareness, 80, 83, 108
Auditory disorders
processing problems, 124, 133–134, 147, 155, 164
Auditory feedback, 73, 75, 80, 91, 108
delayed, 79–80, 286
Auditory masking, 74, 75, 286
Avoidance, 128, 129–130, 157–158
Situation Avoidance Checklist, 5

Bankson Language Screening Test (BLST), 136
Behavior
modification, 149–150
rehearsal, 241–242
therapy, 217–218
Borderline/at-risk-stuttering ranges, 191–192
Breathing
abdominal-diaphragmatic, 222, 223–224
breath control, 226–227
Burks Behavioral Rating Scales (BBRS), 132–133

Carrow Elicited Language Inventory (CELI), 136
Cassette tapes, 73, 77, 79–80, 81, 86, 91, 92, 94, 95, 110

Causes of stuttering
central neurologic integration processes, 178
coordinative disorder, 176–177
genetic, 177
neurophysiologic difference, 177
Chanting, 286, 288
Checklist of Physical Behaviors Accompanying Stuttering, 118–121
Child development, 40–43, 60–61
Choral speaking, 274, 284, 286
Chronicity Prediction Checklist, 8
Client and Clinicians Perceptions of Stuttering Severity Ratings, 6
Client Readiness for Fluency Control Inventory, 30
Clinical dropout or clinical failure in therapy, 74
Clinician, effective, 24, 94, 110
Coarticulatory/resonatory processes, 195
Component treatment
abnormal disfluency modification, 144, 146, 156–157, 158, 164
effectiveness, 162, 165–166
Comprehensive stuttering analysis (CSA), 185–186
Concomitant Stuttering Behavior Checklist, 5
Conflicts, 272
Continuity of vocalization, 81, 107–108
Control
breath, 226–227
feeling of, 11–16
motor, 220–221, 250–252
Conventional speech therapy, 74, 95–103
Conversational speaking activities, 80, 86, 90, 91
Counseling, 78. *See also* Parents, counseling

Data-based ranges of fluency/stuttering, 191
Delayed auditory feedback, 79–80, 286. *See also* Auditory feedback
Desensitization
auxiliary, 238, 241–242
in vivo, 243
procedures, 88, 238–243